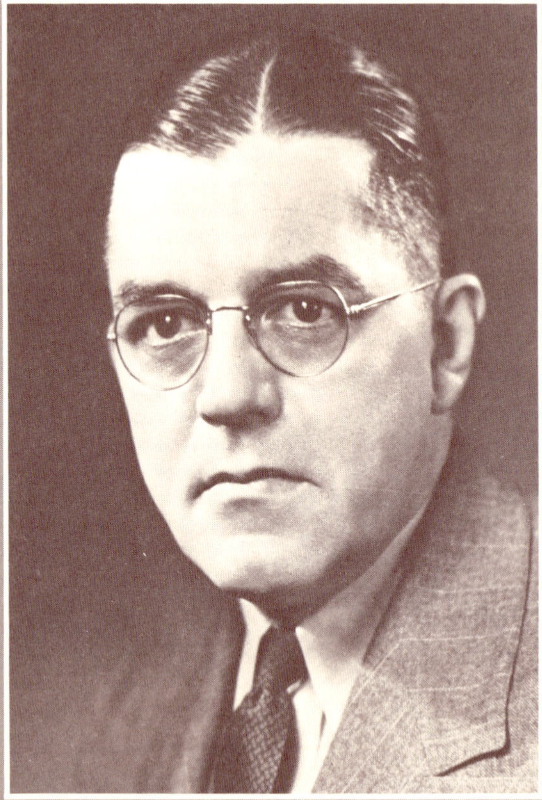

HARVEY A.K. WHITNEY
1894-1957

HARVEY A. K. WHITNEY AWARD LECTURES 1950–1991

Published by the
ASHP Research and
Education Foundation
4630 Montgomery Avenue
Bethesda, MD 20814

This collection is made possible through a grant from Hoechst-Roussel Pharmaceuticals Inc.

Produced by the American Society of Hospital Pharmacists' Special Projects Division.

ISBN: 1-879907-04-6

CONTENTS

VII *The Man and the Award*

IX *Introduction*

3 *Minimum Standards and the Future,* by W. Arthur Purdum (1950)

11 *Work by the Side of Work,* by Hans T. S. Hansen (1951)

17 *Background to Progress,* by Edward Spease (1952)

23 *Hospital Pharmacy Looks to the Future,* by Donald E. Francke (1953)

31 *The Point-Rating Plan—An Opportunity,* by Evlyn Gray Scott (1954)

37 *Responsibilities of ASHP Affiliated Chapters,* by Gloria Niemeyer Francke (1955)

47 *Ethical Standards: Professional Conduct and Responsibilities,* by George F. Archambault (1956)

63 *Hospital Pharmacy—Past, Present, and Future,* by Sister Mary John (1957)

75 *The Authority of Ideas,* by Walter M. Frazier (1958)

81 *What Price Success in Hospital Pharmacy?* by I. Thomas Reamer (1959)

93 *Expanding Role of the Hospital Pharmacist as a Member of the Health Team,* by Thomas A. Foster (1960)

101 *Goals for Hospital Pharmacists,* by Herbert L. Flack (1961)

111 *Where Do We Go from Here?,* by Grover C. Bowles (1962)

121 *To Whom Much Is Given,* by Vernon O. Trygstad (1963)

131 *Compatibility of Professional Success and Satisfaction,* by Albert P. Lauve (1964)

137 *Quo Vadis 20th Century Hospital Pharmacy?* by Sister Mary Berenice (1965)

145 Robert P. Fischelis (1966)

147 *Drugs and the People,* by Paul F. Parker (1967)

157 *As We Move into History*, by Clifton J. Latiolais (1968)

163 *Form and Substance*, by Leo F. Godley (1969)

171 *Commitment and Involvement*, by Joseph A. Oddis (1970)

179 *An Added Dimension*, by Sister M. Gonzales (1971)

187 *On Maturing*, by William M. Heller (1972)

199 *Uncle Harvey*, by George L. Phillips (1973)

209 *A Personal Opinion for Professional Reflection*, by Louis P. Jeffrey (1974)

217 *Enthusiasms*, by Sister Mary Florentine (1975)

225 *The Peril of Deprofessionalization*, by R. David Anderson (1976)

237 *Patient Accountability—Pharmacists' Future*, by Herbert S. Carlin (1977)

245 *The Patient's Pharmacist*, by Allen J. Brands (1978)

253 *Moving towards the 21st Century*, by Milton W. Skolaut (1979)

261 *Need for a Theoretical Base for Pharmacy Practice*, by Donald C. Brodie (1980)

271 *Pseudopharmacy Practice and the Future*, by Kenneth N. Barker (1981)

287 *Clinical Pharmacy in the 1980s*, by William E. Smith (1982)

301 *A 20–20 Vision: Alternative Futures for Hospital Pharmacy*, by Warren E. McConnell (1983)

315 *Old Dreams, Young Hopes*, by Mary Jo Reilly (1984)

327 *Research: Cornerstone of Pharmacy Practice*, by Fred M. Eckel (1985)

339 *The Art of Growing Professionally*, by John W. Webb (1986)

345 *Intimations on a Profession: Retrospect and Prospect*, by John J. Zugich (1987)

355 *Leadership in a Clinical Profession*, by Joe E. Smith (1988)

365 *Taking Charge of the Profession*, by Wendell T. Hill, Jr. (1989)

371 *Interdependence in Pharmacy: Risks, Rewards, and Responsibilities*, by David A. Zilz (1990)

383 *To a New Beginning from Converging Paths*, by Harold N. Godwin (1991)

393 *Index*

THE MAN AND THE AWARD

Harvey A. K. Whitney (1894–1957) received his Ph.C. degree from the University of Michigan College of Pharmacy in 1923. He was appointed to the pharmacy staff of University Hospital in Ann Arbor in 1925 and was named Chief Pharmacist there in 1927. He served in that position for almost 20 years. He is credited with establishing the first hospital pharmacy internship program—now known as a residency program—at the University of Michigan in 1927.

Harvey A. K. Whitney was an editor, author, educator, practitioner, and hospital pharmacy leader. He was instrumental in developing a small group of hospital pharmacists into a subsection of the American Pharmaceutical Association and finally, in 1942, into the American Society of Hospital Pharmacists. He was the first ASHP President and co-founder, in 1943, of the *Bulletin of the ASHP*, which in 1958 became the *American Journal of Hospital Pharmacy.*

The Harvey A. K. Whitney Lecture Award was established in 1950 by the Michigan Society of Hospital Pharmacists (now the Southeastern Michigan Society of Hospital Pharmacists) to honor the first Chairman of the American Society of Hospital Pharmacists. Responsibility for administration of the Award was accepted by the American Society of Hospital Pharmacists in 1963, and since that time it has been presented annually to honor outstanding contributions to the practice of hospital pharmacy. The Harvey A. K. Whitney Lecture Award is known as "hospital pharmacy's highest honor."

INTRODUCTION

The idea of publishing this collection of Harvey A. K. Whitney Lecture Award addresses was largely an outgrowth of the establishment of the Donald E. Francke Memorial Library at the ASHP headquarters building in 1982. The purpose of the Francke Memorial Library is to chronicle the evolution and development of institutional pharmacy in the United States. When the steering committee was formulating plans for the Library, it listed this collection of addresses among the various publications that should be acquired. It is not difficult to understand why this collection came to mind. The men and women who wrote these addresses played prominent roles in the development of hospital pharmacy in this country. Collectively, the addresses constitute a condensed chronicle of this development. They portray the history and culture of institutional pharmacy practice up to the present time.

All but one of the 42 addresses presented since 1950 are included in this volume. The address by Dr. Robert P. Fischelis (1966) was never published, and we must conclude that he did not prepare a finished manuscript. All but three of the remaining 41 addresses were published in the *Bulletin of the American Society of Hospital Pharmacists* (through 1957) or the *American Journal of Hospital Pharmacy* (since 1958). The unpublished addresses are those by Donald E. Francke (1953), Gloria Niemeyer Francke (1955), and Sister Mary John (1957). Since Don Francke was editor of the *Bulletin* during those years, only he could tell us why they were not published; we were, however, able to obtain copies.

Publication of the Whitney addresses has been made possible through a generous grant by Hoechst-Roussel Pharmaceuticals Inc. to the ASHP Research and Education Foundation. The grant provides for distribution of complimentary copies to past award recipients, residents in ASHP-accredited pharmacy residency programs, and other selected individuals. The Foundation hopes that this volume will help young practitioners understand and appreciate the history and culture of their profession.

HARVEY A. K. WHITNEY AWARD LECTURES

1950

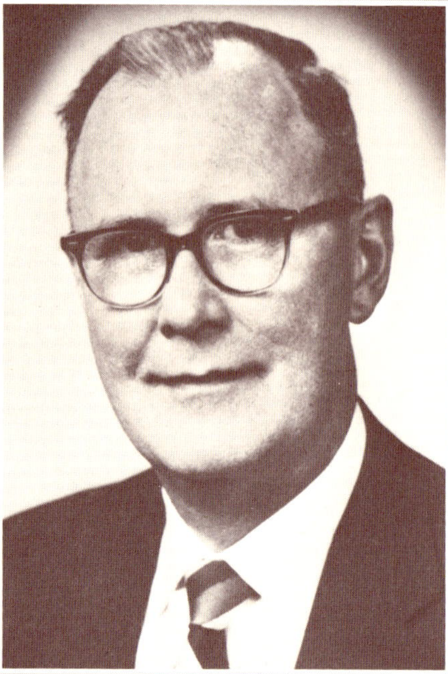

W. ARTHUR PURDUM

"Revision will take place and the level of our practice will be raised."

MINIMUM STANDARDS AND THE FUTURE

Hospital pharmacy has made great progress since Harvey Whitney became the first chairman of the American Society of Hospital Pharmacists a relatively few years ago—greater progress, in fact, than any other specialized branch of our profession. To cite tangible evidence of the growing interest in and respect for our specialty, I mention the creation of the Division of Hospital Pharmacy by the American Pharmaceutical Association with a $10,000 budget for its first year of operation, the recent introduction of undergraduate and graduate courses in hospital pharmacy by a number of our universities, and only last week the recognition by the United States Pharmacopeial Convention of a delegate from the American Society of Hospital Pharmacists at future conventions.

In large measure, this progress parallels the remarkable growth of the ASHP. The underlying reasons for such rapid development were the adoption of fundamentally sound objectives for the Society and the fulfillment of them. What are the principal objectives and how are they being achieved? We are pledged to improve and extend the usefulness of the hospital pharmacist to the patient, to the hospital, to members of the allied health professions, and to the profession of pharmacy; to assist in providing for the future an adequate supply of qualified hospital pharmacists; and to promote the dissemination of pharmaceutical knowledge.

This latter objective, that is, the interchange of information, is already developed to a high degree. This is taken care of in part by the information service offered by the Division of Hospital Pharmacy in Washington and is available to all pharmacists. Another medium is the well-established annual institute on hospital pharmacy, which originated in Ann Arbor less than five years ago. Last, but certainly our most potent medium, is our *Bulletin*. Much credit is due Don Francke for this fine publication; and while numerous bouquets have been tossed in his direction in the past, the most recent compliment is the eagerness of large manufacturers to advertise in this journal.

Hospital standardization was born in 1918, and the proud parents are the American College of Surgeons. Its object is to foster better hospital care in all its phases, and the results obtained far more than justify the effort expended. In that year, 692 hospitals of 100 or more beds were surveyed and only 12.9% were approved. By 1926, the figure was well above 90% of those inspected and it has been climbing steadily towards perfection since that time.

Not until 1935, at the suggestion of Dr. Malcolm T. MacEachern, former director of the ACS, was a standard written for the hospital pharmacy. This was prepared by Edward Spease, at that time dean of the Western Reserve University School of Pharmacy and the only man other than Harvey Whitney who holds honorary membership in the ASHP. He was assisted by Robert M. Porter, then chief pharmacist at the University Hospitals of Cleveland. The standard was adopted very soon thereafter by the ACS and is still recognized today by that body. It was an excellent standard in 1935, but pharmaceutical practice has changed in 15 years and there is definite need for a revised standard today. We now have this new standard, and all of you have had opportunity to read it in a recent issue of *The Bulletin.* In this standard lies the key to our first objective: improving and extending the usefulness of the hospital pharmacist.

In what respect is the new standard an improvement over that currently recognized by the American College of Surgeons? The old standard permits a hospital to obtain pharmaceutical service from a nearby drugstore whereas the new standard requires that: "There shall be a properly organized pharmacy department under the direction of a professionally competent, legally qualified pharmacist. . . ." In the small hospital, pharmaceutical service from a nearby pharmacy no longer suffices. No longer shall a nurse be in charge of the "drug room." In fact, no longer shall there be a "drug room." Under the new standard, the drug room is being elevated to the plane of a pharmacy with a competent pharmacist in charge, even though his services may be on a part-time basis. He may be a nearby pharmacist or preferably a full-time hospital employee who has been assigned additional professional or administrative duties.

A chapter on policies, not appearing in the old standard, now vests in the pharmacist the authority to develop and carry out the administrative policies of the department. He shall also develop, with the assistance of the Pharmacy and Therapeutics Committee, the professional policies of the department, and he is responsible for their implementation. In keeping with good administrative practice, it is natural that all policies should secure the approval of the hospital administrator.

The section on personnel has been perhaps the most controversial of the entire standard. When it originally emerged from the committee at the time of the 1948 convention, it required that: "...the chief pharmacist shall be a diplomate of a hospital pharmacy specialty board." (It was anticipated that these requirements would include graduate study leading to an M.S. or a Ph.D. degree in pharmacy and the completion of a recognized hospital pharmacy internship.) It was soon quite obvious that the good intentions of the committee were misunderstood and not appreciated, to state the case mildly. We of the committee envisioned for the future a group of specialists in hospital pharmacy who had become fellows of the yet to be organized "American College of Hospital Pharmacists." This was incorrectly interpreted by a number of protestants as a squeeze play on the part of a few to form an exclusive fraternity. Actually, the statement was written into the standard by a committee member holding a three-year degree, and it received the blessing of another member who is a two-year graduate. The committee's oversight was our failure to append a statement recognizing experience in lieu of advanced education. In its final form, this section requires that the department have an ample number of qualified personnel to furnish pharmaceutical service of the highest quality. Furthermore, steps have been taken to make secure the positions of those pharmacists who graduated during the days of the two- and three-year courses.

The chapter on facilities assures the pharmacist of adequate pharmaceutical and administrative equipment in a well-lighted and well-ventilated area in order to perform properly his many and varied duties.

The scope of the pharmacist's responsibilities has been expanded to a considerable degree. The old standard charged the pharmacist with supervision over eight specific functions whereas the new makes him responsible for 15. Among his added duties, he must maintain a pharmaceutical and therapeutic information service for the hospital staff, he must establish and maintain a satisfactory system of records, he should cooperate in the teaching of courses to student nurses and assist in the medical intern training program, and he should file periodic reports on the progress of the department with the hospital administrator.

The Pharmacy and Therapeutics Committee is an important and influential body in the operation of a hospital. The judicious selection of therapeutic and diagnostic materials plays a major role in patient care—not only is the patient's physical welfare affected but his pocketbook as well. The decisions of this committee also play a major role in the economical operation of the pharmacy. The responsibility of the committee with regard to professional policy was recognized in the old standard. However, the old standard also charged the committee with supervision over the purchase and issuance of all drugs and pharmaceutical supplies which function is purely administrative, and the new standard places this responsibility on the shoulders of the pharmacist in charge. A most important new requirement of the Pharmacy and Therapeutics Committee is that it develop a formulary of accepted drugs for use in the hospital.

Our other principal objective concerns our assistance in providing an adequate number of qualified hospital pharmacists for the future. We all appreciate that there is an acute shortage of well-trained personnel. What can be done to alleviate this shortage? Part of the answer lies in our colleges of pharmacy. The school not offering a course in hospital pharmacy should make one available to its students. The ASHP, through a special committee, has already written a syllabus and is now prepared to assist those colleges interested in inaugurating such a course. Where possible, the course should be taught by a practicing hospital pharmacist. This course is not expected to produce finished hospital pharmacists, but it can serve the very useful purpose of stimulating the student's interest in our branch of pharmacy. After this interest has been aroused, the final solution to the problem lies in the creation of more training programs—programs which can qualify under the proposed *Minimum Standard for Pharmacy Internships in Hospitals.* This standard has undergone major revision since it was first published in *The Bulletin* approximately 18 months ago, and the committee feels that we now have a satisfactory and workable standard. The revised version was presented to the Society at the time of the Atlantic City convention in 1950.

This standard recognizes two types of internships: nonacademic and academic. Each consists of a minimum period of training of 1920 hours in the hospital pharmacy. In addition, the academic internship requires one year of graduate study leading to an M.S. degree. The minimum number of hours has been reduced from 2100 to 1920 at the request of pharmacists in government service so that the entire training period can be scheduled in one federal work year of 48 weeks of 40 hours each.

Because we are always seeking to enlist the very best people available, applicants must have a better than average scholastic standing, be of high moral character, and be in good health. The training hospital shall be a general hospital of at least 200 beds and shall have an active outpatient department. The minimum of 200 beds has been criticized as too high by a number of interested individuals. It was the consensus of opinion in the committee that smaller hospitals for the most part would not have adequate facilities to offer the broad training required for these trainees. The pharmacy department of the training hospital must comply with the requirements of the *Minimum Standard for Pharmacies in Hospitals* and shall include among its activities outpatient prescription service, dispensing to hospital divisions and inpatients, the manufacture of pharmaceuticals, and departmental administration.

The supplemental elaboration to the standard spells out many details not given in the basic standard itself and is intended to be a guide for pharmacists offering training programs and for examiners. Certain sections, no doubt, will be subject to criticism, but no standard ever developed in the past or to be developed in the future will be completely satisfactory in the eyes of all concerned. It is almost a certainty that no pharmacy or training program exists that can earn a perfect score. Nevertheless, we must all strive for as high a rating as possible.

Even though we have come a long way during the short history of the ASHP, our forward movement must continue; there are still jobs to be done.

At the present time, the new standard for the hospital pharmacy carries the approval of the ASHP, the APhA, and the American Hospital Association. Before the end of this year we hope to receive the approval of the American Medical Association and the approval and adoption of the standard by the American College of Surgeons.

Speaking before a sectional meeting of the American College of Surgeons about a year ago, I found fault with the point-rating system for hospitals on three counts. First, and of least significance, was the allocation of only 10 points to the pharmacy out of 1000 for the hospital. Since then, pharmacy's points have been increased to 20. Of greater consequence was the fact that only three questions had to be answered satisfactorily to earn these points. No pharmacy can be evaluated properly on this basis and, during the past year, several additional questions have been added. The questionnaire is still inadequate, and another should be written based on the new minimum standard. My chief objection was that pharmacy is found among the adjunct and service divisions of the hospital rather than with the essential divisions where it should be. Today we are still recognized as a complementary service department, and we must continue our efforts until pharmacy is regarded as essential.

I would like to see the standard for internships reviewed and approved by the Executive Committee of the Society at an early date and forwarded to the Division of Hospital Pharmacy with the recommendation that the Division undertake the responsibility for organizing the procedure of accreditation and act as the accrediting body for hospitals offering such training. One tool needed by the Division to carry out this function will be a questionnaire or checklist based on the standard, and I hope that this can be accomplished in the near future. Those of us who offer training programs now must arrange to meet or exceed the requirements of the standard, and it behooves all of you who can qualify and are not offering internships to initiate such programs as soon as possible.

Several months ago, Don Francke presented an excellent editorial in *The Bulletin* entitled "Needed—a Standard of Practice." While we now have an excellent minimum standard to control the board practice of pharmacy in hospitals, I concur with Editor Francke that a detailed standard of practice will prove of great value to the hospital pharmacist, and I urge that such a standard be written.

As time passes, we will recognize our new standard as insufficient, revision will take place and the level of our practice will be raised another rung on the ladder of progress. We should keep in mind the future creation of that specialty board, mention of which was withdrawn from the standard because of current opposition. Such a board will serve as an incentive to all of us to improve ourselves in order to earn what I hope will be a highly coveted diploma.

What will be the ultimate effects of these standards? While we are only one wheel in the hospital machine, through better pharmacists, better facilities, and better management, we can expect to render a more efficient and economical service to the hospital, to the other medical care professions, and, above all, to the patient.

A final consideration is the threat of compulsory national health insurance. Our public servants in Washington have made John Q. Public well aware of the high cost of medical care. The paying hospital patient is indignant over the high per diem cost of hospital care, and it is true that these costs have risen considerably in recent years. But he overlooks the important fact that advances in the pharmaceutical and medical sciences have substantially reduced the term of his stay in the hospital. He also overlooks the fact that he now pays $75 for a $35 suit of clothes and $1.50 for a $0.60 cut of beef. I am opposed to the federal program for the socialization of medical care and believe that we as pharmacists can assist in forestalling this dangerous enemy of free enterprise by doing all within our power to supply the highest type of pharmaceutical service at the lowest possible cost.

Compliance with the minimum standards will assist immeasurably in realizing these goals. We must not wait for an accrediting agency to require observance but rather, in the interest of immediate improvement in pharmaceutical service, we should begin our own program of self-enforcement and have our house in order before the inspector arrives at the door.

At the time he received this award, W. Arthur Purdum was the Chief Pharmacist at Johns Hopkins Hospital, Baltimore, Maryland.

1951

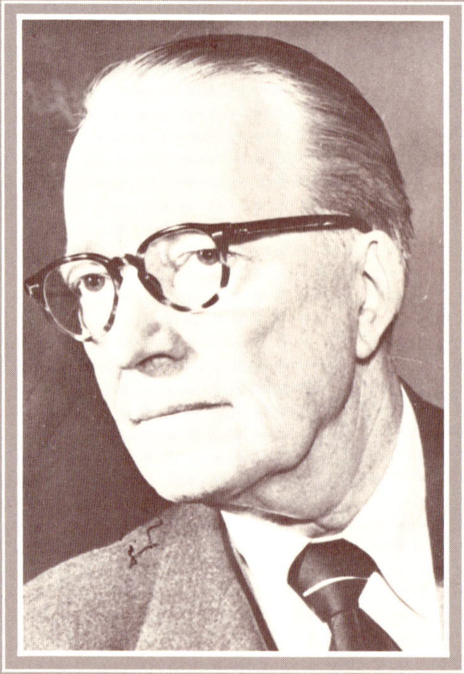

HANS T. S. HANSEN

"It is only through work that we find happiness and a measure of success."

WORK BY THE SIDE OF WORK

I have never been a very good storyteller, so I have avoided the use of stories in opening remarks. Tonight, however, I am going to use one. It is not humorous and it is one you have all heard many times, at least I hope you have. Some who have children have told them this story.

It is the story of Adam and Eve and the Garden of Eden. God created these two and gave them this beautiful place as a home. They could enjoy all the pleasures and comforts that anyone could imagine but, you recall, there was a little restriction placed on them. I have had the idea, for some time, that God looked upon his handiwork and questioned their fitness for this life in the Garden, so he willed that they disobey and eat of the fruit from the tree of good and evil. The God of the Old Testament is a stern, wrathful, and sometimes cruel God, so many theologians agree that this curse of earning their bread by the sweat of their brows was a punishment. I would rather think that it was a blessing, a blessing that has been man's salvation.

Work has been the butt of many a joke and story. We all say we hate work but we don't mean it, for it is only through work that we find happiness and a measure of success, and it is immaterial what kind of work you do, just so you like it and take pride in it. Sometimes I wonder if pride in work is a thing of the past. I remember as a boy watching a carriage maker varnish carriages; such time and care he put into this final process. Rubbing and polishing each succeeding coat, stepping back to admire but with a critical eye as well for his craftsmanship. I wonder if we pharmacists can step back and, with a critical eye, admire any or all of our finished prescriptions.

The work I want to talk about this evening is not the work that furnishes us our daily bread; some of this other work may, however, be the means of having cake with our daily bread. I want to explore two areas of work with the thought in mind that the Michigan Society of Hospital Pharmacists might investigate these two areas and spearhead a movement of development. Your group has pioneered before for hospital pharmacy.

Through the efforts of Harvey Whitney and yourselves, hospital pharmacy received the impetus that has brought it to its enviable position in pharmacy today. I am convinced, in spite of what other groups in pharmacy may think or say, that pharmacy's standing among the health professions today is due, in large measure, to hospital pharmacy. In making this statement I am not unmindful of, nor do I want to belittle, the work of other groups in pharmacy; but I guess I am a bit prejudiced. However, in our admiration for the present-day pharmacists, we should not forget our wonderful heritage including such men as Serturner, Robiquet, Brandes, Scheele, Balard, and Pellitier.

Even though hospital pharmacy has made great strides in the past decade, there still remains much to be done. We cannot stop in our efforts; times change; and unless we accept changes and adjust hospital pharmacy to these, we are through as an important department in the hospital. A few weeks ago, I had the opportunity to attend a conference on Human Relations in Administration in the hospital. It was brought out that the hospital pharmacist is pretty much alone in the hospital picture. Other workers, because of their greater numbers, can get together within the hospital, talk over their problems, and air their gripes. The lecturers suggested that this was corrected to some extent by membership in local, district, state, and national pharmaceutical societies and associations. Here one meets with fellow pharmacists and, like the walrus and the carpenter, talks of many things, of prices and hours and penicillin—of records and the administrator and why the hospital is so full and whether interns and residents really know the score. All this may satisfy a need or a want and give the hospital pharmacist a feeling of solidarity. It is good but it is not enough; that feeling of being alone will persist until the hospital pharmacist fits his job into the hospital as a whole.

We are, I am sure, in agreement on pharmacy's importance in the hospital. But does the hospital pharmacist take advantage of this opportunity, of this importance of himself and his department? You may say: "Of course he does. Why, doesn't he fill all orders and prescriptions; doesn't he keep good records; doesn't he keep abreast of all that is new, pharmaceutically speaking? He keeps his department neat and clean, opens on time and closes on time. Has he not satisfied the implied need, required when he was appointed chief of the department?" When he closes on time, he goes home with the feeling of a job well done, satisfied that he has earned his daily bread. But he is not, and never will be, a part of the whole picture if he continues so. He must change, he must work at work by the side of work.

Work that, for the time being at least, does not return wages. You ask: "What is this work?" In every hospital, we find many and varied activities, all apart from the actual care of the patient but nevertheless a part of the whole. These are the medical staff meetings, clinical pathological conferences, medical departmental meetings, activities of the nursing department, capping, graduation, refresher courses, alumna activities, activities of the woman's auxiliary, the hospital's drives for funds. You say you doubt your welcome. Don't worry about that; there is more to do than they can find workers for. If you once begin to take an active part, you will enjoy it and the new friendships found. Do this to a degree that no function is complete without the presence of the pharmacist; make yourself indispensable. It will mean work, but rewards will be there as well.

May I suggest another activity? University and large teaching hospitals should and do carry on research that, many times, includes the services of the Pharmacy Department. But size is not the determining factor. If your hospital does not do any clinical research, that does not prevent you from doing some of your own. This probably cannot be clinical in nature, but there are many other areas for such research. How about a little study on the value of records? We all keep many of these; and unless some use is made of a record, it is wasted effort. To illustrate, let us assume that a study of the value of records was to be made as to their value in the control of the use of barbiturates in hospitals. This would require the use of a questionnaire sent to cooperating hospital pharmacists. It would bring out facts such as the following, and this is true.

This is the story of two hospitals; they are located in the same suburban area and have approximately the same bed complement, the quality and quantity of the medical staff are almost identical, and the clienteles are about alike as to economic status, ranging from the lower income groups through to the highest bracket. Both have good pharmacists and pharmacies. In one hospital, the pharmacist, a few years ago, put his distribution of barbiturates on a record control as strict as the one for narcotics. In the other, the distribution is more or less comparable to floor stock drugs. The one with the record control uses about 10,000 doses annually of one of the more popular trade name barbiturates. The other, without any controls, uses 50,000 annually. It is not necessary to elaborate on the economic significance of this. I can imagine the open-armed acceptance by hospital administrators of such a study. I have had the opportunity of talking to future hospital administrators at two schools for the past few years. It has been my observation that they accept the fact that if they employ a good hospital pharmacist, they will have a good professional service. But the portion of the lecture that elicits most questions is that on the economics of hospital pharmacy.

I would like to see the Michigan Society of Hospital Pharmacists initiate a program of education among hospital pharmacists on the importance of the business or economic side of hospital pharmacy. Make this a real basic program. See to it that it is outlined in our *Bulletin*; but when results are to be published, let there be feature articles in hospital journals. As long as hospitals operate on the present philosophy that the adjunct departments shall carry the load, so long will administrators be interested in the economies of these adjunct departments. This philosophy has carried on from the days when hospitals were places for the poor to come to die. No attempt was made to operate at cost. Each year, charity carried the load. As medical science developed and new therapy as well as diagnostic aids was introduced, hospitals became places for rich and poor to go in order to regain health; but the concept of charity remained and adjunct services had to carry the burden. This thinking is wrong. Such a philosophy should be discarded; but as long as it prevails, the hospital administrator will welcome a pharmacy department that produces a good revenue.

Your department should be one of the best of adjunct departments, and this does not have to be at the expense of the patient if you develop sound business principles. Why not, in this connection, develop a study of economic waste in the use of therapeutic agents? This could be on the basis of misuse, use after need was gone, use of high priced specialties when USP and NF preparations would serve. This study will require the help of your medical records department, and they should be willing to assist you as it is part of their duty to assist in all research projects.

I have mentioned records before. I suppose unused records and statistics would paper many a hospital's walls. Maybe that is why so many hospital pharmacists abhor records. I have talked to many, and I believe they would use records that fit their particular pharmacy. Why not then develop a basic set of records that could be adjusted to fit most general hospital pharmacies? How about a hospital pharmacist writing a text on materia medica that would fit into the educational program of the student nurse? He knows better than most professional people what a student nurse should have in this field. How about a hospital pharmacist developing a handbook for medical interns, conducting a time and motion study, developing a program of better human relations and many other things?

The last area that I would like to call to your attention tonight, and suggest that hospital pharmacists explore, has nothing to do with pharmacy as such, but you will be better hospital pharmacists if you will do so. Not only better hospital pharmacists but better citizens as well as better human beings. One thing professional people are so apt to do is to live their whole lives within the bounds of their profession. This is natural and is, in some respects, an interesting life but it is also a very narrow life. I heard a director of a professional department state that he insists and sees to it that his technicians spend some of their leisure time in cultural pursuits. He is convinced, from observing this over a period of years, that he has better technicians. This particular area of activity I would now suggest is the community in which you live and work. You owe your community something; and if you pass up this responsibility, you will have missed something in life. There are many channels through which you can achieve this: the church, schools, service clubs, and political organizations. The real worthwhile folks in the community are those who are busy with the art of living. Don't spread yourself too thin; select one of these avenues and give it some of your time.

In suggesting the last area for us to explore, it is my hope that we can, in a small measure, attempt to level off this lopsided civilization of ours. Scientifically we are way up on the top of the mountain of civilization, but spiritually and socially we are still at the foot stumbling around in the morass. It may be 1951 A.D. scientifically, but spiritually and socially it is, let us say, 500 B.C.

At the time he received this award, Hans T. S. Hansen was the Administrator at Grant Hospital, Chicago, Illinois.

1952

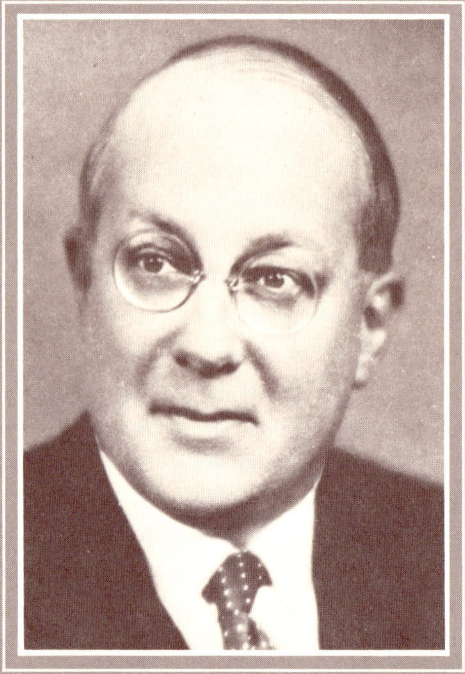

EDWARD SPEASE

"I felt that if professional pharmacy was to exist. . ., it would have to be in the hospital."

BACKGROUND TO PROGRESS

When invited to receive the H. A. K. Whitney Lecture Award, it was with a great feeling of happiness and appreciation that I accepted; but it was also mixed with some feeling of trepidation.

The joy and appreciation stemmed from the fact that in all your activity and progress, I had not been entirely forgotten. It is usually the case that one must be seen now and then, and one must be fairly active to be thought of often. The feeling of trepidation naturally arises within me when I am expected to present an address, the day being gone by for me to write of scientific things such as steroids, hormones, antibiotics, and perhaps such new drugs as hydrazinophthalazine, whose names are difficult for me. My paper must be mainly reminiscences, with the hope that some of them may be of help, to at least the younger among you, and it may be a bit of an inspiration.

You have progressed so far and so fast in hospital pharmacy that I even find it a bit difficult to keep posted about what you are doing.

My interest, not *in hospital pharmacy* as there was none but *in pharmacy in hospitals,* dates back perhaps 40 years or more, longer than I like to remember now. It was inspired, doubtless, by a summertime job in a village where there was a small hospital. It was from that time on I visited hospitals whenever I could, just as I have always visited pharmacy schools and drugstores.

I expected to see true professional pharmacy in hospitals and was much disappointed that it did not exist there. The more I observed and heard about the growing tendency towards commercialism in drugstores, the more I felt that if professional pharmacy was to exist, let alone grow to an ideal state, it would have to be in the hospital where the health professions were trained. That is the reason why I joined an organization where there was a medical school and hospitals that were connected with a teaching institution. It is an easy picture to visualize in a teaching hospital but more difficult to see in hospitals remote from teaching centers. Good pharmacy is as important in hospitals away from teaching centers as it is in the teaching and research hospital. It can be developed to a high degree of perfection there too, if the pharmacist can get the picture in his mind.

I also learned much from the hospital pharmacists who were pioneers in urging better professionalism in pharmacy. Many of them came regularly to conventions of the American Pharmaceutical Association where I met them and then later visited in their hospitals. Among these were William Gray of Presbyterian in Chicago and Irwin Becker of Michael Reese in Chicago. They were often together at meetings and always talked about professional pharmacy. Then there was Edward Swallow of Bellevue in New York City, who wrote constantly for the *National Drug Clerks Journal.* Ivor Griffith, now president of the Philadelphia College of Pharmacy and Science, was a hospital pharmacist at one time.

There were doubtless others whom I did not know, probably because they did not come to meetings or did not make themselves well known. I advise strongly attending all meetings of your profession, and you must never cease to urge your hospital to pay your necessary expenses to at least the annual meeting of your Society.

I never secured much help for hospital pharmacy from retail druggists, who often knew little about hospitals and probably thought of some of them as competitors. I never could arouse a very enthusiastic interest in hospital pharmacy among the leaders in our pharmaceutical organizations, though I talked to many of them about it.

My first real contact came when I told our director of hospitals at University Hospitals in Cleveland about my ideas. His first question was where could I go or where could he investigate this idea. We were forced to conclude that we could not find out about it all away from home. So he suggested that I come into our hospital several days each week and try to learn where pharmacy and how pharmacy could fit into the scheme of things. This I did for about a year. I placed a second man in the pharmacy who later became the hospital pharmacist. He was an exceptional person and could take notes; and in two or three evenings together each week, he gave me much information, both good and bad. His name was Paul Raymond Hudson, and he is now connected with Veterans Administration Hospitals.

We progressed from this point, even then giving practice to our seniors in the School of Pharmacy at Western Reserve in the hospital pharmacy until the hospitals moved to the campus when we then drew up an agreement between the hospitals, the school, and the university. In this agreement, I became directing pharmacist and my hospital pharmacists were put on our faculty.

About our first step after that was to establish a manufacturing and control laboratory in the school for the hospitals. This soon brought about the teaching of hospital pharmacy, first to undergraduates and later to graduate students. All received supervised instruction in the hospital pharmacy as well as in the manufacturing and control laboratory, and of course we developed regular courses in hospital pharmacy.

The next step was the selection of a Pharmacy Committee and a drug policy for the hospitals. An outgrowth of this was the development of a hospital formulary. These developments did much to establish our standing with the medical and administrative personnel. It was not long after this that Harvey Whitney developed the idea of hospital pharmacy interns and so we followed suit. We were able to get a small salary for an intern and placed him to live with the medical interns and residents. This first intern was Roger K. Lager, who later became the hospital pharmacist. He did much for our idea because of his close association with the younger medical men. Another idea that I got from Harvey, because of his pharmacy-controlled brace shop, was that of putting all professional stores under pharmacy control. We took them from the General Stores and placed a man in charge who could do some minor repairs.

We tried to aim at a policy of having all medicines and devices used by the hospital for the care of the patient under the pharmacy department. After all, this was no different from what existed in drugstores in the early days. Under our agreement, all pharmaceutical research was assigned to the pharmacy, and we had just been assigned a laboratory in the hospital for this purpose when I left in 1940.

The first minimum standard for hospital pharmacy was written upon the request of Dr. Malcolm MacEachern of the American College of Surgeons. He visited us, surveyed our work, talked to the medical members of the Pharmacy Committee, and then asked us to work up our standards and present them to a meeting of the American College of Surgeons in San Francisco. As such a trip was expensive, we asked Dr. Troy C. Daniels, a friend of ours and dean of the University of California School of Pharmacy, to read the paper. The standards were then adopted and printed in the *Bulletin of the American College of Surgeons.*

I think our greatest success from an educational standpoint, and from the standpoint of prestige, was the acceptance of hospital pharmacy by our graduate school and the placing of our staff upon the graduate faculty where I became chairman of the work. I had 13 graduate students in hospital pharmacy when I left Cleveland in 1940.

This is a very brief sketch of our activities and does not tell you anything about the "blood, sweat, and tears" of the doing. From a personal viewpoint, I think I was most fortunate in the pharmacists I had during the whole period of our activity, and they are the ones who really did the job and developed and carried out many of the ideas. These men and women are all in positions of responsibility today. Most of them are still in hospital pharmacy, though three are in hospital administration. One, Robert M. Porter, is administrator of the Baby's Hospital in Columbus, Ohio; another, Roger Marquand, has recently been appointed administrator of Cleveland's new Chronic Hospital; and a third, John Miller, is administrator of the Dover Hospital. The success of these young people is due to their knowledge, ability, and marked industry, coupled with a talent for making friends and being liked by people.

I think the most important faculty of a good hospital pharmacist, after a thorough knowledge of his subject, is to be able to create respect for himself and to make and keep friends.

It is of immense satisfaction to me to see the standing of the hospital pharmacist of today and to realize the fact that perhaps half, or more, of our hospitals have hospital pharmacies.

I am not unmindful of the help I received in early days from the Catholic Sisters, many of whom were students of mine. Many of them are still in hospital pharmacy, though several are administrators of their hospitals. They did, and are still doing, yeoman work in the cause of true professional pharmacy. One of them went to India and built a hospital there at Rawalpindi and is now building another in Karachi.

Like Hans Hansen, I too believe that professional pharmacy of today owes much of its standing and prestige to the stimulation given it by the hospital pharmacy movement.

It has been gratifying indeed to see the present attitude of the American Pharmaceutical Association towards hospital pharmacy, and I am certain that much of the recent reputation of professional pharmacy is owing to its affiliation with hospital pharmacy; and from my viewpoint, it is nothing short of miraculous to know that a leader in hospital pharmacy is the president of the great American Pharmaceutical Association. I have also been pleased by the writings and interest of the executive secretary of that Association in hospital pharmacy. One must not go further without expressing congratulations and thanks to Gloria Niemeyer.

The younger ones of you will find the going now far easier than we did. You have someone now in the ASHP to give advice on every problem you may have. You have precedents of things done to draw upon when you wish to do something. These things may be obtained by sending a letter to the editor of *The Bulletin*, or to such other hospital pharmacists who are known to you, or to Gloria Niemeyer in Washington. Even the older ones of us will always be willing to give as many answers as we can to one trying to do something. I have been amazed by the questions I have had over the years, even since I left the active work, and I have appreciated the letters that have been answered for me, and the visits too I have received from hospital pharmacists, and yet I am off the beaten track.

The individual pharmacist must not only read pharmaceutical journals and *The Bulletin* of the ASHP but also should read at least one journal in general medicine. He must read hospital magazines and be familiar with all new movements in the hospital field.

He must know the functions of each department in the hospital, what it is doing and why, and then do some thinking and see if there is any place where he fits in, to the end that the patient is better served. Hospital administration is always interested in economics and in savings; and while service comes first, savings make an impression upon the administrator.

Above all else, make friends with the administration and some important person in every department—more than one if possible. You must be known, respected, and recognized by your hospital colleagues if you are to succeed. Always be on the lookout for opportunities to recommend economies and better service. You do not need ever to be a pusher-in, but well-thought-out suggestions are always well received. Find time to take part in all movements of the hospital wherein people must help to make them a success for the name of the hospital.

Be sure to submit an annual report of the pharmacy to the administration, whether it be asked for or not. This justifies your better service which you have rendered. Do not confine it to savings alone but also point out service.

In closing, let me again thank you for the honor bestowed upon me, for perpetuating the name of my old friend and colleague Harvey A. K. Whitney, for the meeting and seeing you all again as old friends and the many new ones, and may I add I shall always be glad to hear from any of you and my latchstring is always out for you.

Inasmuch as this is probably the last time I shall ever address a body of pharmacists, I am going to quote one of my father's poems that expresses so well just how I feel today, and then from the church I shall sign my *Nunc Dimittis:*

An Instant of Retrospection

So many happy hours have been
Along my slight career,
That while I'm sitting calmly in
The deep'ning twilight here
I somehow feel a quick regret,
A sudden throb of pain,
A thought that makes my lashes wet,
That naught can come again.

At the time he received this award, Edward Spease was retired. He formerly was Dean of the School of Pharmacy, Western Reserve University, Cleveland, Ohio.

1953

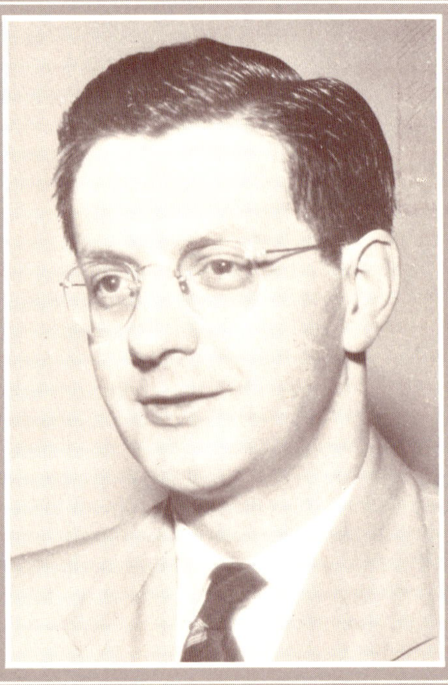

DONALD E. FRANCKE

"Hospital pharmacists can take justifiable pride in the fact that they are leading the way."

HOSPITAL PHARMACY LOOKS TO THE FUTURE

The first 10 years of the American Society of Hospital Pharmacists are now recorded history. In a great measure, the results of the past decade will ever stand as tribute to the inspiration and creative efforts of Harvey A. K. Whitney in whose honor the Michigan Society of Hospital Pharmacists has created this Lecture Award. Harvey Whitney's achievements and his influences continue to leave a permanent mark on all of us who now practice hospital pharmacy, and we know it will continue for years to come. I consider myself particularly fortunate to be one of those whose efforts have been inspired by Mr. Whitney's teachings. His sponsorship of the ASHP, his staunch support of the APhA, his pioneer work in hospital pharmacy internships, as well as his multitudinous efforts on behalf of hospital pharmacy, have been an inspiration to countless numbers in this field, as well as to me. He may well view with pride the ASHP as it begins its second decade of progressive activity.

During the past 10 years, hospital pharmacists have made a record which is recognized by all within our profession. But they are not ones to rest upon well-won laurels. While recognizing advances of the recent past, they are more interested in planning for the future. And they agree with Emerson when he said: "This time, like all other times, is a very good one if we but know what to do with it."

As hospital pharmacy looks to the future, I hope I may be bold enough to suggest a few areas to which increasing attention should be given. These suggestions will not contain much that is new. In fact, as one attempts to find new approaches and new ideas, he is reminded of the words of the former president of Fordham University who said:

All true civilization is 90% heirlooms and memories—an accumulation of small but precious deposits left by the countless generations that have gone before us. Only the very proud or very ignorant people imagine that our muddle headed present can begin everything all over again every day.

Tonight I shall limit my discussion to three points of what are in their entirety much larger problems. These are the expanding field of hospital pharmacy, the increase in professional responsibilities of the hospital pharmacist, and the increase in his professional consciousness.

Why is the field of hospital pharmacy expanding? Let us first look at hospitals in general for, after all, that is where hospital pharmacists function.

Hospitals are big business. In fact, they are the nation's fifth largest industry, yielding rank only to such industries as food and steel.

Let us look further at hospitals:

Hospitals	6,637
Beds	1,529,988
Bassinets (one live baby born in a hospital every 10 seconds)	92,000
Census, daily	1,300,000
Number admitted (one out of eight in the United States)	17,000,000
Employees	1,000,000
Investment	8 billion
Operating budget	3.5 billion
Pharmaceuticals	0.25 billion
New beds needed	850,000

Health insurance:

Total more than 80 million—over half by Blue Cross

Aged:

12 million over 65

In 1980, number will double to 24 million

This is the framework within which the hospital pharmacist functions. To say that pharmacists in hospitals play an important part in total medical care is to be conservative.

But there is very good evidence that the field of hospital pharmacy itself will expand greatly during the next few years. We know that today hospitals with less than 100 beds comprise our largest group of hospitals. But I believe this picture is changing. For example, 871 hospitals with between 50 and 99 beds reported that they were increasing their bed size in 1952 by an average of 66 beds per hospital. You can see what that will mean. In effect, it will mean that we shall have almost 900 new hospitals where full-time pharmacists will undoubtedly be employed. Of course, I don't know where these pharmacists will come from. But it is of great significance to hospital pharmacy, to the colleges, and to pharmacy as a whole that these potential positions are available.

Further than this, 1535 hospitals with less than 50 beds reported an addition of an average of 28 beds per hospital in 1952. The effect of these figures on the future of hospital pharmacy is more difficult to evaluate because all of these hospitals are still less than 100 beds. On the other hand, today 20% of all hospitals under 50 beds and 38% of those between 50 and 99 beds do employ a pharmacist. Thus, it is not difficult to predict that of these 1500 hospitals, several hundred more will be adding pharmacists—or at least the potential is there.

There is also another large area in which expansion has taken place. A total of 933 hospitals of between 100 and 249 beds have added an average of 146 beds each during 1952. If we think in general terms of one pharmacist per 100 beds in a general, short-term hospital, then it is clear that several hundred new positions will open.

The total impact of these developments is difficult to judge precisely. However, I think we are relatively safe in predicting that there are now between 1000 and 2000 new potential jobs in hospital pharmacy.

Thus, hospital pharmacy is an expanding field, and it is a specialty which has become increasingly important to the APhA, to hospitals, and to colleges of pharmacy, as well as to manufacturers of pharmaceuticals. It is a field full of opportunity, a specialty which is only now developing its potential, a profession which has great promise for a brilliant future.

This expansion of opportunities in hospital pharmacy places obvious obligations upon the ASHP, the Division of Hospital Pharmacy, local chapters, colleges of pharmacy, and hospitals themselves. It calls for more publicity on the opportunities in our field; it means that we should devote more attention to the training of pharmacy interns; it means greater opportunities for graduate education in hospital pharmacy; it indicates a greater role than ever before for the hospital pharmacist in the distribution of drugs and an increased opportunity for hospital pharmacists to play an important role in pharmaceutical education of the future. I shall discuss none of these tonight.

One of the significant trends in hospital pharmacy today—and one which will become even more firmly established in the future—is the active role played by the hospital pharmacist in the evaluation and selection of drugs used in the hospital.

It is principally through his role as member and secretary of the Pharmacy and Therapeutics Committee that he carries out these responsibilities. Today, more than ever before, there is a great deal of interest in the Pharmacy and Therapeutics Committee, and an increasing number of hospitals are actively promoting the work of this committee. For some time, requests for information on the related subjects of the Pharmacy and Therapeutics Committee and the hospital formulary have formed one of the largest single categories of information requests handled by the office of the Division of Hospital Pharmacy.

Now the pharmacist has always, in fact and by tradition, been a consultant to the physician in matters pertaining to drugs. Why then do we say that there is an increase in professional responsibility when this type of activity is nothing particularly new? It seems to me that the difference today, as it will be in the future, is one of degree rather than of new function. We know too that those pharmacists, whether in retail or hospital practice, who have served as consultants to physicians are the ones who have enjoyed the greatest professional prestige. There are several reasons today why hospital pharmacists have greater opportunities to act in a consultative capacity.

One of these is the tremendous advance in therapy accompanied by the introduction of a great number of new basic drugs. So rapid have been these advances that it is said that 90% of the prescriptions written today couldn't have been filled 10 years ago. Is it any wonder that physicians have a difficult time keeping up with new advances?

But this is not the only reason why physicians and hospital pharmacists are working together more cooperatively. Another is the great number of product duplications and combinations introduced constantly. For example, these are the figures for 1951: firms, 86; products, 332; basic drugs, 35; duplication of basic drugs, 74; and combinations, 221.

These figures represent only those products introduced in one year. If we attempt to determine the cumulative effect of this practice for even a three-year period, we are confronted with a most confusing and chaotic situation. Over a period of but a few years, hundreds of combinations and duplications come and go, but it always seems that more come than go. And, of course, it is impossible for the physician to find his way alone through this labyrinth of complex and oftentimes controversial materia medica. He needs the assistance of the pharmacist and, to an increasing extent, those in hospital pharmacy are filling this need.

We see today that there are stirrings of a more objective approach towards sound drug therapy, and in this movement the hospital pharmacist plays an increasingly important role. In a recent article in *The Bulletin*, J. S. Mordell discussed very well the hospital pharmacist's role in the support of sound drug therapy. He emphasized that the success of the program depends in large measure on the professional stature of the pharmacist. Mordell stated:

> *To some pharmacists, as to some physicians and dentists, this type of operation may mean a departure from deeply rooted pathways of thought and action. It calls for a new perspective in the handling of drugs. It calls for basic knowledge not only of technical pharmaceutical functions but of drug actions and use and the differences and shortcomings which may exist among drugs.*

It seems to me that this trend, which is gaining momentum constantly, offers great opportunities for us as pharmacists to increase our professional responsibilities. Through our cooperative efforts with our colleagues in the medical profession, we can increase our value as professional men and women with resulting benefit not only to pharmacy but also to medicine, to our hospital, and to the patient. These are indeed goals towards which we should continue to strive. And as time moves on, I am confident that the hospital pharmacist will, through the efforts of the Society and its network of affiliated chapters, occupy an increasingly important position not only in the selection and procurement of pharmaceuticals but also as a valued consultant to the physician.

Of all groups in American pharmacy, none has increased in professional consciousness and stature during recent years more than have hospital pharmacists. Why is this? Of course, there are many reasons. One of them is the professional advancement which has come about through the development of the American Society of Hospital Pharmacists and the cooperative efforts of its members and local branches. Surely the Society with its 35 affiliated chapters and more than 2000 members, widely scattered but still working for the same prime objective, has been and continues to be an important reason for increased professional stature.

But it seems to me that there is even a more fundamental reason. And this I believe is the loyal support that hospital pharmacists give to the American Pharmaceutical Association. As you know, each active as well as associate member of the ASHP is required to be a member of the APhA. Local chapters of the ASHP have similar provisions in their constitutions and by-laws, and, as a group, they are very cooperative in enforcing this rule.

At first thought, this may appear to be a subject worthy of little emphasis. But actually it has many ramifications. To appreciate fully the implications of this strong support of the APhA, we must note one of the fundamental errors of American pharmacy. This is the error of poor professional organization, of uncoordinated activities, and of the failure of the American pharmacists to support their national professional organization. You will recall that when the American Pharmaceutical Association was founded, members of that organization went back to their home states to form state associations. These men very naively assumed that the state associations would be closely affiliated with the national organization. How sadly they were mistaken we know full well today. Hindsight is always more clear than foresight, but still it is very difficult to understand how a national organization could develop over the course of the century with so little effort given to sound organizational structure.

It is not a question of lack of organizations. Today we have at least 18 organizations which serve pharmacy nationally; nine of these are classified as professional in character and activity while the other nine are commercial. The aims and activities of these 18 organizations are uncoordinated and oftentimes in conflict. As a result, the quality and quantity of professional accomplishment are low. Not only this, but we must remember also that scarcely more than one-half of America's 100,000 pharmacists are professionally minded enough to maintain membership in any pharmaceutical association.

It is my firm conviction that American pharmacy will not come into its own until we have a majority of our pharmacists actively supporting their national professional organization. Someone has defined an organization as a medium for the efficient movement of groups of men towards goals to which they aspire. How can we move American pharmacists towards professional goals until we enroll them in our Association? Only when this is done will the Association, its ideals, its ethics, its concepts of professional service become ingrained in all who practice our profession.

The state of affairs in our country is, of course, in sharp contrast to those in European countries where every pharmacist who practices must be a member of his national professional organization. As a result, pharmacists are united in their professional objectives and are powerful when they wish to sponsor a program for the welfare of the profession. For example, the National Health Service in Great Britain will eventually establish a number of clinics. But so far the Pharmaceutical Society of Great Britain, of which every British pharmacist is a member, has seen to it that patients have their prescriptions filled in an established local pharmacy. They have also required these local pharmacies to meet rather rigid requirements. A similar situation exists in France where the National Order of Pharmacists has persuaded hospital pharmacists not to fill prescriptions for outpatients in order that pharmacists as a group may more fully practice their profession. We recognize, of course, that similar attempts have been made in this country. But these have been characterized by efforts to gain certain advantages without any attempt to correct underlying difficulties.

The basic difficulty of American pharmacy has been well stated in the Pharmaceutical Survey:

Unity of purpose requires a unified utilization of power. This requirement pharmacy has not met. . . . Throughout the survey there has been an accumulation of evidence indicative of the handicaps for the professional unity and professional progress of pharmacy due to the absence of any one recognized agency that speaks to us upon matters of fundamental policy.

Historically, the American Pharmaceutical Association should be the key organization, and under certain circumstances it does represent pharmacy. Yet no more than one-seventh of the pharmacists of the country are members of this organization. Consequently, the scope and speed of its influences are limited.

It seems to me that hospital pharmacists can take justifiable pride in the fact that they are leading the way for other groups in pharmacy to correct some of our gravest errors. By requiring membership in the American Pharmaceutical Association, they have served notice on American pharmacy that they are concerned not only with hospital pharmacy but with the welfare of the profession as a whole. It is relatively easy for specialists such as hospital pharmacists to be selfish in organizational matters and to build their own organization up, at the same time forgetting the total welfare of the profession. This is the general pattern that too many in American pharmacy follow. But it is truly exceptional and heartening to see a group like the ASHP place the welfare and strength of the profession of pharmacy above and beyond that of hospital pharmacy.

Again let me quote from the Pharmaceutical Survey:

The profession must contain a far greater proportion of members who are ever sharply jealous of the high reputation of the profession and who, by energetic cooperation, are determined ever to protect that reputation.

Hospital pharmacists as a group have met this challenge. But as we look to the future, we see that if we are to continue to add strength to professional pharmacy in America, we must redouble our efforts to see that every hospital pharmacist is a member of the APhA and the ASHP. Membership in the national professional organization is the first step in increasing professional consciousness of any pharmacist.

As hospital pharmacy faces the future, let us recall the words of John Stuart Mill who said:

History shows that great economic and social forces flow like a tide over communities only half conscious of that which is befalling them. Wise statesmen foresee what time is thus bringing and try to shape institutions and mold men's thoughts and purposes in accordance with the change that is silently coming on.

The unwise are those who bring nothing constructive to the process, and who greatly imperil the future of mankind, by leaving great questions to be fought out between ignorant change on one hand, and ignorant opposition to change on the other.

Let us in hospital pharmacy anticipate the future and prepare for it. With vision, with courage, with a true recognition of our opportunities for greater service in public health, let us aim high in hope and work as we fulfill our obligations as members of an important segment of the public health team.

At the time he received this award, Donald E. Francke was the Chief Pharmacist at the University of Michigan Hospital, Ann Arbor, and Editor of *The Bulletin of American Society of Hospital Pharmacists.*

1954

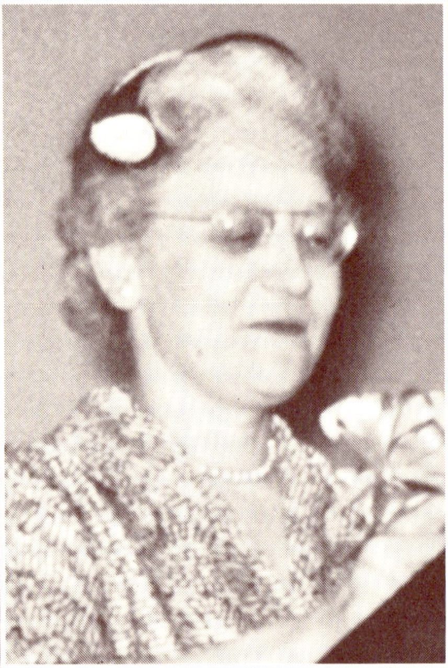

EVLYN GRAY SCOTT

"United strength should be the guarantee of the future progress of pharmacy."

THE POINT-RATING PLAN— AN OPPORTUNITY

In America during the past 10 years, as you are all aware, there has been a phenomenal growth in the number of hospital patients. This increase in hospital patients has necessitated an increase in available hospital beds, which were provided either by remodeling or by new hospital facilities.

During the same period, cost per patient day has more than tripled; a new factor has to be dealt with in the payment of patient bills—hospital insurance companies; diagnostic aids have multiplied; and the therapeutic measures have become complex. Pharmacy plays some part in most of the therapeutic facilities of the modern hospital. In today's overall complex hospital picture, pharmacy finds itself involved with an increasing budget, finding adequate storage for many more heat- or cold-sensitive drugs or chemicals, helping hospital personnel through the maze of confusing drug names, helping with the selection of basic drugs so that adequate care may be given a patient without unduly adding to the cost per patient day, providing sufficient supervision for the pharmacy technical staff, and many other involved problems that any of you could add to the list.

Hospital pharmacists have looked forward to the time when the administration of hospitals and pharmaceutical educational faculties would be aware of the part pharmacy should contribute to the nation's hospitals. The time has arrived, and why aren't we as satisfied as we had expected to be? For the reason that there are many more places to be filled with competent hospital pharmacists than there are pharmacists available.

An adequate basic college degree in pharmacy should provide sufficient groundwork upon which to build the specialized training needed to cope with today's hospital pharmacy. For the recent graduate of pharmacy, the hospital pharmacy internships provide this specialized training. But there are not enough such plans nor enough graduates enrolled in them to supply our hospitals' needs. Then how can the situation be aided until the above condition changes? Self education of the present hospital pharmacists will aid us now. And how can we do this? One of the aids that has helped in the past 10 years has been the specialized professional publications—both periodicals and books. Probably the one of most general help has been our Society's *Bulletin. The Bulletin* as we have it today is the result of the devoted care and time given it by Mr. Don Francke and Miss Gloria Niemeyer.

Another aid has been the institutes and refresher courses for hospital pharmacy held all over the United States. Part of the success of the institutes and refresher courses has been due to the great amount of time and thought given to them by a great number of people interested in hospital pharmacy. Conventions and local meetings of pharmacy groups have aided not only by their programs but because of the opportunity afforded for pharmacists to become acquainted with others of their profession and so more easily exchange ideas and enthusiasms.

In going back to the hospital as a whole, when we look for one single thing that probably has contributed more than any other one factor in providing the American people with the best hospital care to be found in the world today, we find standardization programs such as that started by the American College of Surgeons years ago. Now we in pharmacy have been very fortunate in having some foresighted pharmacists who were aware of what hospitals should be getting from their hospital pharmaceutical service. Two such people were Mr. Edward Spease, one of the recipients of the Harvey Whitney Award, and Harvey Whitney for whom the Award was so appropriately named. Mr. Spease was instrumental in formulating the original *Minimum Standard* which was adopted by the American College of Surgeons. The concepts found in this standard are the same as those in our present *Minimum Standard.* There is one difference; the concepts have been expanded. I imagine at the time of the original writing Mr. Spease hoped there would not be too many, when they read them, that would think he lived in an ivory tower instead of the practical world of teaching hospital and active pharmacy college.

Your own Mr. Whitney established the hospital pharmacy internship at the University of Michigan. I believe that the examples they set and their teaching programs inspired and influenced so many other pharmacists that it was possible to develop the groundwork necessary, over the past years, to have made possible the development of the present *Minimum Standard for Pharmacies in Hospitals.* We are fortunate and should be ever grateful that precepts of what constitutes modern hospital pharmacy were developed long enough before this great upsurge in modern hospital care so that hospital pharmacy is ready to present a united front based on sound concepts when carrying out the objectives of the pharmacy in a hospital.

As has been mentioned, we cannot wait for sufficient special formal training such as internships of hospital pharmacists but must turn to self education. Three aids have been mentioned—first, *The Bulletin*; second, the institutes; third, conventions and meetings. And now a fourth is added, the Point-Rating Plan to implement the *Minimum Standard*. This plan was worked out by Mr. Ray Kneifl, Executive Secretary of The Catholic Hospital Association, with the help of a committee made of Catholic Sisters who are hospital pharmacists. The plan was for the aid and education of the Catholic group of hospitals. The universality of the plan was recognized when the American Society of Hospital Pharmacists accepted this plan at the Philadelphia Convention in August 1952.

To me, the Point-Rating Plan represents more than a tool to implement the *Minimum Standard*—rather it represents an opportunity for every hospital and hospital pharmacist to become aware of where he and his hospital pharmacy stand as regards the standards for hospital pharmacy in the United States. This affords the opportunity for one to locate the strong points as well as the weak, where more emphasis must be placed, where we are to look for help, and where we shall be able to help others. And why is this such an opportunity? It is an opportunity to help yourself. We can foresee in the not too distant future the need of a standardization body evaluating the pharmacy department of the hospital. Until then, we have the opportunity of correcting and improving our own weak points. But regardless of this, most of us like keeping up to a mark; but sometimes we get a little confused as to what is the mark. I suppose that it works something like competition. We sometimes need to get a stimulant from an outside source to keep up our spirits. So we need a measuring tool, and now we have one for hospital pharmacy—the Point-Rating Plan.

There comes a time during feverish activity, shortage of time, ever increasing responsibility, piling up of unread literature, and endless conferences when we must find time to stop and survey our results to see if we are still on the road towards our goal. This appraisal is absolutely necessary if we are to keep forging ahead with our other partners in the hospital team. Even if one feels he cannot spare the time to attend conventions and institutes at distant places, one need have no doubt as to how well he or his department measures up in the field of good hospital pharmacy. Here is a rating plan one can study, alone if necessary and at his own convenience. The results would be more objective if he could do it with someone else who has some understanding of hospital procedures. Using the plan alone, the pharmacist might be too modest in his scoring—then he does his hospital and himself an injustice. On the other hand, he does an injustice to both if the scoring is too high, because then a false sense of security or performance prevents expending the necessary thought and energy to correcting the weak spots. Should the rating be too low at first, here is the opportunity to become aware of which areas need reinforcement. A low score does not necessarily place the blame on the pharmacist, because this score might be the result of conditions that only the administration can remedy. The pharmacist should feel that he has the backing of the whole American Society of Hospital Pharmacists as he presents these points to the administrator.

We are all too busy; we need the stimuli of something such as the Point-Rating Plan to make us stop and think about our overall plan. Working hard does not excuse us from obtaining the expected and necessary results. Pharmacy is no longer working alone, no longer can it be hidden off in a far corner because the past few years have taken pharmacy off of its island of isolation. Partnership in the public health team carries the responsibility of constantly keeping abreast of pharmaceutical progress. So we need to review our past and present performance if we are to decide what we need to do today and tomorrow to keep our part of the partnership in good order.

There are some things about the Point-Rating Plan which look a little formidable at first glance. For instance, there are a lot of pages with a lot of print. There is the temptation to put it aside and do something about it another time. You know, the time that never comes. One needs to remember that this rating was designed to fit all hospitals—large, small, specialized, or general—and to be applied by skilled pharmacists with varied experiences or the neophyte, and to be understood by many types of administrators. To fit such a great array of things and people, an explanation that is extensive is needed. By the time anyone has gone through such explanation and definition of terms and checked the rating sheets, a much clearer picture of what comprises hospital pharmacy is provided, even if a rather complex one. Is there anyone who still thinks that hospital pharmacy is a place to retire or an easy berth? Then here is an outline to disillusion quickly that innocent.

This plan is not meant to be static. There is no reason it should not be worked over to try to simplify or clarify it. In fact, the plan in its present form is simpler than the form first presented in the July–August (1952) issue of *The Bulletin.*

The categories of the Point-Rating Plan are specifically numbered to show which minimum standard they are implementing. The total possible basic points is now 2000 so that each 20 points equals 1%. This makes the figuring simple. There probably could be some way to summarize the plan so that we would have a long and short form—something like the government has with its short and long tax blanks.

In conclusion, the Point-Rating Plan affords the opportunity for every hospital pharmacist to see the maximum possibilities of hospital pharmacy in all its ramifications and the inter-relationship between the various categories; with this understanding, all hospital pharmacists should be able to have a feeling of kinship to every other hospital pharmacist. This united strength should be the guarantee of the future progress of pharmacy in its special field of hospital pharmacy.

At the time she received this award, Evlyn Gray Scott was the Chief Pharmacist at St. Luke's Hospital, Cleveland, Ohio.

1955

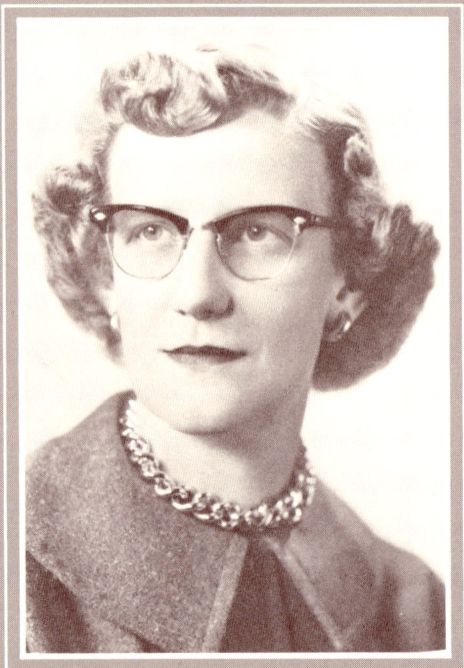

GLORIA NIEMEYER FRANCKE

"How much we need leaders in hospital pharmacy!"

RESPONSIBILITIES OF ASHP AFFILIATED CHAPTERS

One of the significant developments in the growth of hospital pharmacy has been the springing up of organized groups throughout many parts of the country. Fortunately, these local organizations have aligned themselves closely with the American Society of Hospital Pharmacists, each affiliated chapter having a constitution and by-laws patterned after those of its national organization and each requiring membership in the national professional groups—the Society and the American Pharmaceutical Association. In so doing, these groups of hospital pharmacists have also subscribed to the objectives of the APhA and the ASHP. The very fact that these chapters are closely affiliated with the national organizations—having the same ideals, the same goals—gives hospital pharmacy great strength.

With this strength has come a need for the national organizations and the individual affiliates and members to take certain responsibilities in order that one unit, one common goal and concord, will exist.

The need for affiliated chapters established in local areas throughout the United States is evident. In fact, organization of local groups of hospital pharmacists preceded formation of the national Society. In a survey of hospital pharmacy organizations in the United States in 1939, we find that already 11 local or regional groups were active. In this survey, the author pointed out that among the "hospital pharmacy associations now existing in the United States, a feeling of isolation predominated. Thus the main purpose of this survey is to cement each group, each association together, enlightening each as to how the other functions. . . ." As pointed out by Dr. Alex Berman in *Ten Years of the American Society of Hospital Pharmacists*, this implied that only a national hospital pharmacy association could weld together the disconnected regional hospital pharmacy groups and dispel the "feeling of isolation."

Thus, the American Society of Hospital Pharmacists had its roots in these already established local groups. Leaders of these chapters became the first leaders in the Society.

We who are in association work are often asked to enumerate the services made available from the national organizations—or what do I get for my membership dues? We like to think that tangible benefits are provided, but is not membership in your own professional group more meaningful than what you get out of it? For years, we have been talking about what the Society can do for you, and now what about the responsibilities of the affiliated chapters and the individual members to the Society? With unity comes progress. Only by carrying out our responsibilities in our affiliated chapters and the Society will we be able to move forward towards the betterment of hospital pharmacy and the entire profession.

With the growing needs in hospital pharmacy, the national organization must be ready to assume an ever important role in the profession. Hospital pharmacy must have a voice in matters concerning practice in this specialty. Major problems facing the profession today—education, substitution and duplication, cost of drugs, international problems related to drug distribution, and many others—all affect hospital pharmacy practice. In all of these, we must look to the ASHP chapters for help.

Development of the affiliated chapters of the ASHP has been a significant contribution to the total organization. Probably in no other specialty in either the hospital field or pharmacy has such a small group made such great strides in so few years. Your own Michigan Society has played a part in this progress. But, above all, there has been a growing need for adequate pharmaceutical service in the nation's hospitals. Increases in the number of hospital beds and the trend towards centralization of medical care increase the need for your services as hospital pharmacists.

So tonight let us look at this development from the standpoint of our own organization and its affiliated chapters. From time to time, we must evaluate our contributions in relation to the profession as a whole and assume our share in its strength. We need to examine continually the present concept of our organization, measuring accomplishment against objective, practice against idea, and, perhaps from time to time, redefine our goals.

Before considering the responsibilities of our affiliated chapters in relation to our objectives and goals, let us for a moment look at the Society from the "local level." At the 1955 Annual Meeting, it was reported that the Society has 43 affiliated chapters. Of these, three are regional groups and 40 are state or local organizations. An additional three groups have recently applied for affiliation. These chapters represent a great part of our membership and must accept certain responsibilities in the national organization.

And now with this brief background, *what* can the chapters do to strengthen our Society, hospital pharmacy, and the profession? What part should they play in the national organization? And above all, what are their responsibilities?

It has been said that "organization begins when people combine their efforts for a given purpose. The first principle of organization is coordination, which is the orderly arrangement of group effort to provide unity of action in the pursuit of a common purpose."

Organizations cannot be put into narrow categories. The Society's local groups follow no one set pattern. The national organization has not attempted to set up a program to be followed by all chapters. Still, great contributions have been made by each group. We must expect a type of disorder in organization—a multitude of expressions and ideas—differences of opinions. Or, as the poet has said: "The chaos is come of organized disorder." From these expressions, we must determine attitudes and define our common goals.

At first I thought I would attempt to outline for you some of the projects which have been carried out by the ASHP chapters. But much of this has been reported through *The Bulletin*, and I would prefer to spend the time discussing briefly our greatest need in hospital pharmacy—leadership.

Further, I could mention some of the responsibilities as outlined in the Constitutions and By-Laws and elaborate on why affiliated chapters must keep the national organization's office informed about their activities, why membership in the ASHP and the APhA should be a requirement for membership in the local group, et cetera. But these are fundamental responsibilities with which you are all familiar.

And so it seems quite apropo tonight for us—at this H. A. K. Whitney Award Lecture—to appeal to you and all the affiliated chapters for leadership. Mr. Whitney *led* the way in so much that is ours today. As stated in *Ten Years of the American Society of Hospital Pharmacists:*

> *Harvey A. K. Whitney has inspired all who practice in this specialty by his leadership and untiring efforts in bringing about a national organization for hospital pharmacists. As the first chairman of the American Society of Hospital Pharmacists, one of the first editors of* The Bulletin *and a leader in establishing the internship programs, hospital pharmacists will always recognize his role in the advancement of their specialty during this era.*

We must keep in mind that every leader is not necessarily a national figure. True, it is probable that those who become leaders in local groups will find their way to working in activities on a national basis. Some become disillusioned with working with a national group. Projects move more slowly, and by nature the American people expect everything to move forward fast and in great proportions. Hospital pharmacists are no exception.

Just to stir our thinking and in the hope that Society members will be giving some thought to the need for leadership in the ASHP, we might mention some of the qualities of a good leader and translate these into action in the ASHP and our affiliated chapters.

Although tonight we are thinking primarily of the need for leaders in hospital pharmacy, actually every enterprise in life is bound up with leadership—the problem of providing able individuals to help others achieve useful goals.

How much we need leaders in hospital pharmacy! And here the local chapters of the ASHP *must* play an important role. We need people who know *good* hospital pharmacy practice. We need people who are familiar with the problems of hospital pharmacy. We need people who have worked with hospital pharmacists and who are familiar with the activities of the ASHP. We need hospital pharmacists—members of the Society—who actively support the American Pharmaceutical Association and know something about its affairs. But above all, we need people with a sense of professional pride, those who accept their role in the Society as being a part of their role as a professional person, not on the basis of what do I get but what can I give.

Recently, when thinking a great deal about leadership, particularly in the Society, I found these qualities outlined. They appeal to me and, though modified somewhat to apply to our organizations, they carry the message which I would like to bring to you tonight.

The *first quality* of a good leader is a harmonious or sympathetic relationship with the group he is working with. There must be an appreciation of what the individuals in the group are doing—and with this goes a measure of confidence, sincerity, integrity, and humility.

A *second quality* is ambition—not for ourselves but for the cause, our profession. Those who have this quality take pay for their work, but they do not work for pay. I guess that is like saying: "I would gladly work without pay if I could but afford it."

A *third quality* is knowing where you want to go with your group—you must have a goal. I heard a story once which illustrates this very well. A teacher advised the students in her class to "learn to play the game of life." One boy spoke up and said: "But how can we teacher when we don't know where the goalposts are?" And so it is in the Society activities. We must define our goals.

The *fourth quality* is that the good leader will face opposition creatively. He must be tactful, tolerant, and understanding of the other person's point of view. The following quotation, taken from John Erskine's *The Complete Life*, points out the importance of seeing the other person's point of view:

> *The body travels more easily than the mind, and until we have limbered up our imagination, we continue to think as though we had stayed at home. We have not really budged a step until we take up residence in someone else's point of view.*

And *five*, the good leader must have skill and inspire confidence. This might be translated into knowing your job and your organizations. Here, hospital pharmacists have not always taken every opportunity to learn about what is going on in the Society. When hospital pharmacists are appointed or elected to positions of responsibility, they are not always adequately prepared to accept. They have not taken the necessary time to learn about the details of organization, the activities of the committees, et cetera. Attendance at Annual Meetings and institutes and attention to publications all contribute to knowing your Society, its objectives, and what it stands for. This would apply as well to the day-to-day work in your pharmacy.

A *sixth quality* of the good leader—and to me the most important—he must have enthusiasm. In Proverbs, we read: "Whatsoever thy hand findeth to do, do it with all your might, heart and soul."

And in organizational work, it is important that the good leader have a realistic sense of the lethargy of people. Truly, we cannot drive. Timing is important, and the leader knows that people do less when pushed.

We could stop here since with leaders having these qualities, we are bound to succeed. Perhaps we all cannot be leaders, but I am sure that all of us have at least some of these qualities.

These qualities of leadership must be translated into action in the American Society of Hospital Pharmacists and its 43 affiliated chapters. Specific application falls into many categories, and I am outlining some of the ways in which your affiliated chapter can provide even greater contributions.

These qualities of leadership can very well apply to our ASHP chapters. They also apply to the national organization, although the very roots of our Society are in the local groups and in your individual efforts.

The leader in the local group recognizes the fact that his chapter is made up of hospital pharmacists who have varied backgrounds in education and experience. These people have reached the position they now hold by traveling different roads. One, there are those who have followed the same educational program which all undergraduate pharmacy students follow and then simply accepted a position as a hospital pharmacist where they learned by doing. Two, there are those who have followed the usual undergraduate course with a master's program along with specialized training in hospital pharmacy. And three, there are those who have taken what might be called the straight internship, that is training which is not combined with graduate work in a school of pharmacy. We know that in each case the road traveled has some merit, and it is difficult to evaluate one method over the other.

Too, in the leader's relationship with the group, he recognizes the fact that the members are practicing in different types of institutions—government, nongovernment, large, small, specialized, et cetera. Consequently, the problems vary from one institution to another and may call for an appreciation of what your fellow member is doing.

With these understandings, the leader will inspire confidence, sincerity, integrity, and humility—the first quality of a good leader.

Application of the second quality—ambition—is perhaps not too rare. Those who have ambition for the profession will make every effort to help others improve their pharmacy service. There are perhaps hundreds of ways in which this can be accomplished through your local meetings. Providing regular programs, special seminars, panel discussions, and continuing projects and working with the various committees all contribute towards this end and, in turn, foster ambition among the other members. Too, encouraging new people to enter hospital pharmacy, fostering establishment of internships, and working with the schools in providing courses in our specialty all contribute towards providing better pharmacy service. Here we must recognize that progress in the profession is based on advancement of education and training of the future hospital pharmacists.

We have talked about goals in a general way. I keep thinking of the lines from a poem: "Keep your goal in sight and labor toward it day and night." In Society work, we have two types of goals. First, the long-range objectives which are set down in our Constitutions and By-Laws and which usually remain the same; and second, the immediate goals which can be accomplished this year. Our long-range objective—providing pharmaceutical services which will contribute to better patient care—provides a basis for our total Society program. Projects in local groups must be keyed to the needs of members in the different areas. Thus, in defining our goals in the Society from year to year, we look to our leaders to analyze the greatest needs in hospital pharmacy. In your local groups, this requires diligent leadership; but here there is a great opportunity to serve your local Society, the national groups, and the profession.

We have also mentioned that the good leader will face opposition creatively. Opposition in hospital pharmacy, as in any group, is inevitable. It is a sign or symptom of an unmet need. View it as an opportunity and find out what the need is. Sometimes understanding can be brought about in a simple manner by offering the opportunity to discuss the problem at hand. Perhaps this sounds a bit too elementary when actually we know that facing opposition requires the greatest of statesmanship, diplomacy, and all that goes to make for good leadership. Sir Winston Churchill, one of the greatest leaders of our time, is known for his facing opposition in spite of all else. On the occasion of Churchill's 80th birthday last year, John Masefield paid tribute to this great leader with this four-line verse:

This Man, in darkness, saw; in doubtings, led;
In danger, did; in uttermost despair
Shone, with Hope that made the midnight fair
The world he saved calls blessings on his head.

Skill and confidence come from knowing. Nothing can replace knowledge and diligent work. Only a few years ago, Mr. Hansen, recipient of the 1951 H. A. K. Whitney Award, spoke to you on "Work by the Side of Work." His message applies very well to all we are saying tonight. Here, I would like to emphasize the importance of your knowing something about your profession. To understand the relationship between the various specialties in pharmacy, to know of the work of the American Pharmaceutical Association as well as your own Society, to follow the trends of the colleges and boards, to have some understanding of the role of industry in the profession will give you the background needed in order to fulfill an important role in your chapter and in the Society.

In the ASHP, we have two problems relating to communication, that of the local affiliates keeping the national group informed of activities and, secondly, the national Society keeping you posted. Our publications, the Annual Reports, the conventions and institutes, and our close contact with the officers in each chapter all serve as mediums for communicating ideas. The one provision which has been made for representation in the Society is the House of Delegates, which meets each year in connection with the Annual Meeting. One of the responsibilities of a local Society is that some one of your Executive Committee members attends the ASHP Annual Meeting so that we know what you are doing and you know what we are thinking. The delegates from the chapters must be informed on the activities being carried out on a local basis, the thinking of hospital pharmacists in their local areas, and be ready to express themselves on matters of policy affecting the Society. Equally important is that they return to their respective chapters with new ideas and details of the discussions so that there can be coordination of the activities on the national level with those on the local level. Leaders must take the responsibility for reviewing the Annual Reports and bringing anything of particular interest to the attention of the group.

Too, a delegate to the ASHP meetings can further expand his background, his usefulness to his local chapter, by giving attention to all phases of the total APhA Convention program.

This method of representation—the House of Delegates—in the ASHP has been set up for a purpose. If we are to function properly, if we are to be a body representing all hospital pharmacists in the country, we must be certain that affiliated chapters assume their rightful role. Otherwise, the entire organizational setup breaks down and it becomes impossible for either the national or the local groups to carry out their responsibilities.

We should mention that some of the greatest contributions to better pharmacy practice in hospitals have been made by small groups where the members have worked closely together. Of particular note are groups such as the Utah Society of Hospital Pharmacists. Organized but a few years ago, this group has banded together to form a strong state organization in which I believe every hospital pharmacist in the state is affiliated with the APhA and the ASHP, as well as the Utah Society. Their efforts in working out a pricing schedule and studying problems related to floor stocks and other phases of hospital pharmacy practice have been major contributions.

Local chapters must have active committees and, when possible, coordinate activities with those of the national committees. In some few cases, we have had an opportunity to work closely with the affiliates on projects, and the results have been rewarding. I believe that when we were working on the *Minimum Standard*, it was sent to all of the chapters for comments. The response was good, and the results of the comments were compiled for consideration when the final draft of the standard was worked out. Such efforts can produce fruitful results.

Numerous affiliated chapters have carried out projects and worked closely with the Society's committees. This one activity alone has opened the way to greater participation by a large number of members. Some of the work which has been carried out by affiliated chapters far outranks anything being done by the national group. Among the projects carried out in recent years are the following: promoting or sponsoring some type of continuing educational programs—seminars, institutes, etc.; sponsoring a student visitation program; studying application of the *Minimum Standard for Pharmacies in Hospitals* with particular reference to the Point-Rating Plan; compiling a list of common household poisons along with antidotes; and a large number of special projects for which there has been a need in specific areas.

We would hope that each affiliated chapter would carry out some type of continuing project. Although suggestions have come from the national group from time to time, this is really something which can best be developed by the members of the individual chapters. The national organization should, of course, give some leadership and coordination to the projects. This has been accomplished, to a degree, by our Committee on Special Projects.

We have emphasized the responsibilities of affiliated chapters in the organization. There are possibly even greater areas in which each individual hospital pharmacist can participate. It is accepted that everyone cannot go to all the national meetings. But we do want representation from all groups and, through the delegates, reach a large segment of our membership.

The role which the greater number of our members are taking—that of improving pharmacy service in their individual hospitals—cannot be overlooked. By sharing your thoughts and knowledge, by carrying out your day-to-day work as a professional person, and by striving towards our fundamental objectives, hospital pharmacists are contributing immeasurably to progress in the organizations and in the profession as a whole. After all we have said about leadership and work in organizations, we still realize that the greatest possibility for progress lies with the individual practitioner in hospital pharmacy.

If we can but carry forward these simple ideas in a small measure, we shall expand the influence of hospital pharmacy in these United States many times—good leaders, participation by all hospital pharmacists, a means of communicating our ideas, and a spirit of unity will join us together.

We again pay tribute to Mr. H. A. K. Whitney whose leadership brings us here tonight. To those others who have been recipients of the Whitney Award—Spease, Hansen, Purdum, Francke, and Scott—we owe a debt of gratitude.

To all of you—members of the Michigan Society of Hospital Pharmacists—I express my appreciation, not only for this honor tonight but for all you have done for hospital pharmacy. I am ever mindful of the role of the affiliated chapters and individual members in the national organization.

At the time she received this award, Gloria Niemeyer Francke was Secretary of the American Society of Hospital Pharmacists and Assistant Director of the Division of Hospital Pharmacy, American Pharmaceutical Association, Washington, D.C.

1956

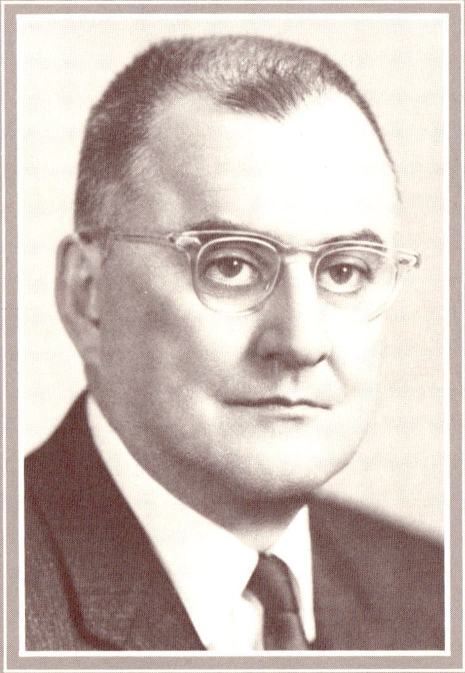

GEORGE F. ARCHAMBAULT

"Where to now, hospital pharmacists?"

ETHICAL STANDARDS: PROFESSIONAL CONDUCT AND RESPONSIBILITIES

Professional conduct is a term we hear repeatedly. What does it mean? Why is it important to us as professional practitioners? What is a profession?

After much reading and contemplation among the writings of ancient and modern philosophers and thinkers on this subject, I conclude that a profession is an occupation of man dedicated in some way to his physical, his mental, or his moral welfare. A profession is generally recognized and respected for several distinguishing characteristic qualities. For example, each profession has an organized body of knowledge and prescribed formalities for using it and for imparting its essential data to those who wish to join. A profession has a literature of its own, both in ever growing basic and refined texts and in dynamically current approved journals published regularly. Each profession demands desirable background prerequisites and cultural and educational achievement. These must be satisfied for admission and maintained for as long as the individual remains a member.

Each profession has its governing or regulatory body composed of its own members, which provides the leadership and the means of participating with other professions in discharging its overall responsibilities of service, being ever vigilant that the obligations towards progress and the technical and scientific advances that time brings become part of its total effort. And finally, individuals seeking the services of a professional person are not in a position to judge the quality of the service given. Rather, they must rely on the reputation of the individual practitioner and the standards of conduct maintained by the profession as a whole. As we say in law, the principle of *caveat vendor*—let the seller beware—applies, not *caveat emptor.*

We hospital pharmacists belong to a true, noble, and blessed profession. For we practice in a setting devoted exclusively to the care of the seriously ill and injured. We represent that specialty of pharmacy that concerns itself with the evaluation, the selection, the control, and the utilization of drugs in hospitals. This encompasses the supplying of medications for inpatient and outpatient use, the preparation of sterile medications, volume compounding, prepackaging, drug formulation, and research. Hospital pharmacy, we know, serves as the focal point in the dissemination of drug therapy information to the hospital staff.

The Constitution of the American Society of Hospital Pharmacists, Article 1, Section 2, reads:

> *The objectives of the SOCIETY shall be (a) to provide the benefits and protection of a hospital pharmacist to the institution which he serves, to the members of the allied health professions with whom he is associated, and to the profession of pharmacy; which they will receive through the skill and art of qualified hospital pharmacists; (b) to improve the qualifications and usefulness of hospital pharmacists through high standards of professional ethics, education and attainments; (c) to assist in providing for a future adequate supply of such qualified hospital pharmacists; (d) to promote research in hospital pharmacy practices and in pharmaceutical problems in general; and (e) to increase the dissemination of pharmaceutical knowledge by providing for interchange of information.*

Dr. Hugh Muldoon so ably said in "The Strengths of Pharmacy," his inspirational Remington Medalist address of 1953: "Specialists in hospital pharmacy form another group in which we (pharmacy) take great pride. These men and women practice their profession in its purest form since in their service the profit motive does not enter."

Applying the definitions and tests for professions as written by man since time immemorial, one arrives at this one unmistakable conclusion—hospital pharmacy is truly a profession. But nowhere in the various fields of pharmacy, be it manufacturing, community practice, pedagogy, journalism, or name what you will, is there to be found a truer form of professional pharmacy than exists in our specialty of hospital pharmacy.

The word "ethics" is derived from the Greek *ethos*, which no doubt meant the same as its Latin equivalent *mores* did to the Romans—"character and approved group habits or customs." Webster defines ethics as "the science of moral duty; broadly, the science of ideal human character." Poland defines ethics as "the science of the role of right and wrong"; Hill says ethics is "the science of putting order in man's free acts"; and Horne, another authority, states that "ethics is the science of human conduct. It is not primarily a descriptive science telling us how men do behave, but a normative science telling us how men should behave."

Ethics relates to all manner of deeds and habits which concern men, either as private individuals or as members of the social whole.

Ethics is that science that points out definite standards and ideals of life in accordance with the natural law. It helps one to answer that most important question: "What ought I to do?"

One studies ethics primarily to understand oneself in relationship to duty. Duty is what one may not violate though he can, that moral obligation from which just men can never retreat.

Concerning professional ethics, Richardson in his text *The Ethics of a Profession* states: "after all the arguments and disputations, after all the theory and doctrine, after all the study and analysis, the conclusion of the whole matter is this, that a professional man does not live unto himself alone and what he does carries an influence far and wide. Every unworthy deed is a power for evil. Every good deed helps the world."

In short, then, professional ethics and conduct mean simply adherence to ideals, to customs, to habits, and to traditions of service to mankind which the members of a profession build up through the years. To be "unethical" is to violate these accepted "mores" of the group. Professional ethics and conduct are the morality of the profession, the "right way" of practicing the profession. Customs or "conduct codes" are not set by outsiders but by the groups themselves, and the conduct of the individual members of a profession is approved, frowned upon, or tolerated, depending on how ethically strong is the profession itself.

This leads us directly into the professional codes, the codes of ethics or codes of conduct of the individual professions, one of the major identifying characteristics of a profession. These, when properly enforced, unquestionably play a large part in determining the moral fiber and strength of a particular profession and its members.

Mayer and Ross, in *Ethics and the Modern World*, inform us that the main goals of the professional codes are:

1. To insure high qualifications of those who are admitted to the profession.
2. To stress the service motive; professions thus are guided by the ideal of contributing in an unselfish manner to the public good.
3. To develop a spirit of exclusiveness.
4. To protect the public. Unethical behavior is taboo. Codes guide the policy and conduct of those in the profession who need this positive professional sanction in moments of temptation.
5. To prevent governmental regulation of the profession. Most professions believe in the spirit of laissez-faire; they hold that government interference destroys initiative. If the profession tolerates abuse, then the defenders of the people may need to move in.
6. To regulate the relationship between the members of the profession. For example, the Code for Educators determines the respective responsibility of teacher and administrator. Through its Code, the American Medical Association attempts to prevent unethical practices between competing physicians.

Let us for a minute or two cull sections of the codes of some of the health professions that are of particular interest to hospital pharmacists.

First, the *Principles of Medical Ethics of the American Medical Association*, adopted in 1848 and as revised December 1953. This code consists, as you know, of four sections: (a) the responsibilities of the physician to the profession; (b) the relationship of the physician to the patient; (c) the duties of the physician to his colleagues; and (d) the duties and responsibilities of the physician to the medical profession and to the general public. Section 3 of this code states:

Pharmacists. Physicians should recognize and promote the practice of pharmacy as a profession and should recognize the cooperation of the pharmacist in the education of the public concerning the practice of ethical and scientific medicine.

Second, the *Code of Hospital Ethics*, adopted in 1941 and endorsed by the American Hospital Association and the American College of Hospital Administrators:

Item 16. Professional Codes of Ethics. It is the duty of the hospital insofar as the hospital personnel and regulations can render assistance, to aid and support the members of all professional groups in their observance of the code of ethics of their respective organizations.

Item 25. The Relationships of the Administrator to Vendors. The administrator should bear in mind constantly that, in his relationships with the representatives of the supply houses or commercial organizations, his hospital is almost inevitably concerned. Therefore, his relationships should be courteous at all times and of such nature that under no circumstances will the hospital be involved or obligated in any way. Particularly important is it that the administrator refrain from becoming under personal obligation to a firm or its representative as would be the case by the acceptance of personal gifts or unusual social favors. Personal commissions or rebates should never be accepted. The administrator should not give a testimonial for public use and should not authorize or otherwise permit the public use of his name or photograph in the endorsement of commercial services, equipment, materials, drugs, or other supplies.

Gifts or donations should not be solicited from business houses on the basis of making a return for business granted. Unless required by law to do so, the administrator or his staff should not disclose the price to a competitor of a firm submitting prices. Orders placed in good faith should not be cancelled or the goods returned without legitimate reason.

Requests for special extensions of credit should be definitely arranged before any merchandise is ordered.

How fitting and how proper might this section also be for one of the sections of a special code of ethics for hospital pharmacists.

Let us reflect here on pharmacy's own Code of Ethics, as developed by the American Pharmaceutical Association in 1852 and as revised in 1922. Much of this Code applies equally to the hospital practitioner of pharmacy as it does to the community practitioner. Consider if you will, however, the desirability or need for a special code for hospital pharmacists. There is much that needs to be stated, much that is missing in our overall pharmacy Code, much that is vital to good hospital pharmacy practice and which should be stated officially. For those of you who wish to study this matter in detail, I refer you to the complete Code of Ethics. Suffice for us now to note the preamble of the Code and its areas of coverage. The preamble states:

> *The primary obligation of pharmacy is the service it can render to the public in safeguarding the preparation, compounding, and dispensing of drugs and the storage and handling of drugs, and medical supplies.*
>
> *The practice of pharmacy requires knowledge, skill, and integrity; therefore, the State laws restrict the practice of pharmacy to persons with special training and qualifications, and license to them privileges which are denied to others. Accordingly, the pharmacist recognizes his responsibility to the State and to the community for their well-being, and fulfills his professional obligations honorably.*

The Code of Ethics for pharmacy then goes on to cover:

1. The pharmacist and his relations to the public.
2. The pharmacist and his relations to the other health professions.
3. The pharmacist and his relations to fellow pharmacists.

Now, what of the professional ethics and code of conduct of individual hospital pharmacists? What are the *mores* or standards for hospital pharmacists? Do we have stated positions for "conflicts of interest" situations? Hospital pharmacy in the United States dates back to 1752, to Jonathan Roberts, the first hospital pharmacist in colonial America, who practiced at the Pennsylvania Hospital in Philadelphia, a hospital founded by Benjamin Franklin. Unfortunately for our specialty, it was not until 1920, when the American College of Surgeons began its hospital standardization program, that hospital pharmacy began to emerge and grow as a professional specialty. In 1956, 36 years later, with over a third of a century of experience behind us, it is time for the leaders of hospital pharmacy to give serious thought to this subject of ethics and to a professional code of conduct designed particularly for us, the members of this professional specialty.

Professional codes, we know, are inspirational. They are aids to the young in a profession. Codes afford inspiration to the oldsters of a profession, like myself. They help to maintain a high moral tone of those in active practice.

An appropriate code for us would spell out the principles underlying our duties, our responsibilities, and our rights as individual hospital pharmacists. These principles of conduct would be considered as they concern our relationships with our trustees, our administrator, our medical and dental staffs, our pharmacy committee, the rank and file personnel, visitors, the hospital itself, the general public, and the community. They would delineate our relationships with other pharmacists, both the hospital and community practitioners, with our co-workers in nursing and in the paramedical disciplines such as the medical record librarian, the social worker, the dietitian, and others of the hospital family. They would crystallize our obligations to the young of hospital pharmacy, to the pharmacy student, to the drug research firms of the country, and to the medical service representatives and other vendors. And, finally, but not of least importance, these principles would include statements of our proper rights as members of a profession. Shouldn't we take a stand now, for example, as to what is and what is not substitution in hospital pharmacy practice? Isn't this an important ethical matter?

If you, the leaders of hospital pharmacy, will pause and reflect on the desirability of an enforceable code of ethics for our specialty, a code that expresses the social conscience of our group, that expresses the convictions shared in common by us all, I would feel indeed as though another valuable contribution to our profession is in the making through this Harvey A. K. Whitney Lecture.

Dr. Mason Gross, Provost of Rutgers University, in his address to the Fourth Annual Rutgers Pharmaceutical Conference, placed particular stress on self-policing as a prime responsibility of a profession. Dr. Gross stated:

> *A profession is a profession... when it is self-regulating in the sense that it has a code of ethics which determines for its practitioners their social obligations and their moral responsibilities, and... when it does not turn over to others to determine what its moral obligations are, but assumes full responsibility for discovering and for enforcing these obligations itself.*

Louis Kazin of *Drug Topics*, in his column "Your Pharmacy and Mine" recently chided the pharmacy profession with his editorial, "It Is High Time to Police Ourselves." Kazin pleads with pharmacy to establish an impersonal, objective approach for handling violations of its overall code by the application of suitable sanctions at state levels. I plead likewise for hospital pharmacy to develop and adopt a well-thought out, enforceable code.

I am proud to say that up to now there has been no national adverse publicity directed at hospital pharmacists. Hospital pharmacy, we know, hopes to keep things this way. But suppose we should become faced with some of the problems of the community practitioners of pharmacy where, because of a few, many are suspect. Would it not be lifesaving for us to have our disciplinary mechanism, our code of conduct, in order? Tsanoff, in his text *Ethics* (1955), speaks of this prostituting of pharmacy from its offending side as follows:

In considering ethical practice in medicine our attention naturally turns to the standards and principles in the manufacture and distribution of medicines and drugs. We may appreciate the conflict of commercial and professional motives in a trained pharmacist with some medical ideals who is also a plain trader in drugs and patent medicines. The public danger in the sale of impure and deleterious drugs promoted by nation-wide advertising has roused social reformers within and outside the profession to check this evil by more stringent legislation. The stubborn resistance to this reform shows how strongly entrenched corrupt business is in this auxiliary branch of Medical Service in our Society.

And note, this was written not in 1852 but in 1955.

As a boy, I was taught by my good Vermont Dad that: "There is not so much good in the best of us, nor so much bad in the worst of us, that it behooves any of us to speak ill of the rest of us." I am sure all of us have been taught not to be "busybodies." However, the non-enforcement of a code makes of that code a mere pleasantry at best and possibly a hypocrisy of that profession. Individuals of a profession who bring it into disrepute must be subjected to professional discipline, and the respectable members of the profession must accept this responsibility. Taeusch states, in his text *Professional and Business Ethics*:

This is a professional obligation, an unpleasant, distasteful but nevertheless essential part of a profession. It consists of the courage to purge the profession by eliminating from it the unfit members. . . Every professional man is in a real sense his brother's keeper to the extent of being an example of the right mode of conduct and thereby indirectly admonishing his less conscientious fellow member. Every professional organization is further the keeper of its members by being obligated to exclude from its membership such as those that fail to keep the faith.

Pharmacy's Code is fairly definite in its statement concerning the proper conduct of pharmacists. "The pharmacist will expose any corrupt or dishonest conduct of any member of his profession which comes to his certain knowledge, through these accredited processes provided by the Civil laws or the rules and regulations of pharmaceutical organizations, and he will aid in driving the unworthy out of the calling." But note, the actual action of discipline remains, where it should be, in the local or state atmosphere.

The fear of washing "dirty linen in public" by the respectable member gives courage to the less properly motivated in any profession. Witness the courage of the American Bar Association when, last January, it made public a proposed new code for disciplining its unethical lawyers. The proposal, to operate at state levels, sets forth these sanctions:

1. Permanent disbarment.
2. Indefinite suspension from practice.

3. Public censure.
4. Private censure.

The commission, by a lawyer, of any act contrary to honesty, justice, or good morals, whether the act is committed in the course of his relations as an attorney or otherwise, and whether or not the act is a felony or misdemeanor, constitutes a cause for discipline, the code states.

So I repeat, what of the professional ethics and code of conduct of the individual hospital pharmacist? What is he teaching, by example or otherwise, to those following in his footsteps in this, the most professional of all pharmacy pursuits? What are some of the specific problems that might tempt the not so ethical hospital pharmacist? Does he sanction the nonprescription sale or giving away, by lax controls or otherwise, of barbiturates, amphetamine, and other even more dangerous, more habit-forming drugs? Does he treat subordinates in his department as he would wish to be treated, that is, with a firm, definite, fair policy? Or is he indecisive or wavering in his decisions, constantly changing the rules to fit the "last in" objector; or worse still, is he reluctant to make decisions? Is he mindful of his overall professional responsibilities, keeping an eye on the leadership and the possible future leadership of the local chapter and the national Society? Is he alert to prevent what Dr. Jack Masur, Assistant Surgeon General of the U.S. Public Health Service, refers to as "the fostering of a gerontocratic elite of ancient and outdated leaders bent on retarding progress to preserve their own tenure" or leaders who are trapped by timidity or ultraconservatism?

Does he approve, by conformance or by nonobjection, unethical actions in hospital administration, actions unknown to the clinicians whereby drug economies are effected at the expense of the patient, possibly actions that encourage the purchase of substandard, subquality, or unknown brands of drugs? Does he, jointly with his administrator or purchasing agent or by himself, enter into nonethical relationships with his vendors? Does he, in collusion with his administrator or unknown to his administrator, allow nonprofessional individuals (pharmacy helpers) to engage in duties that state law demands be performed by licensed pharmacists only? I refer in particular to certain acts of compounding and dispensing and the filling of nursing station medication containers where no immediate direct pharmacist supervision is exercised.

And again, does he, in hospital charity cases, engage or condone in the cutting of prescribed prescription quantities without the consent of the physician? Isn't this a serious ethical matter? And again, how does he handle mistakes in dispensing or compounding? They do occur, we know, for pharmacists are but human. Does he seek to place the blame on the nurse, the patient, the physician, the manufacturer, or does he obtain and promptly report the facts? Does he act quickly to prevent further possible damage or loss of life? Does he evaluate honestly the error and determine where the fault lies? Does he attempt to set up corrective measures to prevent a recurrence of the error? Ethics and morals are involved. What do his subordinates think of him as they watch him handle these situations? Are they proud of him and of us? Or do they have names for us that we would rather not hear because we do not discipline the man? Does he follow the "Good Book," the Ten Commandments, and the Golden Rule in protecting not only the property of the hospital but also its good name? And what of the good names of those on the hospital team and the good name of the patient? Does he have a proper attitude towards his responsibilities and duties of professional secrecy concerning diagnosis, prognosis, and medical records? Is he loyal to his institution?

As a group and as individuals, are we recognizing our responsibilities in connection with the geriatric problem of the nation? (There are over 18 million individuals now over 60 in this country, and 5.3 million are said to have a chronic disease in our national population of 164,764,230.) Meeting the pharmaceutical needs of the aged, the disabled, and the chronically ill will require special types of hospital, outpatient, and home care pharmaceutical services. Also, the projection of better pharmaceutical service into the nursing homes and other long-range illness domiciliaries is imminent.

Will we be found lacking professionally because of a want of preparedness, a lack of a plan in this area? Already, criticism has been aimed at the medical profession for their alleged negligence in moving into the preventative aspect of medicine. Robert MacIver, in his treatise "The Social Significance of Professional Ethics," states: ". . .the medical profession has incurred to many minds a serious liability, in spite of the devotion of its service to actual patients, by its failure for so long to apply the preventative side of medicine, in particular to suggest ways and means for the prevention of the needless loss of life and health and happiness caused by the general medical ignorance and helplessness of the poor."

Let it not be said that hospital pharmacy failed in its responsibilities towards the geriatric problems of the nation. How about the small hospital that is unable to support a pharmacist? Are we seeking means of providing adequate pharmaceutical service for patients in these hospitals?

Let us look again at the daily action of the hospital pharmacist. Is he teaching our young that our profession is a live, a dynamic, an ever changing one; that hospital pharmacists are in conscience morally obliged and committed to continuous study, to reviewing their professional texts, and to studying current professional literature; that hospital pharmacists must never cease to seek the latest knowledge in drug therapy? Isn't this one of the more important duties and responsibilities of the drug therapy consultant of the hospital—the hospital pharmacist—a duty from which he cannot, he dare not, shirk and still hope to maintain a clear professional conscience? Pharmacy's Code speaks to this point for all pharmacists when it states: "the pharmacist strives to perfect and enlarge his professional knowledge. . . he keeps himself informed regarding professional matters by reading current pharmaceutical, scientific and medical literature, attending seminars and other means."

Let our code, is we decide to have one, remind us that like the physician, the dentist, and the nurse, the work of the hospital pharmacist is of such a nature that he is obligated in conscience to require and maintain sufficient knowledge and skill to discharge these professional and moral functions. Important functions? The people of this country believe so, for before one is allowed to serve in our sphere of pharmacy or that of the community practitioner, he must devote years in formal study (four now and soon five) and then be examined by peers, appointed by state officials, to insure that he is capable of executing properly this public trust.

We hospital pharmacists, unlike our esteemed colleagues of the pharmaceutical profession who practice as private individuals as the community practitioners of pharmacy, serve in institutions as public employees. As such, we are subject to supervision and direction which normally constitute restraints on unethical conduct not present in the case of the community practitioner of pharmacy. Like the hospital-employed physician, dentist, and nurse, the hospital pharmacist recognizes that administration may state "where" and "when" to practice but never "how" to practice. This is an important concept that must not be lost sight of. In the final analysis, this "how" is the practice of pharmacy for which the state has licensed the individual, not the hospital, not the administrator, not the Board of Trustees. The hospital pharmacist stands alone before his peers, be it a Practice or Grievance or Ethical Standards Committee or a State Board of Pharmacy, for any unethical acts or questionable professional practices, regardless by whom suggested or ordered.

Let us not misunderstand this position and responsibility. An employer (the hospital) has the right to control the activities of the staff member (hospital pharmacist). However, the hospital pharmacist is responsible professionally, morally, and legally for his own acts. Besides following the administrative directions of the hospital and professional instructions of physicians, hospital pharmacists have the additional moral responsibility, one binding in conscience, of cooperating with all who are concerned with the welfare of the patient—the dietitian, the nurse, the medical record librarian, the social worker, the technicians, and others on the hospital team.

Earlier, I mentioned the rights of professional men and women. Let us explore this area. Do we, by our acts and deeds, indicate that the hospital pharmacist is "worthy of his hire"? "Probably as much harm is done to professional life and society," says Taeusch, "by the failure to assess sufficiently high fees and secure a large enough income [to us—salaries] to provide the necessities of professional dignity as has been done by overcharging." Are we hospital pharmacists, as a group and as individuals, too servile to demand proper financial recognition? Isn't this a moral obligation of hospital pharmacists? It has been said that "any professional man who fails to take all pertinent economic items into account in his charges and fees is a menace to his profession, and conceivably to the economic order."

What of the ethics and code of conduct that are to be expected of a national professional society, the local branches, and our leaders? Much that I have already cited concerning the ethics of the individual hospital pharmacist is applicable here. There are no real distinguishing features in many areas between the responsibilities, the duties, and the rights of the individual and those of his Society. The cardinal virtues of prudence, justice, honesty, fortitude, and temperance apply to group action as well as to individual action.

Our national leaders, for they are the voice of the Society, and the leaders of our local chapters act, we know, with the prime object of the Society's *existence* in mind. This objective is the promotion of better care for the patient through better utilization of our talents. If this be not true, then our Constitution and By-Laws and our actions here this week would be but fraudulent statements and acts, and we, hypocrites. We must not, we cannot, be a group interested primarily in what we can obtain for hospital pharmacists. We must, to be a true profession, be a group interested in that which is morally right and ethically good for pharmaceutical service in hospitals. We must not be interested in that which is politically expedient, selfishly beneficial to our membership, or personally advantageous.

A great part of the stability of any professional group is due to the spirit of sacrifice, earnestness, and loyalty—in a word, the motivation which characterizes its members. It has been my privilege these past 10 and more years to know intimately the leaders of hospital pharmacy in this country, its oldsters, its middle agers, and its youngsters. Hospital pharmacy has nothing to fear, considering the wealth of leadership among us, from dreaded professional stagnation or the fostering of the "gerontocratic elite." Our leaders are forced to and wish to move up, to serve, and to move on to function in an advisory capacity, making way for the arriving generation of leaders. This is as it should and must be. When the day arrives that the young and the middle-aged leaders do not cast a critical, auditing eye on the oldsters, when they do not review and weigh that which is being done by the national Society, its publication, and the local branches, then on that day hospital pharmacy has lost an important self-examining element and may well pay the fearful price—the lessening and then the loss of professional status.

Of other specific Society responsibilities, may I point out that a moral responsibility rests upon ASHP leaders and those in local chapters to carefully guard the conditions of membership into the group, as well as the general requirements for good standing, and to see to it that these standards are adhered to. Further, it is their duty and ours to develop proper cooperative relationships between other professional hospital groups such as the American Hospital Association, the Catholic Hospital Association, the Joint Commission on the Accreditation of Hospitals, and the American College of Hospital Administrators, as well as to continue to foster the development of an exacting professional consciousness among our membership.

Our Society already reveals itself as one standing for a high concept of professional ethics. It must also indicate its awareness of any existing malpractices and take action for the correction of these conditions. In my opinion, the Society should even now be turning towards the development of an adequate, self-disciplining program as a means of enforcing, at local and state levels, the as yet unwritten but known standards of conduct of hospital pharmacists. The recently announced self-disciplining point-rating plan of the Bergen County Pharmaceutical Association of New Jersey might well be the ideal starting point for such a study.

I repeat, unless we assert the necessary modicum of self-government, we cannot claim to be a profession. Our national Society and our local branches must be vigilant to ferret out and curb unethical practices in hospital pharmacy. The status of any profession is never static. "Nothing is permanent except change," and so it is with a profession. It has its ups and downs, as its members swing from the spiritual to the materialistic and back. Adherence to principles cannot be taken for granted; there will always be those few who are willing to sacrifice principles for self-gain and self-prestige. This occurs most often when the leadership fails to truly lead or when it lacks the courage to punish those who seek to break from that which is right and proper. For a truly inspirational example of outstanding leadership in this area by a national society, I cite the November 1955 report of the American Medical Association's Judicial Council to its House of Delegates. Here is the American Medical Association's answer to a move to change the principles of American medicine to the extent that it would not be unethical for a physician to own a drugstore or sell drugs and appliances. The Council spoke to its membership by first quoting from its Code of Ethics: "The prime object of the medical profession is to render service to humanity;. . . ." Then the Council asked, "Is this outmoded, empty phrasing, or is it our birthright?" Another part of the Code was then quoted: "Reward or financial gain is a subordinate consideration." The Council again asked: "Is this poppycock or principle, a slogan or integral part of our real security?" The Council then reiterated that, "Principles do not change; rules of conduct and laws may change, but principles do not." Proud indeed must be the true physicians of America as they see their Association take this stand.

What of some of the other moral responsibilities of our Society? Let me name but a few of the more important. You, the leaders of hospital pharmacy, know how well the Society, the Division, and the local groups are functioning in these areas and whether any action is necessary or desirable.

I raise the question of fellowships in the Society, the placing of its stamp of approval on proven, capable hospital pharmacists in a manner similar to the Board specialties of the medical profession.

I raise the important issue of *enforceable* standards for internships and graduate programs, standards that will give us true internships and not programs that beg the name of internship by demanding a large number of hours of repetitious labor in bulk compounding or manufacturing of sterile and nonsterile preparations, routine tasks that have little teaching value in relationship to the number of hours invested. Instead, let us seek true standards for real teaching programs, programs taught with the aid and cooperation of the medical staff and others of the hospital team. Programs that, in addition to the training given within the four walls of the hospital pharmacy, rotate the intern through the other departments of the hospital such as internal medicine, dermatology, surgery, pathology, radiology, and the various phases of hospital administration such as finance and personnel. Are we properly discharging this, one of the greatest of our moral responsibilities, through the present proposed standards, or is hospital pharmacy merely establishing standards to fit some of the intern programs now in existence? Is this to be our goal?

I raise the issues of sufficient intern programs for pharmacists interested in hospital careers and the promotion of proper research activities for hospital pharmacy. Should we have guidance programs through special institutes for pharmaceutical educators, programs of a nature that will focus on what needs to be better taught and the proper perspective by educators towards intern programs and graduate hospital pharmacy programs?

Some of our educators, we know, have not yet thought to compare postgraduate hospital pharmacy intern training with medical, dental, dietetic, and other hospital intern programs wherein the experienced hospital team serves as preceptors for that needed experience sought by all young, inexperienced members of the health professions. If this group of educators is correct in their assumption that formal graduate programs are needed and necessary for hospital pharmacists and that the so-called "nonacademic internship" is undesirable, then we must ask what is wrong with our undergraduate pharmacy courses. Are they sufficiently good to allow for the community practice of pharmacy and not good enough for hospital pharmacy practice? And again we must ask: "Is the internship plan as advocated for graduate physicians, dentists, dietitians, and others not proper for pharmacists?" There are 11,048 medical internships in 850 teaching hospitals today, all approved by the American Medical Association; 319 dental internships in 137 hospitals, all approved by the American Dental Association; 662 dietetic internships in 59 hospitals, all approved by the American Dietetic Association; and but 34 pharmacy internships.

We need more hospital pharmacy internships; we need the cooperation of the pharmaceutical educators in this regard. What finer way is there for the profession of pharmacy to advance with its five- and eventually its six-year programs than to move forward with hospital intern programs in many of the 850 teaching hospitals of the nation? These are programs designed to have the pharmacy intern rub shoulders with his medical, dental, dietetic, and other intern brothers and sisters; programs designed to have the young of pharmacy see patients ill in bed, on the operating table, in the recovery room; to witness drugs being prescribed and used and to witness their dramatic action. What better way is there to conclude one's formal pharmacy education? This must be one of hospital pharmacy's long-range responsibilities. We must carry this message to Garcia, to the pharmaceutical educators not yet alerted to this teaching potential.

Lastly, in this area of Society responsibility, let us be reminded that some 200 bills directed towards health care are introduced at each session of Congress. We have an obligation to the public to create soon a legislative section in our Society that will study each bill introduced and its implication on our specialty and on patient care.

So, I ask: "Where to now, hospital pharmacists?" Max Reinhardt once said: "Always act the part—and you can become whatever you wish to become." It is an accepted truism that each member of a profession represents that profession to his community.

In the final analysis, the value each of us as individuals places on our profession will determine the place of the hospital pharmacist in American society. If we wear our professional cloak with pride and with dignity, if we behave professionally and realize the valuable and fundamental contribution our specialty has made in the improvement of patient care since the "renaissance of the twenties," we shall continue to establish in the minds of the American people our rightful place as one of the true health professions.

My only purpose in speaking tonight on this subject is to start us, all of us, thinking seriously in this area of our rights, our duties, and our responsibilities. I hope what I have said will stimulate ethical discussions back home at the local branch meetings and that from the "grass roots" that has made hospital pharmacy the fine professional specialty that it is today will come ideas and ideals in the form of better hospital pharmacy practices and resolutions to the House of

Delegates of the ASHP. I ask: "Are we proud of the ethical practices of hospital pharmacy as they are?" Can we make our *mores* better and, if so, how? How about our young, and the young in the years to come? Hospital pharmacy and hospital care await our answer. What you, and you, and I, as individuals and as a group, think and do about our specialty of hospital pharmacy, about our responsibilities, our duties, our rights, and an enforceable code of conduct in the years ahead will decide whether hospital pharmacy remains a profession or becomes a mere job of work, a combination of technician–tradesman.

(For the complete list of references cited, please see page 455 of *The Bulletin of the American Society of Hospital Pharmacists*, Sept.–Oct. 1956.)

At the time he received this award, George F. Archambault was the Pharmacist Director and Chief of the Pharmacy Branch, Division of Hospitals, Bureau of Medical Services, U.S. Public Health Service, Department of Health, Education, and Welfare, Washington, D.C.

1957

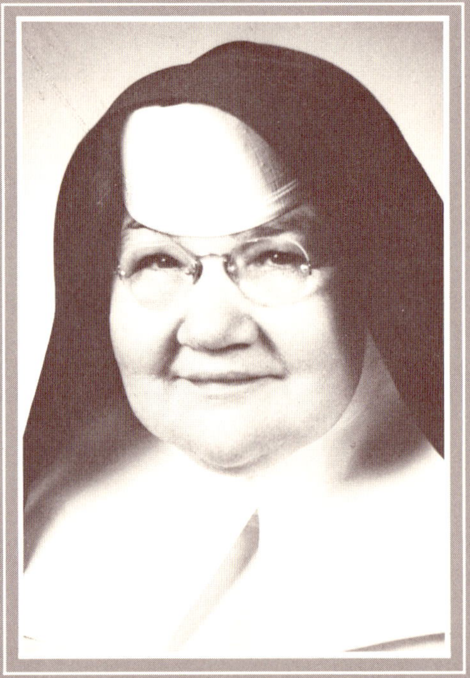

SISTER MARY JOHN

"Accept the challenge and develop it."

HOSPITAL PHARMACY— PAST, PRESENT, AND FUTURE

I would like to talk to you informally about hospital pharmacy as I have known it in the past and in the present—and about my aspirations for its future. Although unbelievable progress has been made through the years, I remember hospital pharmacy when there was little progress.

After graduating from a school of pharmacy, I was assigned to one of our 150-bed hospitals. I was to serve an apprenticeship under a retail pharmacist who was to spend part of the day in the hospital. Strange to say, when this pharmacist, who filled the hospital's prescriptions, was asked to supervise my work, he refused. He said that "hospitals should not have a pharmacist." Even when we had another registered pharmacist coming in, the doctors would request that their prescriptions be filled by the first mentioned pharmacist. Well, since I also did X-ray and clinical laboratory work, I came in contact with the medical staff and soon won their confidence. Without my mentioning the subject, the monopoly in prescriptions ceased to be a problem.

At that time, there was little to do in the pharmacy, or rather I did not know how to do it. It was taken for granted that the surgery would make both the surgical fluids and intravenous solutions. I taught pharmacology and chemistry to the student nurses and attended summer school sessions to complete requirements for a degree.

One day, after Mother Provincial heard Dr. Crile extol the nurse anesthetist, she asked me if I knew anything about anesthesia. Without knowing what she had in mind, I remarked that I had had a course in anesthesia in France but never received a certificate. Another Sister and I were soon starting our course at the University Hospitals of Cleveland, and we enjoyed it immensely. The Director of the School of Anesthesia said: "Sister, as long as you are a pharmacist, I will give you permission to spend your free time in the pharmacy because Dean Edward Spease can teach you how to save money for your hospital." I appreciated this opportunity and learned much about hospital pharmacy during the year. For instance, only three barbiturates were stocked: phenobarbital, sodium pentobarbital, and sodium amobarbital. No new drugs were stocked without permission from the Therapeutics Committee. I saw intravenous and surgical solutions prepared where they should be—in the pharmacy. I know, possibly as well as anyone, the monumental work that Dean Spease has accomplished for hospital pharmacy in the Cleveland area.

To the younger members of ASHP, I would like to say, do not be discouraged if you are assigned to an area where the pharmacy service is not on a professional level; accept the challenge and develop it. When Dean Spease started his career in hospital pharmacy, he said:

> *I visited hospitals whenever I could. . . . I expected to see true professional pharmacy in hospitals and was disappointed that it did not exist there.*

He spent a year observing hospital pharmacy and then accomplished the following. He appointed a pharmacist to work under him who took notes of good and bad points. He visited the University Hospitals two or three times a week as the administrator had suggested. He then gave the seniors practice in the hospital pharmacy. He established a manufacturing and control laboratory in the School of Pharmacy and made tablets and liquid preparations for the hospital's use after an agreement was drawn up between the hospital, the School of Pharmacy, and the University. Hospital pharmacy was then taught with supervised instruction to undergraduates and later to graduate students. Dean Spease then selected a Pharmacy and Therapeutics Committee and wrote up a drug policy for the hospital and also a formulary. His formulary worked because drugs in the formulary were covered in the inclusive per diem rate and any drug sent out for was charged above the inclusive rate. These developments greatly increased pharmacy's prestige with the medical and administrative staff.

When Mr. Harvey A. K. Whitney developed internships in pharmacy, Dean Spease did likewise, as he did in developing professional stores and research. Dr. Malcolm MacEachern had requested that he write the first minimum standards for hospital pharmacy, which were adopted by the College of Surgeons. This great pharmacist and Mr. Whitney have done so much to stimulate the hospital pharmacy movement that is responsible for much of its prestige and standards today; they deserve honorary doctorates for the legacy that they have left to hospital pharmacy. Few of you present here know of the blood, sweat, and tears that went into this work.

The blood, sweat, and tears were also shed by the able leaders who followed them. Mr. Thomas Reamer as secretary and I as treasurer remember the tottering financial structure of the second, third, and fourth years of the ASHP. We all enjoyed reading *The Bulletin*, which at that time was mainly a donation in time and money of Don and Gloria Francke. I trust the time will come when they will be reimbursed for their efforts. According to Samuel Johnson: "Books are tools absolutely necessary to the arts and professions." Well *The Bulletin* is absolutely necessary to us and has undoubtedly given more help and prestige to the ASHP than any other factor.

In reviewing the work done by Dr. Donald A. Clarke during the early life of the ASHP when he was its able Chairman of Minimum Standards, I find that although we have advanced, we have not covered all of his admonitions. He maintained that:

> *A basic plan must be established. . . . The question of salaries must be settled. . . the exchange of students for gaining wider sectional experience. . . certain prerequisite undergraduate training subjects must be included in the four year pharmacy course. . . the basic training must be sufficiently high to assure to the hospitals of the country pharmacists of sufficiently high caliber. The applicant for a hospital pharmacy internship, in order to meet the needs of the medical and allied sciences, must possess the type of intellect for this proposed advanced training.*

Mr. Whitney developed the idea of hospital pharmacy internships, and the young men who spent a three-year training program with him are the dedicated leaders of hospital pharmacy today. What makes them so outstanding is their willingness to impart their knowledge to others. Any newly manufactured product is at once accepted by our medical staff after I inform them that I obtained the formulation from Mr. Phillips. I, for one, am greatly indebted to them. I remember on one occasion when I was admiring the model hospital pharmacy at Ann Arbor, comparing its 100-gallon formulation to be prepared to my 20, Mr. Whitney remarked: "Sister, I started in with only a large spatula."

In 1945, Mrs. Evlyn Gray Scott of Cleveland persuaded me to take an extra intern that she had available. I explained that we were not yet making intravenous fluids and I do not think, as I remember this very fine girl, that I was well prepared for the program at that time. One must have enough help for the routine work without the intern so that the chief pharmacist or educational director is free to mold the intern, as did the preceptor of old, so that at the end of the year the intern has covered the required curriculum and his basic knowledge represents what the chief pharmacist has taken years to acquire.

Although the intern can attend the many useful lectures presented to the nurses and doctors, I think that a textbook covering the theory to be taught would be helpful. Of late I have used the material from Pharmacy Institutes and have questioned the interns on MacEachern's *Hospital Organization and Management*, Walter's

Aseptic Treatment of Wounds, and Underwood's book on sterilization, which they are required to read. This work, plus following Mr. Flack's *Manual for Internship*, is a full time job for both preceptor and intern, but it is stimulating. Because of the time and effort involved, only those who intend to remain in hospital pharmacy for a reasonable time and who are of high intellectual ability—alert, interested, and conscientious—should be accepted.

The intern should be well trained in *professional relations*. He can acquire this training by observing how his preceptor deals with the medical staff, because the physician is confused by the multiplicity of trade names for the same drug. He is glad to learn that the cost of prescriptions to patients can be reduced 30 to 50% by prescribing the generic name. The intern can observe that this problem is placed on the agenda and presented to the Therapeutics Committee, which he should attend as well as the staff meeting where it is passed on. He can follow you, his preceptor, to the nursing office and see how you convince the educational director that the use of generic names in charting medications will raise standards and that the student will only have to remember one name. The doctor has already given you permission, individually or at a staff meeting, to label medicine generically; if he wishes it, you will include the trade name in parentheses on the label.

Some time ago, the secretary of the American College of Apothecaries stated:

> *Excessive duplication should be avoided. It is costly and potentially dangerous to all concerned. It raises the cost of medical care and how much more of this increase the public will take without demanding socialization of our health professions is problematical. The use of generic names is completely consistent with the professional training given the modern-day pharmacist and is an ethical approach wherein he may be able to reduce an excessive and in certain cases an unreasonable inventory.*

Generic nomenclature is found only in medical literature and taught in schools of medicine and pharmacy.

Education of the resident medical staff in the use of medications should be the duty of the pharmacist. Since substitution is illegal, the doctor must be kept informed, preferably by the Therapeutics Committee. By all means, the generic name must meet the specifications of the *USP*, *NF*, and N.N.R. Stock control is likewise very important, as are the commercial aspects of cost accounting and pricing to sell because the hidden costs of indirect expenses are often ignored:

> *According to the National Cash Register Statistics, it costs 8% per month to stock any medicine regardless of whether it is manufactured or purchased from a manufacturer. An item doubles in cost if not sold within a year.*

The intern must be taught how to spend the hospital dollar and that placing orders once monthly in larger quantities will lower the price. As Sister Mary Florentine of Mount Carmel Hospital stated:

After checking Abbott, Lilly, Parke Davis, and other manufacturers, we found that the average price of capsules or tablets stood like this:

5000	*100%*	*$100.00 ($20.00 per 1000)*
1000	*100% + 20%*	*$ 24.00 ($24.00 per 1000)*
100	*100% + 20% + 50%*	*$ 3.60 ($36.00 per 1000)*

In other words, you can purchase 10 brands of 100 for $36 or one brand of 5000 for $20 per 1000. With permission of the doctor, duplication can and must be controlled. A shift in emphasis from compounding and dispensing is due, and the pharmacist of today must be equally skilled in imparting comprehensive professional information to the allied health professions. When the doctor learns that the pharmacist is protecting the patient, he is grateful. Public relations is most important.

Central supply training makes the preparation of sterile products easy. Several of our interns have worked part time in central supply during their four years of pharmacy study, which is a big help to an already crowded curriculum. The chief pharmacist and the intern then need only to take a weekly inventory together, with an explanation to the intern of new procedures that have been adopted. Writing out specifications for equipment is also good training for the intern who later wishes to supervise central supply.

The intern must be taught the use of procedural manuals. I agree with Dr. George Archambault that "there is an essential need for the value of establishing and circulating within a hospital, and in particular, within the Pharmacy Department, a *procedural manual* for a Pharmaceutical Service, a manual spelling out in detail the Department's administrative policies, regulation, and *modus operandi.*"

The intern must also be taught the value of Mr. Kneifl's Point-Rating Plan. According to my dear friend, Evlyn Scott:

We cannot wait for sufficient special formal training such as internships of hospital pharmacists but must turn to self-education. Three aids have been mentioned—first, The Bulletin; *second, the Institutes; third, Conventions and Meetings; and now a fourth is added—the Point-Rating Plan to implement the* Minimum Standards. . . . *To me, the Point-Rating Plan represents more than a tool to implement the* Minimum Standards—*rather it represents an opportunity for every hospital and hospital pharmacist to become aware of where he and his hospital pharmacy stand as regards the standards for hospital pharmacy in the United States.*

Since we follow the new curriculum, it may seem that the intern is a liability to the hospital, but he is really an asset. With his interest to explore and with the curriculum now to guide, the chief pharmacist is kept up to date. For instance, we eliminated expensive germicides that were not germicidal under actual conditions of use. A survey of the amount of gauze needed to protect a clean wound resulted in saving gauze and adhesive. I remember Mr. Weidle of St. Louis showing me a product in his Olive Street Store that he had made popular because it was good. I remarked that we did not have a need for it and he said "create the need." I have followed his advice. For instance, we have replaced "Tucks" by adding 1% diothane to witch hazel and 0.05% PCMX, using medium-sized cotton balls. We have an improved anesthetic and bacteriostatic episiotomy dressing covered by Blue Cross. We dispense about 3000 tubes each annually of sterile breast ointment and a diaper rash cream that is effective. We have dispensed about 14,000 bottles of a skin lotion that we think is superior because of its castor oil base. We have developed a sterile placenta paste which is very healing to burns, decubitis, and skin grafts, and we sell it to other hospitals and pharmacies. We also prepare an artificial sterile spinal fluid with the pH adjusted to that of normal spinal fluid, which it replaces; it is used in other hospitals of the city because we created the need.

Research studies pay dividends that would not be possible without the intern's assistance. Our interns learn the value of the hospital dollar by purchasing under supervision. At present, we are both being trained to use Mr. Godley's Pricing Folder, so there is never a dull moment.

I also would like to tell you about my experience with a cosponsored formulary. About two years ago, a former president of the Academy of Medicine of Toledo and Lucas County was complaining about the high cost of prescriptions and was of the opinion that his patients were being overcharged. He was indignant when told by our intern, who had been a medical representative, that doctors were responsible. This intern told him that pharmacists had to fill prescriptions as written and that if the generic drugs could be used the cost to the patient often would be less.

The doctor, remembering his training at a great university medical center, had learned the value of a formulary from Mr. Whitney, whose opinion he respected highly. He decided that the Academy of Medicine should have its own formulary, and a committee was formed of four physicians and four pharmacists. The chairman of the Formulary Committee was a pharmacist before he studied medicine. He and the three other physicians were interested in rational therapeutics. One professional pharmacist, one general pharmacist (an officer of the O.S.P.A.), one hospital pharmacist, and one professional-relations pharmacist comprised the committee. The last named, who had completed an internship in hospital pharmacy at Mercy Hospital in Toledo, was assigned the difficult task of bringing medicine, pharmacy, and the hospitals together. This task entailed many obstacles because the 33 hospitals comprising the Toledo Hospital Council have "open staffs." The Academy president, who still was not convinced that the hospitals and drugstores were not overcharging, wanted the Academy of Medicine to retain control. This suggestion proved to be a good one since the Toledo Society of Hospital Pharmacists several years ago had spent a year compiling a formulary which was used by all of the Toledo hospitals. But its only use seemed to be as a reference book. The president requested that a copy of the Academy of Medicine's formulary be on each physician's desk so that he could look up generic names when writing prescriptions, at each nursing station for the same purpose, and also in each drugstore for reference in filling prescriptions generically.

This adamant ultimatum by a brilliant physician, dedicated to his patients, was what made the formulary work. Practicing medicine under pressure, he had found it difficult to differentiate between the drugs of proven value and the numerous duplications of questionable value. I was informed that I was a member of the committee representing the hospitals, as well as the secretary and treasurer of the Academy's Formulary Committee, and should attend a meeting at the Academy on a certain evening. When informed that I could not attend at night, they decided to meet at the hospital.

After the Academy of Medicine approved the idea of having its own formulary, cosponsored by the hospitals and the Lucas County Pharmaceutical Association, the committee was ready to work. Should we use a formulary already written? A better one was available from Dr. Francke, but the consensus of opinion was that a loose-leaf formulary was needed. We obtained an outline from Dr. Francke and followed it to a great extent. I was asked to assist with the work because I had a formulary almost ready for publication.

The next president of the Academy of Medicine was likewise formulary minded and wrote the following Foreword:

The Academy of Medicine of Toledo and Lucas County is very proud to be co-sponsor with the Lucas County Pharmaceutical Association, Professional Pharmacists of Toledo, and the Toledo Hospital Pharmacists, of this formulary which will fill a need of the Doctor, Pharmacist and the Hospitals of this area.

It is devoid of advertising, has been published as a non-profit enterprise and as a public service.

We wish to congratulate the committee of both professions for their tremendous effort.

This professional combination was instituted to bring all professional units together to work as one health and medical team. The objectives were to reduce inventories; pass on economic benefits to the hospitals, pharmacies, and patients; and recommend and urge the prescribing of generic and/or chemical titles as listed in the formulary.

Also, its use would influence hospital pharmacists to become associate staff members in their respective hospitals and to discuss various phases of the formulary at general staff conferences. Administrators were interested in our formulary because:

The accrediting and approval body for the nation's hospitals, the Joint Commission on the Accreditation of Hospitals, requires that the hospital have an active Pharmacy and Therapeutics Committee which shall develop a formulary of accepted drugs for use in the hospital. Chief Pharmacists. . . find this responsibility essentually delegated to them.

The task is tremendous. In areas where the physicians are not interested in having their own formulary, I suggest that the *National Formulary* service be used. We may adopt it when a new book is needed.

The hospital pharmacists in our area were not quite ready to assume the responsibility for the public relations work that was needed, so our public relations pharmacist committee member took over and to date has discussed the many ramifications of the formulary with the following groups:

1. The Toledo Hospital Council represented by the administrators of the 33 hospitals of the area.
2. Nurses and head nurses at different hospitals.
3. Resident staffs of physicians at different hospitals.
4. General staff meetings at the different Toledo hospitals where the use of generic names has been adopted.
5. The Lucas County Pharmaceutical Association and branches of the Ohio State Pharmaceutical Association at local and state levels.
6. Church groups. (Recently, he addressed a Methodist group of women at a luncheon, and not only were generic names discussed but the time-honored profession of pharmacy as well, and the integrity of the retail pharmacists of Toledo.)
7. The American College of Apothecaries.

The work is divided among the Academy of Medicine Formulary Committee members. For instance, the medical chairman, who teaches pharmacology to the nurses at Toledo Hospital, has more than 80 books in use in that institution and the Nurses Alumnae Association. He represents the Formulary Committee at Academy of Medicine meetings and has talked to the graduate nurses of Toledo. Another medical member has made the book official for Maumee Valley Hospital by being an active member of its Therapeutics Committee. A pharmacist member, who is an official of the Lucas County Pharmaceutical Association, is responsible for a copy of the formulary being placed in each drugstore and has the assignment of seeing that the public benefits by generic prescriptions. He teaches in the School of Pharmacy and would like to have the book used there, but I have not had time to write a "teaching supplement." You can see from this report that the public relations pharmacist has had too big a load for a volunteer contribution; now that the groundwork has been laid, other arrangements will be made.

As I see it, the young doctor has a lot of money and time invested in his education and has been taught the use of generic names only in medical school and literature. The hospital pharmacist, in cooperation with the Therapeutics Committee, should see that the intern's education continues at the same level. Our Formulary Committee agreed with this suggestion. It obtained the approval of the Academy of Medicine's Executive Committee to sponsor, by its Public Relations Board, four lectures annually at the Academy of Medicine for the resident staffs of the Toledo area. Each lecture will be repeated so that everyone is familiar with the use of the formulary. These lectures will be given in the evening by the public relations pharmacy committee member. The Academy's Public Relations Board is sending letters to administrators and chiefs of staff of the area's hospitals to this effect.

What of the future? It is in God's hands, but He expects us to use our abilities to improve the service for humanity. I predict that autoclaves will become obsolete; sterilization will be done by radiation in a few seconds without heat. We are beginning a new era. The expansionist trends in hospitals of tomorrow and even of today include a separate pavilion for ambulatory cases, which will require less expensive nursing care. There will be patient dining rooms and recreation rooms. More medical cases will increase the volume of drugs dispensed and paid for by a third party who will want prices to reflect costs. Hospital revenue must be equal to expenditures without overcharging, so unnecessary expenditures must be curtailed.

It is the pharmacist's major duty to maintain rational therapeutics in his hospital. He must keep himself well informed about drugs so that he can withstand the flood of unsubstantiated claims often made for new products. A doctor's degree is almost mandatory for the chief pharmacist. He will then be able to evaluate critically and with authority. The chief pharmacist needs more physiological and advanced organic chemistry so that he can explain the pharmacological action of a drug from its structural formula. To challenge scientifically, one needs an equality of knowledge. The doctor, so skilled in the basic sciences, is still vulnerable to the high-pressured salesmanship of even nonpharmacists. The pharmacist, to maintain rational therapeutics, should have a Doctor of Pharmacy degree. I have a manufacturing pharmacist, a Baroness from the royal family of Holland who studied medicine and pharmacy in a seven-year combined concurrent curriculum, which she believes has been increased to eight. According to Baroness I. von Plessen:

In Europe, Medicine and Pharmacy have equal prestige. Medical Technology, but not Pathology, is included with Pharmacy so that the Clinical Laboratory supervision is divided between the Doctor of Pharmacy and the Doctor of Medicine, who has charge of Pathology. Both are on an equal status.

What, may I ask, would be better for our numerous small hospitals than to have a doctor of pharmacy trained to supervise medical technology, central supply, and pharmacy? This highly trained pharmacist should command a good salary. Medical technology is being taught in many universities. After some persuasion, our respected Dean of the School of Pharmacy is in favor of a course in central sterile supply and also in the preparation of parenteral solutions being included in the fifth-year curriculum.

In parting, let me extend my sincere gratitude for receiving the Whitney Award since there were worthier members. Let each of us dedicated to better patient care build up our own area. God willing, hospital pharmacy marches on.

At the time she received this award, Sister Mary John, R.S.M., was the Chief Pharmacist at Mercy Hospital, Toledo, Ohio.

1958

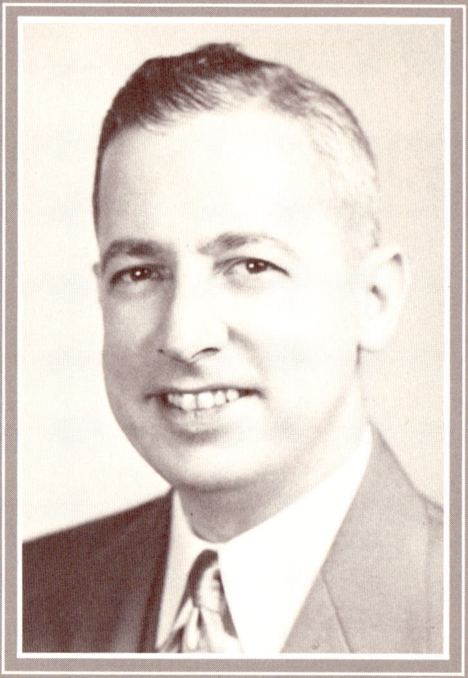

WALTER M. FRAZIER

"The ideas of Harvey A. K. Whitney originated in the application of knowledge, experience, ability, and dedication."

THE AUTHORITY OF IDEAS

To be the recipient of an honor such as the Harvey A. K. Whitney Award causes one to reflect on his indebtedness to those who have been responsible for this recognition. This award provides the opportunity for me to transmit the honor to my colleagues, to those who have generously given me ideas to use and who have inspired me to use them, and who have given me the insight to understand the true meaning of pharmacy and the vast possibilities for a full and pleasant professional life in the practice of hospital pharmacy.

I recently read a little book entitled *Memoirs of Childhood and Youth* by Albert Schweitzer. He says: "The ideas which determine our character are implanted in mysterious fashion." Dr. Schweitzer is deeply impressed by the fact that so many people gave him something without knowing it. Continuing, he says:

Such people, with whom I have, perhaps, never exchanged a word, yes and others, about whom I have merely heard things by report, have had a decisive influence upon me. Similarly, not one of us knows what effect his life produces and what he gives to others; that is hidden from us and must remain so, though we are often allowed to see some little fraction of it so that we may not lose courage.

The word "ideas," like other words in our language, often fails to express adequately the meaning which the speaker wishes to convey. To some people, an idea may be a thought, an apprehension, a notion, or perhaps a design. To the theologian or the philosopher, ideas may mean images, ideals, or beliefs. To a professional person or a member of a progressive organization, ideas may mean ideals or opinions or knowledge, or plans in stages of development or implementation.

Norman Cousins talks about the history of ideas in a new book titled *In God We Trust*. He says an idea does not have to find its mark in the minds of large numbers of people in order to create an incentive for change. He observes:

Ideas have a life of their own. They can be nourished and brought into active growth by a small number of sensitive, vital minds which somehow respond to the needs of the total organism, however diffused the parts of the organism may be. These minds sense both the need for change and the truth of the ideas that define the nature of change. When the ideas are articulated and advocated, the popular response is not merely the product of logic reaping its gains, but of a dormant awareness coming to life.

These thoughts cannot but recall the life of Harvey A. K. Whitney. Surely his influence has been decisive. He has influenced our profession in ways far beyond measure, its practitioners in numbers far beyond his knowledge. Mr. Whitney's ideas had a life of their own and they truly created an incentive for change.

The ideas of Harvey A. K. Whitney originated in the application of knowledge, experience, ability, and dedication. These ingredients formed the destiny of his career. His ideas have become ideals in the sense of attainable standards of practice. His systems and practical methods are still patterns of procedure in the operation of pharmacy departments in hospitals.

Mr. Whitney was also influenced by his contemporaries. He traveled in good professional circles. He was recognized as a superior practitioner in the American Pharmaceutical Association, a man whose ideas and opinions were sought by leaders in the various branches of pharmacy. He had unusual ability to recognize good opinions and competence in others. His friendship with Dean Edward Spease was important because both men were pioneers and their ideas fused into mutual assistance and the encouragement of others.

There was a small group of people who represented hospital pharmacy, who knew Mr. Whitney and Dean Spease and understood the ideas and plans which were developing. Mr. Donald A. Clarke, Mr. J. Solon Mordell, Mr. Thomas Reamer, Miss Hazel Landeen, Mrs. Evlyn Gray Scott, Miss Geraldine Stockert, Mr. Russell Stimson, Dean Louis Zopf, and a few others wanted to participate in these plans; they, too, had ideas. Persistence enabled Mr. Whitney to convince other leaders in the American Pharmaceutical Association that hospital pharmacy practice constituted a special activity which deserved a place in the Association.

In an organization of any kind, experience has much to do with ideas. Good ideas and designs become, through good planning, the ideal and accepted standards for action and performance. The authority of ideas is established in convincing manner by James D. Mooney in his great book *The Principles of Organization.*

In his discussion of the advisory phase of staff service, Mr. Mooney points out that leaders in every large organization need information and even staff counsel. Beyond that, he states:

staff function exercises an authority of its own, an authority no less real than line authority, even though it includes no right of command. The line represents the authority of man; the staff represents the authority of ideas. *The true value of a staff official has only one measure, his ability to generate ideas that are of value to line authority, and his efficiency in imparting these ideas to the whole organization. Through this authority in sound and workable ideas, the staff official may frequently advance to important line command. Likewise, advancement in line leadership may often depend on the leader's capacity to generate workable ideas, quite as much as anything inherent in his own right of command.*

During the early years of Harvey Whitney's activity, there was no authority of man in hospital pharmacy. The profession was unorganized. The hospital pharmacist was, indeed, the forgotten man of pharmacy. But Harvey Whitney did possess the authority of ideas. With this authority, he was able to mold an obscure and unrecognized group of professional practitioners into a well-organized professional society. Berman, the historian, has called this: "One of the most dramatic and significant developments in the whole range of American pharmaceutical history. . . ."

The energy and enthusiasm of Mr. Whitney brought about the implementation of ideas which resulted in the founding of the American Society of Hospital Pharmacists. This was only the beginning, however, and he continued to work to build a national organization. He personally visited individuals and small groups to recruit members. It was his idea that every ASHP member should first be a member of the American Pharmaceutical Association. Each step of the new organization was on solid ground and although progress was slow, it was steady and it was inspired.

Creation of a national publication for hospital pharmacists is another area in which Mr. Whitney exercised the authority of ideas. Mr. Whitney bent his energy to the task of unifying all members by joining with Mr. Leo Mossman of the Ohio Society of Hospital Pharmacists to launch *The Bulletin of the American Society of Hospital Pharmacists. The Bulletin* became the greatest source of encouragement and information to the individual member, and it nourished the roots of the growing organization.

Ideas in the sense of ideals or goals give the impression of something of the future or something never attainable for the present. The following passages were written by the psychologist John Dewey in his book *Human Nature and Conduct*:

Every ideal is preceded by an actuality. Ideas, thoughts of ends, are not spontaneously generated. Reason, pure of all influence from prior habit is a fiction. Aims begin as a wish to change. The transformation depends upon the working out of means through study of existing circumstances and this knowledge, joined to a wish creates a purpose. . . The trouble with what sometimes passes for ideals, is that they do not get beyond the stage of fancy, of something agreeable and desirable based upon an emotional wish. . . Idealism must indeed come first, the imagination of some better state generated by desire. But unless ideals are to be dreams, and idealism a synonym for romanticism and phantasy-building, there must be a most realistic study of actual conditions. . . .

Mr. Whitney was an idealist but not an idle dreamer. His imagination was keen, but he was also realistic. His ideals and imagination generated in him a desire for a better state for hospital pharmacy service. Studying the actual conditions which existed in his profession, he perceived the great need for specialized education and training for hospital pharmacists. He took action.

The first internship program for hospital pharmacists was established by Harvey Whitney. His success as a teacher and preceptor is well known. He realized that the future of hospital pharmacy depends on adequate preparation of the men and women who would accept the responsibility for improving the pharmaceutical services required in hospitals. The ideas he developed in the practical application of specialized training grew and were later adopted by other practitioners and educators who became aware of the need for this training and the significance of his work. He was alert to all opportunities for providing new services, and he gladly accepted any new assignments in which the pharmacy department could provide additional or improved service for the hospital. This too was observed and followed by his contemporaries.

Mr. Whitney's authority of ideas for specialized education for hospital pharmacists was not strong enough to overcome the authority of man which was held in his local college of pharmacy. Still the influence of his ideas went beyond his local situation and greatly influenced Dean Edward Spease who, in 1937, instituted graduate work in hospital pharmacy at Western Reserve University. It was to be yet another decade before another college of pharmacy would offer a similar program. The authority of ideas is not bounded by time, the authority of man is fleeting. In time, it is always the authority of ideas which reigns supreme.

Ideas and ideals have a special significance in a profession. Herman Finer, author of *Administration and the Nursing Services*, speaks of the *ethos* of a profession. These are his words:

Every occupation and more particularly every profession has its ethos, that is the fountain of its ethics, or in other words, the values that pervade its practical conduct and attitude to its clientele. Ethos means the animating spirit of any undertaking, whether carried on by one person, or by collective effort. It is the dominating spirit infusing, graduating and adapting all efforts, more or less consciously and sensitizing the practitioners to their tasks. It is composed of (1) a sense of purpose and obligation, (2) an apprehension of a mission, (3) a clear idea of the significance of such purpose and mission in relation to one's own selfish claim for reward and recognition, and (4) a certain moral tension or excitement in their conduct.

The animating spirit of Mr. Whitney was professional service. He had a keen sense of purpose and of his obligation to achieve it. He knew his mission, and he had a clear idea of the true significance of hospital pharmacy. He lived his profession with enthusiastic excitement.

Mr. Whitney was quite aware that thoughts without action are vapor. He knew that to make his ideals of professional service meaningful, he must make them a part of his everyday living.

Thus, in his own department, Mr. Whitney developed the many services offered to the point where his pharmacy actually provided what we strive for today in total pharmacy service. He was appreciated and respected by his medical staff as a true colleague in all allied health services. His ability, ingenuity, and initiative enabled him to adapt the facilities and capabilities of his department to unprecedented service for the patient, the physician, and the other departments of the hospital. His professional achievements continue to be an inspiration to hospital pharmacists. Even those who never knew him are influenced by his ideals, and his dedication now lives in the performance of his colleagues and his proteges.

A few months ago, hospital pharmacy lost an inspirational leader. As it must to all men, death came to Harvey A. K. Whitney. But through his contributions, hospital pharmacy has begun a new life. During his fruitful lifetime, organizational difficulties one by one were met with a determination characteristic of the Whitney influence. His ideas have become the realities we now enjoy. Harvey A. K. Whitney contributed immeasurably to the heritage of every member of the American Society of Hospital Pharmacists. His inspiration has extended the services of the pharmaceutical profession. The authority of ideas still prevails.

At the time he received this award, Walter M. Frazier was the Director of Pharmacy Service at Springfield City Hospital, Springfield, Ohio.

1959

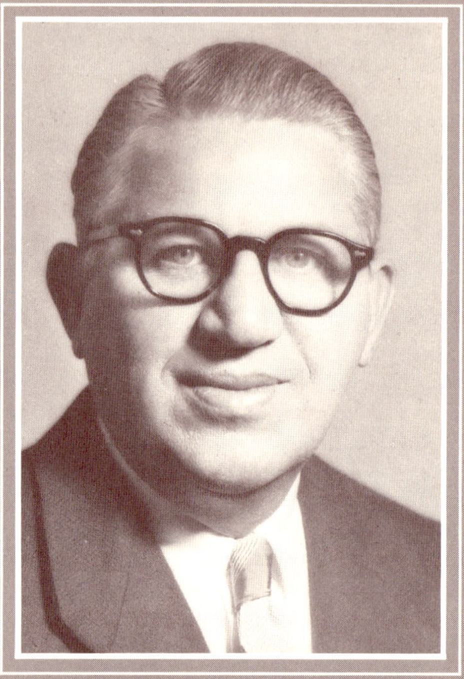

I. THOMAS REAMER

"Service is the key word to our success."

WHAT PRICE SUCCESS IN HOSPITAL PHARMACY?

It is with a deep feeling of humility that I accept the 10th annual Harvey A. K. Whitney Award. I had planned to begin my talk with a few jokes, Bob Hope style *I hoped*; but after witnessing the presentation of the first Whitney–Spease Scholarship Award this morning to Harvey Whitney, Jr., and knowing that I was the person who suggested to the chairman of the Award Committee, Walter Frazier, that such a memorial would be the best approach to a fitting remembrance, I was just as emotional and choked up as Harvey Whitney, Jr.

The presentation of the plaque to the memory of Mr. Whitney by the Michigan Society was well done, but some of the details can be filled in by me. I will attempt to tell of Harvey's contribution by bringing to light for the first time the background of his organization of the Corresponding Society of Hospital Pharmacists and then the Forum of Hospital Pharmacists, and how this led to the beginning of our *Bulletin* and later on to our present *Journal*.

Then I will evaluate a few of the problems which we face, a self-rating chart which could be a guide to professional advancement, and finally a tribute to Robert S. Fuqua, the gentleman who was most responsible for starting me off in the right direction in my professional career.

Before I start with my story I would like to contribute a sure-fire old-fashioned remedy for success in any endeavor. I found it in Dan Rennick's column of the *American Druggist* and it was written by Maury Goldsmith of Belmont, Massachusetts:

Take time to think—*It is a source of power.*
Take time to play—*It is the secret of perpetual youth.*
Take time to read—*It is the fountain of wisdom.*
Take time to worship—*It is the highway to reverence.*
Take time to be friendly—*It is the road to happiness.*

Take time to dream—*It is hitching your wagon to a star.*
Take time to love and be loved—*It is the privilege of the gods.*
Take time to work—*It is the price of success.*

"I know of no way of judging of the future but by its past" is a quote of a great man in American history, Patrick Henry. Therefore, I will now tell you a bit of our early history.

The name Harvey A. K. Whitney has always been associated with whatever success has come our way in hospital pharmacy. I met Harvey for the first time in the summer of 1936, just 23 years ago, in Dallas, Texas, at the annual meeting of the American Pharmaceutical Association. I was encouraged to join the APhA that year by the late Dr. E. F. Kelly, who was my Dean at the University of Maryland School of Pharmacy in Baltimore and who at that time was the Secretary of the APhA. He told me that he had heard some organizational activities might be contemplated at this meeting. It proved to be a true statement of the facts. Hospital pharmacy, an unorganized stepchild of pharmacy, was to be put on the map in 1936. Harvey Whitney contacted me the same morning of my arrival and, with Marvin "Jack" Andrews from the University of Maryland Pharmacy School faculty, we had a breakfast meeting with the President of the APhA, the President of the National Association of Boards of Pharmacy, and other top officials at that time. I was caught in the "net" by a few men who were interested in "success in hospital pharmacy." Our Sub-Section on Hospital Pharmacy in the APhA was born.

At the annual APhA meeting in Minneapolis in 1938, one of the featured speakers for the sessions was unable to attend, and Dr. E. F. Kelly, a wise gentleman of the old school, had heard that one of our hospital pharmacists, J. Solon Mordell, from the Pharmacy Department of Syracuse University was a good speaker. With less than 24 hours notice, Jack Mordell appeared at the General Session of the APhA and told the story of hospital pharmacy. He spoke of the needs of our group and the responsibilities and possibilities, and his talk was the top one of the annual session.

Hospital pharmacy was off to a good start from the point of interest, enthusiasm, and possibilities of organization. I had prepared a paper about our work at the Duke Hospital Pharmacy for the New York meeting in 1937 and was flattered at the attention I received. I was elected chairman to preside at our meeting in Atlanta, Georgia, in 1939, and I well remember asking for funds to help defray some expenses that would be incurred. Dear old Dr. Kelly told me that we could possibly get a contribution of $25 from the APhA if I thought that would be of some help. Needless to say, I took the money and had the thrill of seeing my name in print on our official stationery.

Harvey Whitney was not satisfied with slow growth. He wanted more activity and a speedier accomplishment of our total needs. At our meeting in Atlanta in 1939, we had a display of pictures of equipment contributed from hospitals whose hospital pharmacists I had met in my travels. I had the opportunity to go to the West Coast in 1938 to see our Duke team play football in the Rose Bowl. I visited hospitals in Chicago, San Francisco, and Los Angeles; and when I told Harvey about my idea for pictorial display which, of course, included his own hospital at Ann Arbor, New York hospitals and the Baltimore area group, and the Charity Hospital of New Orleans, with Albert Lauve, whom I visited in 1936 en route to Dallas, Harvey's eyes lit up with satisfaction and he commented: "Why can't we go a step farther—why don't we put these folks to work—why don't we organize a 'Corresponding Society of Hospital Pharmacists'?" We talked to Don Clark of the New York Hospital, Ben Howiler of the University Hospital in San Francisco, Jack Morrison from the University of Illinois Research Hospital, Eldon Roberts from the Medical College of Virginia at Richmond, and, later, to Roger Lager of the Lakeside Hospital in Cleveland and Louis Hickenall of the Cleveland City Hospital, who, Harvey commented, were to be found on the home grounds of that educator to whom we all owe a great deal, Dean Edward Spease of Western Reserve University.

Shortly thereafter the following confidential release was sent to a small group of active hospital pharmacists.

Memorandum

Confidential

It is hereby proposed that there be formed a corresponding society of hospital pharmacists for the purpose of interchanging ideas, routines, formulations, and any other interesting or critical observations that might develop mutual benefits of any nature.

It is further suggested that the membership in this society be restricted to the active roll of members of the A.Ph.A., and loss of membership in the A.Ph.A. implies a loss of membership in the society.

It is proposed that membership in this society be by election by the several incorporating members or their duly appointed representatives. Membership in the society implies an active interest, for example, the submission at frequent intervals of ideas or observations through a corresponding secretary.

It may be suggested that the society actively interest itself in standardizing the hospital formulae. It is not unlikely that observations may be agreed upon, and, this information may be of such character of value that will permit its being passed on to the Revision Committees of the United States Pharmacopeia and the National Formulary.

A further suggestion would be that the society could actively interest itself in the evaluation of new drugs being offered for investigational use. A cooperative endeavor in this direction would certainly reflect to the credit of the several members of the society.

Further, some proposition might be entertained such as taking an active part in columns of these publications that are now engaged in presenting articles on hospital pharmacy. It may be presumed that such activity may be in the manner of submitting comment on published articles, or the publication of articles by the several members, or perhaps with the consent of the society. To further create an interest it is also suggested that the several members take the responsibility of addressing themselves personally to the authors of particularly interesting and pertinent articles favoring hospital pharmacy.

It occurs to this proponent that the adoption and use of an appropriate name for the society might be considered. A name such as the Corresponding Society of Apothecaries *would very well lend itself to the adoption of individual signatures, such as John Smith, C.S.A. Perhaps the curiosity developed through the recurrence of several such signatures of this order might very well provide a desirable impetus toward the development of a rather fecund society. The maintenance of a degree of secretiveness in divulging its character might well lead to some interesting results in furthering membership.*

The feeling obtains that this society might very well be kept small in number during this formative period until the organizational detail can be thoroughly worked out. Accordingly only a small number of individuals are being approached and I feel the list is rather select because of my intimate knowledge of the individuals concerned. Furthermore, I feel that they are a particularly fertile group and for this reason I am earnestly soliciting your most candid criticism of this proposition. While this outline is somewhat sketchy, I believe you will understand what I am trying to accomplish.

Signed: H. A. K. *Whitney*

As a result of the messages received from the CSA, the name of this group of letterwriters was changed to "Forum of Hospital Pharmacists" with Harvey Whitney, as usual, supplying the secretarial energy.

In his Bulletin No. 1, he expressed the following opinions:

1. You can see by the heading the title having the greatest appeal to those voting (of which there is more later). It is relatively unimportant to our cause to attempt to make out a case for any one title, all are respectable, and probably none will stand strict interpretation on the basis of derivation alone. In the main the name will satisfy our purposes and it is to be hoped its existence as a professional tool will be justified by our subsequent interest.

4. This leads up to the proposal of another name for membership, that of Mr. Robert Emmett Church, B.S. Pharm. 1938 (Michigan). Mr. Church served his internship here and had just acceded to the post vacated by Griggs. I believe he will be a worthy addition to our "family" and should bring us the stimulating freshness of youth (and I might add inexperience if Church isn't listening). I am inclined to this latter facetious remark because my own experiences have taught me it is usually revealing to have some one ask "why do you do something this way or that?" It is one sure way to keep in the van for too often we "acquire" a tradition of routine and develop "apothecaries astigmatism."

Harvey asked all of us for a contribution on the following subjects to be printed in the next issue of his *F.H.P. Bulletin*:

Subjects for descriptive report:

1. Home-made "GEL-CAPS" or binders for serum-bottles, etc.

2. Adhesive-remover used.
3. Experiences with manufacture of pollen extracts, vehicle used, etc.
4. Experiences with manufacture of Alumina-gel (Aluminum hydroxide)
5. Experiences with manufacture of "Hydrophilic Bases," with particular reference to elements involved.
6. As modestly as possible your Secretary remarks his election to the Sub-Committee of External Preparations of the N.F. Revision Committee. I am happy to report the selection of Howiler (California) to an Auxiliary Committee for the same group. This "advertising" is meant simply to solicit all of you to work off some "pet peeves" or "pet formulae" by submitting remarks, comment, criticism or formulae to your Secretary. Who knows; we may find it desirable to accept "Morrison's Mucilage," "Clark's Cerate," "Lager's Lager" or even "Reamer's Reamer" might be inserted in the next N.F.

Harvey A. K. Whitney was paying the price for success in hospital pharmacy.

He was thinking, reading, writing, being friendly, dreaming, worshipping, and working.

Not everyone agreed 100% with Harvey at all times. Jack Mordell commented, regarding the contemplated Corresponding Society: "Weren't the aims of this group as outlined by you, the original basis for the organization of the Sub-Section?" "Yes," Whitney answered, ". . . but don't think harshly of me. . . the intimacy I'm attempting to develop with this group, an intimacy you suggested we foster by round-table discussion, has not seemed possible of realization. Recall too, JS, that not all of us can get together year after year and correspondence will lag for want of specific stimulation." Whitney further commented that he hoped that all of this would lead to an increased interest and activity in the APhA. ("They are always in need of papers," he said.)

The seeds planted in the thirties have grown and prospered during the forties and fifties but, in some ways, we see the glaring faults that stare us in the face. We know that our membership growth from 100 or so charter members to almost 3000 reflects a lot of doing. We also know that our *Minimum Standard* and institutes and seminars, our educational and internship program, research and development, public and professional relations, and long-range planning, all of these are on the plus side. But we still need and should demand much more than has been accomplished. Our personnel standards are not what they should be, our educational background needs expansion, our physical plants need overhauling, our salary demands leave much to be desired. Our story and needs are reaching the young administrators who are being trained at this period, but our efforts have not met with proper success in influencing the older group of hospital administrators.

What does a dean of a school of pharmacy think of us? Dean Sprowls of Temple University in Philadelphia, Pennsylvania, had this to say at a seminar last year:

The question really is this: Will hospital pharmacy continue to attract a fair share of the available graduate students? Here the future does not seem too bright. Large numbers of young men cannot be expected to enter hospital pharmacy as a career when the number of worthwhile positions which exist in the field are numbered, perhaps, in the dozens. So long as hospital administrators fail to recognize the services which a well-trained pharmacist can provide, and so long as they think of hospital pharmacy salaries on the same level as those of technicians, so long as law enforcement agencies permit a lower standard of pharmaceutical service in some hospitals than that required at the retail level, this condition will prevail. We must do everything we can individually and collectively to upgrade the position of hospital pharmacists both salary-wise and position-wise; for, only in this way can hospital pharmacy be made sufficiently attractive to be elected by the most qualified students. For those now in hospital pharmacy a special challenge exists. They must make worthwhile contributions through their work so that their value will be recognized, and so that others will be motivated to follow in their footsteps.

I did not realize before I read Dr. Sprowls' contribution what our total responsibility was in relation to our working force. We dispense, he said, 30% of the total distribution of ethical pharmaceuticals. We also do this with less than 5% of the nation's pharmacists. I started thinking about the distribution of drugs in my own hospital and came up with the following astounding facts. My four registered pharmacists dispensed an ethical drug volume equal to that of all the 20 drugstores of our city of Durham, where at least 40 pharmacists are employed. We have the responsibility, we do it with a minimum of help and at the lowest salary level. Salarywise 10 to 30% lower—and responsibilitywise double or more. We not only have the larger volume, but we accept the responsibility of manufacturing mouthwash, soap solutions, eye solutions, parenterals such as dextrose, saline, procaine, etc.; package capsules, bulk ointments, etc.; teach nurses and physicians; prepare formularies, etc.

Success in our profession will not follow our footsteps by complaining. It is not unfashionable though to complain. Our own Medical Director, Dr. W. C. Davison, when he made his 30-year report to the President of Duke University, Dr. Hollis Edens, had this to say: "In our dissatisfaction with the Present—we have no Peers." He also commented in his report: "The only rooms serving the 1930 original purpose are the toilets and the amphitheatre—the cost of plumbing charges has stabilized the former and a hydrogen bomb would be needed to move the solid concrete of the amphitheatre."

How many hospital pharmacies need remodeling? Are we equipped to keep the inventory properly? Do we have air-conditioned rooms to protect our supplies? Do we have large walk-in type refrigeration units so that economies can be effected in large volume purchase of parenteral antibiotics? Many questions enter our minds when we think of some method of checking our work and our facilities to find out if we qualify as good hospital pharmacists. Do you enjoy your work? The following story implies that a job is what we make it.

Remember the old story of the man who approached the three construction workers and asked them what they were doing? The first man sighed: "I am laying brick." The second snapped: "I'm working my arms off for two dollars an hour." But the third man's face lighted up as he said: "I'm helping to build a cathedral."

A recent issue of Lilly's *Tile and Till* contained "The Hospital Pharmacist's Self-Rating Chart." If you can pass this test with a high rating, you will know that you are a success in hospital pharmacy. I will list the 25 questions, and the answers are up to you.

The Hospital Pharmacist's Self-Rating Chart

1. *Do you conscientiously try to dress as a professional man should?*
2. *Are you ever asked to address groups in your hospital on professional subjects?*
3. *Are you a member of the therapeutics committee in your hospital?*
4. *Do you have an organized and up-to-date formulary?*
5. *Do you have a statement of pharmacy policy in written form?*
6. *Is it distributed or made available to all departments in your institution?*
7. *Do you regularly inspect drugs and medications in ward cabinets and other areas outside the pharmacy?*
8. *Do you have an organized file of company literature on new drug products?*
9. *Do you belong to the American Pharmaceutical Association?*
10. *Do you belong to the American Society of Hospital Pharmacists?*
11. *Do you belong to a state or local professional group?*
12. *Have you attended a professional meeting in the past year?*
13. *Do you have any kind of regular conference with your administration?*
14. *Do the staff physicians request much information from YOU?*
15. *Do you get what you consider satisfactory cooperation from the nursing staff?*
16. *Was your last salary increase given to you without your asking for it?*
17. *Have you found any errors in orders for medication in the past week?*
18. *Do you have a system for recording proof of use for hypnotics?*
19. *Do you have an up-to-date inventory of your pharmacy stock?*
20. *Are you familiar with the minimum standard for hospital pharmacy set up by the ASHP?*
21. *Do you have up-to-date reference books in your pharmacy?*
22. *Do you enjoy your work?*
23. *Do you have an accurate accounting system?*
24. *Does your pharmacy run efficiently when you are not around?*
25. *Do you have adequately trained help?*

Did you fail to answer "Yes" to more than five? If so, use this as a guide to professional improvement.

It is obvious that we do not rate a hospital pharmacist a success because of the profit he might show by having only an excellent financial record. Service is the key word to our success, service to the patient, the doctor, the nurse, and the administrative staff.

We do not always receive 100% cooperation from our staff when we try to make changes to overcome obsolete practices. I can recall when our first formulary was being worked out some years ago and we tried to eliminate some old-fashioned names such as Ward Cough Mixture, Schlesinger's Solution, Bladder Mixture, etc. Our committee voted to change Bladder Mixture to H.P.C. Solution which, of course, was an abbreviation for Hyoscyamus and Potassium Citrate Solution. Within a few days, I received this note: "Dear Tom: I do not mean to continue our little argument, but I disagree with you thoroughly that H.P.C. is a preferable name to Bladder Mixture. Bladder Mixture at least denotes that it is a mixture we hope will help the bladder. H.P.C. could be a new government agency to help migratory birds get to Saskatchewan."

We, in the pharmacy, also try to get our physicians to make some changes to improve service to the patient. One area in which we have failed to improve what I believe to be an unsatisfactory situation is the Investigational Drug Policy. The American Hospital Association has made a statement of principles which should be followed. These principles are as follows:

a. Investigational drugs should be used only under the direct supervision of the principal investigator who should be a member of the medical staff and who should assume the burden of securing the necessary consent.

b. The hospital should do all in its power to foster research consistent with adequate safeguard for the patient.

c. When nurses are called upon to administer investigational drugs, they should have available to them basic information concerning such drugs—including dosage forms, strengths available, actions and uses, side effects, and symptoms of toxicity, etc.

d. The hospital should establish, preferably through its pharmacy and therapeutics committee, a central unit where essential information on investigational drugs is maintained and whence it may be made available to authorized personnel.

e. The Pharmacy Department is the appropriate area for the storage of investigational drugs, as it is for all other drugs. This will also provide for the proper labeling and dispensing in accord with the investigator's written orders.

We are asked embarrassing questions when we are not included within the framework of a policy which is a sound one only when the pharmacy department is included according to the policy as stated.

Parenteral fluids were manufactured in an area other than the pharmacy when I arrived on the scene at my hospital. When difficult times were encountered, we accepted the responsibility for their manufacture.

Laboratory stains and reagents were taken care of for a period of time outside the pharmacy. When we were asked to assume this responsibility, we accepted the challenge.

Later on, we were asked to assume the responsibility of screening all chemical orders for all the research laboratories and governmental research projects so that the job of the purchasing agent would be much simpler; we accepted the challenge.

The point that I wish to convey is that we should at all times be ready to accept the challenge of increased responsibility within our hospitals.

In a recent issue of *Southern Hospitals*, June 1959, I read an interesting story of success. It was about a pharmacist whom we all know. He was good at folding powders, he knew the doses for morphine and codeine, he could turn out an excellent suppository, he could tell a good story, he was well versed in the law of pharmacy. But he knew nothing about the sulfas, penicillin, cortisone, or polio vaccine. I shall hold you in suspense no longer, his name was Dr. George Archambault. Alas, the year I refer to was 1931. George has climbed the ladder of success by making a study of every facet of our profession; he has traveled, studied, and lectured and has given his life to the improvement of hospital pharmacy whenever and wherever possible. There are many other success stories that I could bring to your attention. Dr. Archambault does not need my help to make you aware of his accomplishments; but another story needs to be told.

Early in the summer of 1925, I became tired of filling 25 to 30 prescriptions a day in a retail drugstore. My hand was becoming blistered dipping ice cream for children who flocked into my store because the "boss" liked to run specials, "2 big cones for 5 cents, a chocolate sundae for 6 cents." I could not become accustomed to a 12-hour day of work. I wanted a more professional outlet for my training in pharmacy. When I mentioned the possibility of getting a job at the Johns Hopkins Hospital, my boss informed me that in a hospital you merely poured from the big bottles into the little ones. I refused to believe him. I visited Mr. Robert S. Fuqua, Chief Pharmacist at the Johns Hopkins Hospital, and he accepted my application. The challenge of hospital pharmacy was ahead of me. I had to learn bulk compounding, soap solutions, parenterals, ointments, toothpaste, laboratory stains and reagents, etc. Robert S. Fuqua came to work a bit late in the morning, perhaps 9:30 to 10 a.m., but he always put out the lights at night and stayed on until 10 p.m. or later most of the evenings. Bob always wanted to improve his formulas; he wanted to make sure that all the techniques used were the best; he was continually making up a "batch" of special solutions for research projects for higher staff physicians.

In 1931 when the opportunity came for me to take over at Duke University, he drove 350 miles over rough roads with me to Durham to look over the new hospital. He helped me draw the plans for all the cabinets needed, he did all in his power to see that I had the proper information to give the best professional advice; and when I wrote back to him for additional help, he always responded. My feeling tonight is that whatever honor is bestowed upon me, I can thank Bob Fuqua for starting me out in the proper attitude and frame of mind to pay the price for success in hospital pharmacy.

There are many others to whom I owe so much: Dr. W. C. Davison, the Director of our Hospital, who is retiring next year, for his wonderful cooperation over the past 28 years; and Don and Gloria and all the wonderful people who make up the ASHP. I could say that I have given a little of myself and whatever talent I may have possessed, but I received so much more in return. I also wish to thank the Michigan Society for having made this wonderful evening possible.

At the time he received this award, I. Thomas Reamer was the Chief Pharmacist at Duke Hospital, Durham, North Carolina.

1960

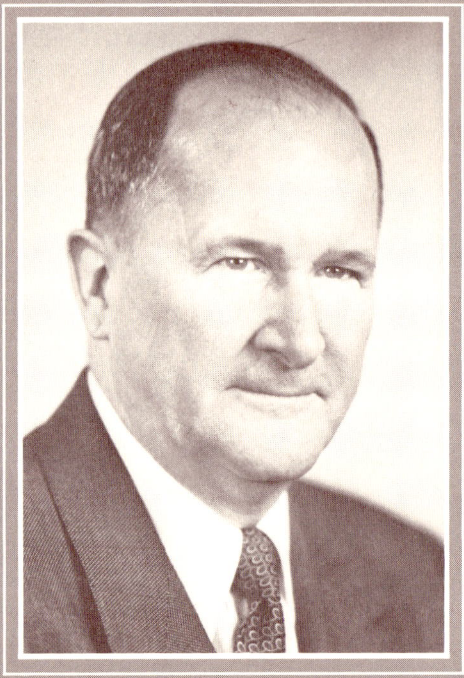

THOMAS A. FOSTER

"You, the hospital pharmacy group, face some of the greatest challenges."

EXPANDING ROLE OF THE HOSPITAL PHARMACIST AS A MEMBER OF THE HEALTH TEAM

It is with deep appreciation to the hospital pharmacists of this country, to the Michigan Society of Hospital Pharmacists, and, in particular, to its Selection Committee that I accept this high honor.

It is difficult for me to express the feelings of satisfaction, pride, and humility that I experienced when informed that I was to be in this spot tonight—that I was to be the 1960 recipient of the Harvey A. K. Whitney Award. I wish to thank each of you most sincerely for this recognition of my work which comes, as many of you know, at the termination of my government career.

Cognizant of the fact that recipients of this award are expected to present a Harvey A. K. Whitney Lecture, I have, after much thought, selected for my subject the "Expanding Role of the Hospital Pharmacist as a Member of the Health Team." My remarks will be projected to the two decades just ahead. My remarks will also be confined to the accomplishments and the expanding roles, as I visualize them, for hospital pharmacy—this dynamic specialty of ours which is even now making significant contributions towards revitalizing and reprofessionalizing all of American pharmacy.

It is probably trite for me to say that the past provides us with experience from which we should learn and *not* continue to live. My age and experience in pharmacy in several areas and decades possibly give me license to speak of concepts to be envisioned for hospital pharmacists in the years just ahead.

A quote from Robert Louis Stevenson fits my theme tonight: "The world must return some day to the word 'duty' and be done with the word 'reward.'" The meaning of the word "duty" and its close relative "work" is well known to the leaders of hospital pharmacy, as evidenced by their truly great accomplishments of the past two decades. Not only do you know the significant meaning of these two words, but also you know the meaning of those other old-fashioned words "honor," "respect," and "loyalty." Words such as Stevenson's "reward" or new words and phrases such as "payola" and "conflict of interest" are simply not in the vocabulary of your leaders or in your rank and file. This is one of your towers of strength—preserve it well.

Time will not permit me to itemize all the great strides made by this professional specialty—hospital pharmacy—in the past two decades. There are, however, a few highlights that must be mentioned.

The first great step was the organization of the American Society of Hospital Pharmacists.

Another step contributing importantly to your professional advancement was the affiliation with the American Pharmaceutical Association and its professional groups. With your progressive growth, recognition by and affiliation with other professional associations followed—the American Hospital Association, Catholic Hospital Association, and American Medical Association.

Utilizing these affiliations and your own initiative aided greatly in bringing about improvements in status, quality, and stature of pharmaceutical services in hospitals.

I believe it appropriate to name some notable achievements created by long-range planning with these groups and by the Society itself:

1. Publication of the internationally accepted and highly respected *American Journal of Hospital Pharmacy.*
2. *Minimum Standard for Pharmacies in Hospitals.*
3. *Minimum Standard for Pharmacy Internships in Hospitals.*
4. Founding of the very successful and popular Institutes of Hospital Pharmacy conducted under the joint auspices of the ASHP and AHA.
5. The ASHP Formulary Service.
6. Statement of principles relative to the use of investigational drugs in hospitals.
7. Principles relative to the Pharmacy and Therapeutics Committee in hospitals.
8. The proposed statement of principles concerning hospital formularies, which is to be acted on at this convention by your Society.

In our Capital City of Washington, there is carved in marble on one side of the entrance to the great National Archives Building a quotation from a Greek philosopher: "What is past is prologue." I would say to you tonight that the accomplishments I have just enumerated are but a prologue to those which lie ahead for hospital pharmacy and pharmacists, provided you continue to develop and mature future leaders of the caliber of the Whitneys, Speases, Scotts, Franckes, Fraziers, Reamers, and others.

And now to the "expanding roles"—the *six* expanding roles, as I see them for the next 20 years. I recognize, as I know you do, that our nation's geriatric problem will increase greatly over the present 16 million and that our total population will also increase. This is due to the continuously improving methods of treatment of disease affecting human life itself—methods resulting from research in which you as health professionals should play an increasingly important role. These strides in lifesaving care and treatment now contribute and will continue to contribute materially to the welfare of the enormously increasing population.

As for the first of the "expanding roles" I would cast you into, I name "research," for here you have made few, if any, contributions of note to date. In the last two or three decades, you have moved forward to furnish an idealistic service, a complete hospital pharmacy service, including in some instances responsibility for radioisotope medications and central supply. To play your proper and full role as a 1960 pharmacist, you must, and I know you will, move into a research role, especially where you are located in a great medical teaching and research center. You must not lose any opportunities to advance in this vital field.

The second expanded role I visualize for some of you is helping to solve national socioeconomic issues tied deeply into the geriatric and catastrophic disease problems. The best thinking of all health specialties will be needed in order that the American people receive the kind of medical care that is rightfully theirs—the best that modern science can produce. Whether this means health care through general taxation or through a specialized tax, such as Social Security, really matters little, for already both Republicans and Democrats have agreed in principle that the aging population and those with catastrophic illnesses should be a government responsibility.

We, as leaders in the pharmaceutical profession and as civic leaders, must, with others, study carefully the proposed solutions to these problems and insist that the basic principles of our capitalistic system not be violated. This includes not only free choice of physician and hospital but also, and let us not forget this, free choice of pharmacist. It is my considered opinion that if these electives are lost, we as citizens of this great land stand a good chance to lose a part or all of our freedom in the bargain. This fact has been demonstrated in the past, as a reading of the history of other nations tells us so well.

Now for my third specific of your expanding role, let us consider for a moment the leadership part you must play in disaster planning. I refer not only to the plan of the hospital in which you are employed but also to the overall disaster plan for your local community. You are well aware of the hospital disaster plan recommended by the Joint Commission on Accreditation of Hospitals. There is a real need for hospital pharmacists to be *more* aggressive in the formulation of and participation in these plans. Who is better equipped to be a wise leader in the procurement, storage, and distribution of drugs and hospital supplies than you? Then why hide your talents under the proverbial bushel basket?

In this connection, let me refer to a speech made by me at the 42nd Annual Convention of the Catholic Hospital Association in Cleveland in May 1957. I said at that time, and I repeat now, that hospital pharmacists have a definite responsibility in hospital disaster plans. There is not time for elaboration on the duties and responsibilities as they are outlined by the Commission and the American Society of Hospital Pharmacists through your Committee on Disaster Preparedness. Most of you are aware of the details of what your hospital is supposed to do, if and when such an emergency arises.

I should emphasize at this point that the Joint Commission requires hospitals, large and small, handling emergency cases to have a *written plan* for the care of mass casualties. Dr. Kenneth B. Babcock, Director of the Joint Commission, stated in *Hospitals* (August 16, 1956) that such written plans are necessary for the reason that in the case of a severe accident or storm emergency with multiple casualties, the public will immediately think of the hospital. Every hospital should have a routine plan prepared so that all cases can be quickly screened and adequate treatment instituted immediately.

As a hospital pharmacist, your capability in the medical supply area is unquestioned. Your interest in disaster planning would be a real contribution and professional service to your fellow citizens. So, I repeat, in the decades ahead, stop hiding your light under that bushel basket. Go out and make your services available to hospital officials who are responsible for the overall planning—show them what we have to offer. It is a lot of valuable "know-how," let me assure you.

Enough of hospital and local emergency planning. Let us move now to a large element of the problem—total community civilian defense planning and its relationship to national civilian defense activities. It is needless for me tonight to cite the terrible effects of a nuclear attack on our civilian population. Our mobilization and military leaders warn that the potential enemy is capable of delivering such an attack. We must not assume an "it can't happen here and if it does I won't be here" attitude. This country was not founded by our ancestors with that philosophy, nor can we now harbor such thinking and be true to our heritage.

The hospital pharmacist, as an experienced professional and civic leader, must take time now, and certainly in the foreseeable future for at least as long as present international tensions exist, to participate actively and enthusiastically in the civil defense activities of his hospital and also the civil defense activities of his community, city, and state. By his active participation, he can bring proper and sensible pharmaceutical and hospital medical supply planning to these civilian defense programs. Do not be backward; this is a matter of national and human survival. Your country needs your assertiveness in this matter now. Do not allow the local civil defense authorities to overlook you.

Lastly, in this regard, I recommend more active leadership and support at the national level. I suggest intensifying the ASHP's participation with other national associations and organizations in disaster and civil defense planning. I refer to such groups as the AMA, the AHA, the ADA, and the national nursing associations, all of which have very active disaster preparedness committees. This participation should include close cooperation with officials of the national and state civil defense organizations. It is my feeling that the ASHP must provide overall policy guidance and give direction to hospital pharmacist groups at the local level and where most of us participate most effectively.

Now to your fourth "expanded role": this lies in the field of economics. I refer to the hospital pharmacist collaborating with other specialists in the development of intelligent, practicable, and economic prepaid health care plans. In this role, you will lend your influence and support in developing workable systems that include drugs, always bearing in mind provisions that allow for free choice of pharmacists and pharmacy service. Your national association, the ASHP, must here also provide the leadership for your participation in this fast developing activity.

The fifth role I picture for you is one of playing a vital part in formulating public and professional opinions and attitudes on the health issues of the day. For example, what stand are you taking this week as a national group on such matters as:

1. Mail-order prescriptions?
2. Tightening of Food and Drug Regulations relative to hazardous substances and the possible need for national licensing and inspecting of drug manufacturers?
3. The philosophy of formularies and their correct interpretation and use?
4. Proper use of nonprofessionals in civilian and government pharmacy and also in the military and Coast Guard?
5. Full credit for hospital experience as a prerequisite for licensing in all states, not just 36 alone?
6. Generic *versus* trade name debate?

You should establish a position and be so recorded on current and important national issues such as these.

The sixth leadership role that I believe has not as yet been given proper attention by hospital pharmacists, and must be expanded, is your service on the Public Health Boards of your communities. I understand and appreciate fully why you have made little or no advances in this area. I believe it is because you have quite naturally devoted all your energies towards the improvement of professional pharmaceutical services within the hospital atmosphere. This is right and proper, but some of you are now prepared and capable of rendering civic duty. I believe it essential for you to serve your community, if called upon, as a board of health commissioner or council member.

A recent survey indicates that there are approximately 250 pharmacists out of some 110,000 who have given evidence of their recognition of this civic responsibility by accepting appointments (elective or otherwise) to Boards or Commissions of Public Health in their county, city, or state governments.

It is interesting to note that one of pharmacy's foremost educators, and a long-time friend of hospital pharmacy, is truly the dean of this small group of civic-minded pharmacists. I refer to Dean Glenn Jenkins of Purdue University, who has recently been reappointed as one of the members of the Executive Board of the Indiana State Health Department. He now starts his 17th year in this post.

Do you know that now, in 1960, 25 states have pharmacists on their boards of health? In many states (Arkansas, Florida, Georgia, Indiana, Kansas, Kentucky, Louisiana, Maryland, Montana, Nebraska, North Dakota, Oregon, South Carolina, South Dakota, Virginia, and West Virginia), it is mandatory by law that a licensed pharmacist serve on the State Board of Health. In eight additional states, the recognition is voluntarily accorded (California, Colorado, Minnesota, New Hampshire, Tennessee, Texas, Utah, and Washington). Pharmacists also serve in Georgia, Ohio, and Pennsylvania on State Public Health Councils. With your basic education, involving either a course in public health or public health subjects taught in a variety of courses such as biology and microbiology, you are indeed most able and capable of serving your state and community in this capacity; for in your college courses, insecticides and rodenticides were objects of study, as well as the control of communicable diseases and the analysis of water, milk, and food. Water- and milkshed sanitation problems and their solutions are also not unknown to you. How many hospital pharmacists will be serving their communities and states in this work in the next 20 years? Now is the time for you to make a start in this direction.

In looking over the past lectures of Harvey Whitney Award recipients, a statement by Hans Hansen in his 1951 address particularly impressed me. I quote: "You owe your community something and if you pass up this responsibility you will have missed something in life."

I have gone further than this tonight in stating my belief that a pharmacist owes much to his profession and his community. In the days ahead, you hospital pharmacists, having but recently fought for and established your professional position within the hospital, must carry the fight to the broader horizons that I have mentioned. By so doing, I promise, you will significantly aid in restoring pharmacy to its original full professional stature.

Finally, looking back on the progress of the past 20 years and looking into years just ahead, I envy you, for yours is the challenge to move forward in these activities of research, professional influences on public opinion, civilian defense, public health, community disaster planning, and overall policymaking for the total profession. You, the hospital pharmacy group, face some of the greatest challenges offered to American pharmacists; and in the coming decades, I predict, as leaders of the profession of pharmacy, you will have recreated in the minds of the American people the thought that "pharmacy is truly a health profession."

At the time he received this award, Thomas A. Foster was a Medical Supply Consultant in Washington, D.C. He formerly was the Pharmacist Director, U.S. Public Health Service, Department of Health, Education, and Welfare.

1961

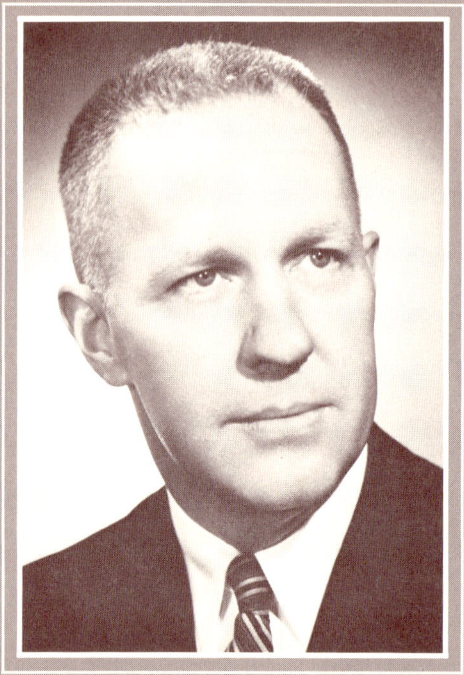

HERBERT L. FLACK

"Hospital pharmacists. . .should seek increased representation and active participation."

GOALS FOR HOSPITAL PHARMACISTS

Fellow pharmacists and friends, it is the privilege of my lifetime to stand before you tonight in the position as recipient of the Harvey A. K. Whitney Award. It is an honor that my associates throughout this great nation have considered my contributions to hospital pharmacy practice such as to merit this award given in the name of one we shall always cherish and respect as the man who developed modern hospital pharmacy practice. I am humbled and pleased that my name shall be associated with that of Harvey A. K. Whitney and the previous award recipients.

To the Michigan Society of Hospital Pharmacists, I offer sincere thanks for making this award available to me. To both the Michigan Society and the American Society of Hospital Pharmacists, I offer sincere thanks for this wonderful award dinner. To you hospital pharmacists and friends, I offer sincere thanks for attending and for giving me the opportunity to discuss what I consider urgent "Goals for Hospital Pharmacists."

When I received the wonderful news of the Award, I suddenly realized that I had inherited an obligation to present a talk that should be both stimulating and brief. I hope this will be so.

Some time before receiving the news of this Award, I had read a brief of the "Report of the President's Commission on National Goals." With the knowledge that I might be repeating some of the goals and desires that President Latiolais, President-Elect Heard, or our distinguished visitor, Dr. Svend Aage Schou, might be presenting, I nevertheless went forward in this direction to present goals for hospital pharmacists as I see the need and opportunity.

A goal for each active member of the ASHP should be to act as an individual recruiting service. This recruitment effort must be developed in two areas. First is recruitment of high school students into our schools of pharmacy, and second is recruitment of above average pharmacy students into hospital pharmacy practice.

There is need for cooperation with the guidance counselor in the senior high school. This cooperation can be obtained through personal discussions, through visitation to the school and discussion with the students about pharmacy in general and its future, or it can be by invitation of selected students to the hospital and hospital pharmacy. In this latter case, the recruitment effort often overflows into the total hospital recruitment picture.

Your recruitment efforts at the pharmacy school level are needed even more where there is no formal hospital pharmacy program or where there is not a specific member of the faculty assigned to discuss this subject. In the present academic year at the Philadelphia College of Pharmacy and Science, Jefferson's Director of Pharmacy Service addressed the freshman class for an hour on hospital pharmacy practice. In the sophomore class, our pharmacists are participating in a hospital pharmacy symposium presented by selected sophomore students who had previously visited our hospital pharmacy and obtained necessary background data. For junior and senior students, the course "Hospital Pharmacy Orientation" has been offered as an elective. This course, carrying two semester credits, provides a one-hour lecture per week and also a weekly two-hour laboratory period in the hospital.

A goal for hospital pharmacists should be the establishment of a formal standard for presenting an orientation to hospital pharmacy practice to the third-year students in the five-year program or to the fourth-year students in the six-year program. There should be established a subcommittee of the Committee on Minimum Standards, which should develop formal syllabi for lecture courses titled "Hospital Pharmacy Orientation," carrying one or two credit hours. There is need also for laboratory periods for this course. These should carry either two or four credit hours, and syllabi are required for each.

Ten years ago, in 1951, a special committee under my chairmanship prepared a syllabus for the course "Hospital Pharmacy Administration." This course was to be given to persons majoring in hospital pharmacy practice. This course syllabus needs to be updated and should be modified in light of the syllabus for the course in hospital administration given to students majoring in hospital pharmacy.

Although many educators have adopted the "Hospital Pharmacy Administration" course herein and modified it to the needs of junior and senior students, there is need for committee-type thinking and idea exchange to provide the most effective and stimulating orientation to hospital pharmacy practice. There is not the need for detailed subject matter as would be covered in the more detailed courses, "Hospital Pharmacy Administration" and "Hospital Administration."

A goal for hospital pharmacists should be the revision and updating of the *Minimum Standard for Pharmacy Internship in Hospitals.* A further goal should be the establishment of an approval or accreditation program for pharmacy internship and residency programs in hospitals.

Such an approval program has been in the offing for entirely too many years and has not been formalized or made effective. Even after the first year of such a program, there will still be much to be accomplished in weeding out those programs which basically do not provide educational opportunities. Further, improvements will be required in many of the existing programs which have the potential as educational opportunities. It is my opinion that at this moment there are only a few pharmacy internship or residency programs in hospitals that are truly educationally oriented and that give the student a broad perspective in hospital and hospital pharmacy practice.

Since 1947, the Philadelphia College of Pharmacy and Science and the Jefferson Medical College Hospital have been offering a cooperative program in Hospital Pharmacy Administration leading to the Master of Science in Pharmacy degree. These two institutions and comparable institutions in a neighboring city were the first institutions in the United States to offer such a cooperative program. In the years during which this program has been offered, there has been criticism due to the fact that essentially the Master of Science degree in Pharmacy, with the major in hospital pharmacy, has become a terminal degree program.

The Pharmaceutical Survey in 1948 established the need for a six-year program leading to the professional degree of Doctor of Pharmacy. This has provided stimulus to delete the Master of Science degree and to replace it with the professional Doctor of Pharmacy degree. *As a goal for hospital pharmacists,* I would urge adoption of this professional degree for specialists in hospital pharmacy. This could be accomplished through an elective six-year program in the schools now offering a five-year Bachelor of Science program. Schools now offering the professional Doctor of Pharmacy degree should develop an expanded curriculum with major emphasis on hospital pharmacy administration. In this area, there is need for lecture courses of one or two semester credits in the following subjects:

- Hospital Pharmacy Administration.
- Hospital Administration.
- Central Sterile Supply Administration.
- Hospital Pharmacy Seminar.
- Hospital Pharmacy Survey.
- Hospital Accounting.
- Personnel Supervision.

The ASHP presently has an approved syllabus for a course in "Hospital Pharmacy Administration," and I am pleased that I was chairman of the committee that proposed this 10 years ago. This syllabus must be updated, and there must be a syllabus for the several other courses indicated. Here are additional goals for hospital pharmacists.

A goal for hospital pharmacists should be to insure that the Pharmacy and Therapeutics Committee is truly representative of all services in the hospital. Recently I presented a "Review of Pharmacy and Therapeutics Committee Regulations" to the AAAS meeting. The paper indicated that in too many hospitals there was a Pharmacy and Therapeutics Committee that had only two or three physicians as members. It is difficult to assume that such a committee is truly representative of all medical staff services.

At the Jefferson Medical College Hospital, the Pharmacy Committee of the Attending Medical Staff is composed of three physicians, all of whom are department heads. Additionally, however, there has been formed an Advisory Subcommittee to the Pharmacy Committee. This is composed of a physician appointed by the head of each of the 14 departments or services of the medical staff. Every month an agenda is reviewed by each of these individuals, and recommendations are made to the parent committee. Such a committee can carry out additional functions other than the counseling on the basic pharmacy department operations. This becomes a truly representative Pharmacy Committee and, I believe, functions as the ultimate type of operation for which we strive.

The *Statement of Guiding Principles for the Operation of the Hospital Formulary System*, as approved by the Board of Trustees of the American Hospital Association and the Executive Committee of the ASHP, should serve as the basis for a *goal for hospital pharmacists.* In a "Review of Pharmacy and Therapeutics Committee Regulations," which I presented recently, there were many indications that the Formulary System as outlined in this statement of guiding principles is not carried out in all hospitals. In many hospitals, the Formulary System is based on an administrative decree by either the hospital administrator or the director of pharmacy service, thus not permitting the medical staff an opportunity to cooperate in establishment and maintenance of the Formulary System.

This is an extremely undesirable situation and must be overcome immediately. Where a hospital pharmacist observes such a situation in a nearby hospital, he should accept the responsibility to discuss this with the director of pharmacy service in that hospital and to acquaint him with the *Statement of Guiding Principles.* If this provides no relief, then the pharmacist should present the facts to his local hospital pharmacy association for consideration.

A majority of us have a high regard for and are concerned with maintaining the integrity of the Formulary System in our hospitals. We cannot allow any one hospital pharmacist or hospital administrator to discredit the Formulary System.

Over the past few years, I have been privileged to speak on several occasions on the need for a purchasing–quality control program for pharmaceuticals. I present as a *goal for hospital pharmacists* the establishment of such a program.

In many pharmacy publications which present a composite news picture, there appear increasing references to the use of so-called generic equivalents. Just as these discussions have been on the increase, so has there been an increase in the number of small pharmaceutical manufacturing companies which have been offering drugs at extremely low prices. There is no basis for purchase from these companies other than the fast talking salesman's guarantee that no other company offers a lower price.

Pharmacists in state government hospitals have advised me of their concern as to the quality of products purchased by the state purchasing agent and over which the state hospital pharmacist has no control. I have observed a desirable purchasing–quality control program instituted at the Los Angeles County General Hospital, and I understand that a similar program is being instituted at the Philadelphia General Hospital. At the Jefferson Medical College Hospital, the hospital attorney has almost completed his review of a total purchasing–quality control program for pharmaceuticals. I hope to present this information to a future meeting of the ASHP.

There is need to establish a special committee of the Society to study means of adopting a nationwide system whereby hospital pharmacists could evaluate local sources of supply. Through such a procedure, hospital pharmacists could eventually rule out the undesirable sources of supply. There would exist assurances that where a pharmaceutical company in Columbus, for example, offers a good price, a quality product is certain with each purchase since my associates in Columbus would have checked out the control and manufacturing facilities of this company.

At the most recent talk which I gave on this subject, Dr. Lloyd Miller, Director of Revision of the *U.S. Pharmacopeia*, posed the question as to whether the ASHP could carry out such an evaluation program. Here is a man known to all of us who has observed a problem and who is proposing a *goal for hospital pharmacists.*

A goal for hospital pharmacists should be the establishment of a minimum standard for each affiliated chapter of the ASHP. As a basis for this, I would tell you that in the past year, under the able presidency of Mr. Thomas A. Manzelli, the Eastern Pennsylvania Hospital Pharmacists Association has revised its constitution and bylaws. One of the points in the new constitution is that there is only one category of membership, e.g., an *active* member who shall be an APhA and ASHP active member.

A point-rating system is one of the many desirable features of the bylaws. This point-rating procedure is similar to that proposed by the American College of Apothecaries. Points are given for attendance at the association meetings, for committee service, for attending professional meetings in the area or at other locations. There is a point schedule which, if not achieved over a three-year period, will be the basis for loss of membership.

Our local association has a Board of Directors composed of the past presidents plus active members to the ratio of one board member for each 10 association members. The Board of Directors serves with the following responsibilities:

a. *The Board shall be the advisory body of the Association.*
b. *The Board shall hear all grievances, review all of the facts presented, obtain additional information as deemed necessary, and shall make its recommendations to the membership.*
c. *The Board shall supervise and edit the official publication,* The Bulletin of The Eastern Pennsylvania Hospital Pharmacists Association.
d. *Questions which may arise as to the fitness of any member to remain as a member shall be referred to the Board, which shall make an investigation in as private a manner as possible. If the Board deems the facts presented warrant action, it shall notify the accused member by mail at least thirty days prior to the regular monthly meeting at which his case will be presented to the membership. The accused member shall have the opportunity to defend himself at this meeting.*

Another part of the bylaws of this association concerns a survey program of the member pharmacies. The Board of Directors comprises the surveying group and makes recommendations where indicated. Where, in the opinion of the Board of Directors, these recommendations are not accepted or activated by the member, loss of membership may result.

Through increasingly active affiliation with the state and local hospital associations, the Eastern Pennsylvania Hospital Pharmacists Association is attempting to develop the status of its association as a professional body whose basic desire is to see established in all area hospitals a minimum standard of practice for pharmacy service in these hospitals. The day is not far off when it will be a privilege for a Philadelphia area hospital pharmacist to hold membership in this association. Soon we anticipate that the area hospital administrators will *require* their pharmacists to hold membership in this association.

In order to stabilize the chapters where there is a large membership, it is desirable to incorporate as a nonprofit association. This incorporation is aimed at protecting the officers, executive committee, and board of directors against any liabilities that are incurred by the association or any members.

We in Philadelphia believe that no other ASHP affiliated chapter has advanced to this high professional status. As a *goal for hospital pharmacists,* I recommend achievement of similar standards in each local chapter.

Before leaving the affiliated chapters, I would paraphrase a statement made by President Kennedy in his inauguration speech: "Ask not what your association can do for you—ask what you can do for your association." Here is another *goal for hospital pharmacists.*

A previous Whitney Award Lecturer proposed the status of Fellow of the ASHP. As a *goal for hospital pharmacists,* I support this proposal. Once established, Fellowship in the Society would provide a goal for new members. Achievement of Fellowship would be indication that the recipient has contributed significantly towards the development or improvement of hospital pharmacy practice.

In my present position as Assistant Director of Jefferson Medical College Hospital, I am faced with the responsibility to become a member of the American College of Hospital Administrators. Although I am a registered pharmacist and have practiced almost all of my years in hospitals as a pharmacist, I am now practicing as an administrator, with pharmacy service being one of my administrative responsibilities. If I am to make progress as an administrator, I must become a member and eventually a Fellow of the American College of Hospital Administrators. The objectives of this association are indicated partially in the College's Articles of Incorporation as follows:

1. *To elevate the standard of hospital administration.*
2. *To establish a standard of competence for hospital administration.*
3. *To develop and promote standards of education and training for hospital administrators.*
4. *To educate hospital trustees and the public to understand that the practice of hospital administration calls for special training and experience.*
5. *To provide a method of conferring Fellowship in Hospital Administration on those who have done or are doing note-worthy service in the field of hospital administration.*

There are three types of memberships in the American College of Hospital Administrators as follows: Nomineeship, Membership, and Fellowship. I am presently applying for Nomineeship in the College. This status is granted to those persons who have fulfilled all of the requirements for admission to the College as are presented. Membership may then be granted to those persons who have been nominees in good standing in the College for at least two years and who have fulfilled technical requirements for advancement. These requirements include successful completion of both an oral and written examination authorized by the Board of Credentials and in all other respects complying with the constitutional provisions for this status. Fellowship is awarded to persons who have been members of the College in good standing for at least five years and who have been found technically eligible for advancement to Fellowship by the Board of Credentials of the College. To be eligible for Fellowship status, the candidate must have submitted an acceptable Fellowship project. The project may be a thesis, four case reports, a bibliography of four published articles, or any combination of case reports and bibliography totaling four. In addition, the applicant must comply in all other respects with the constitutional provisions of the College for Fellowship.

I have elaborated upon the several areas of Membership and specifically Fellowship in the ACHA because I see in this a *goal for hospital pharmacists.* This goal has been proposed before, and I hope that a special committee will be established to give careful consideration to this. I propose Harvey A. K. Whitney as the first Fellow of the ASHP, although this honor may only be awarded posthumously.

The goals which have been presented up to the moment have concerned our professional practice within the hospital. There are two areas of community participation through which hospital pharmacists can make a contribution because of their professional skill and knowledge.

A goal for hospital pharmacists should be to strive towards representation and more seriously towards participation in activities concerning the operation of health institutions, agencies, and programs. Certainly this takes personal effort and time, but this is a responsibility that we must accept as a professional person. Hospital pharmacists, either representing their specialty or representing the profession as a total entity, should seek increased representation and active participation on local, county, and state public health organizations or advisory units.

As an example, I would cite the Philadelphia story. The County Medical Society has a Committee on Disaster Medicine Health Council. A hospital pharmacist has represented the profession of pharmacy on this committee, together with representatives of the other health professions and services. Hospital pharmacists have been instrumental in founding a joint committee of the several pharmaceutical organizations in the Philadelphia area, with purpose to coordinate the efforts of these organizations for the betterment of the profession. Hospital pharmacists have actively cooperated with the City Department of Community Health in its accidental poisoning prevention program and have given several hundred talks to community groups on this subject. There is more that could be offered for illustration, but time does not permit.

As previously mentioned, in our Philadelphia area some more local hospital pharmacists have offered their services in providing talks to community groups on "The Problem of Accidental Poisoning in the Home." These talks have been well received, and at every talk the hospital pharmacist presenting the talk has been more than reimbursed by the active discussion which has ensued as a result. Hospital pharmacists have participated in other areas of community contributions as in serving on the local school board, in participating in church work, in one or more ways, and there are other areas where hospital pharmacists have made many community contributions. Here is a goal for hospital pharmacists and here is a fertile field in which few hospital pharmacists have attempted to make a contribution.

There are talks to be given to community service groups on the subject of the cost of drugs and the cost of hospital care, the need for polio shots, the value of disaster planning, etc. These are contributions to our profession and to our total hospital picture. They provide challenging enjoyable *goals for* those *hospital pharmacists* who can speak before an audience.

One point that has been proposed in our local area is the establishment of a political action committee. We as hospital pharmacists have another goal in this area, one which has seen the surface barely scratched insofar as our specialty's contribution is concerned.

There are many other areas, but that demon *time*—how it ruins things for the speaker and the audience. In discussing these community and health organization contributions, I am reminded of the recent statement of President Kennedy, which I paraphrase as follows:

You Serve the Profession, Not Yourself—for the Ultimate Benefit of Others. The Persons You Minister to Will Benefit Directly—and You Will Benefit Indirectly.

I hope that I have paid Harvey A. K. Whitney due honor with this talk and with my professional career to date. At this point, I am reminded of the inscription that I noted over the Easter weekend when, with my family, I visited the U.S. Capitol. There in Statuary Hall is a statue of Dr. Crawford W. Long, pioneer in the use of ether for anesthesia. The inscription on the pedestal indicates: *My Profession Is to me A Ministry Unto God.* Oh if we could all believe in such a statement, what a more virile profession pharmacy would be. Here is another *goal for hospital pharmacists.*

Finally, I suggest each hospital pharmacist accept one more statement as a challenging *goal for hospital pharmacists.* In his book called *A Way of Life*, Sir William Osler wrote:

Happy is the man—and happy he alone
He who can call today his own,
He who secure within can say,
Tomorrow, do thy worst—For I have lived today.

At the time he received this award, Herbert L. Flack was the Assistant Administrator at Jefferson Medical College Hospital, Philadelphia, Pennsylvania.

1962

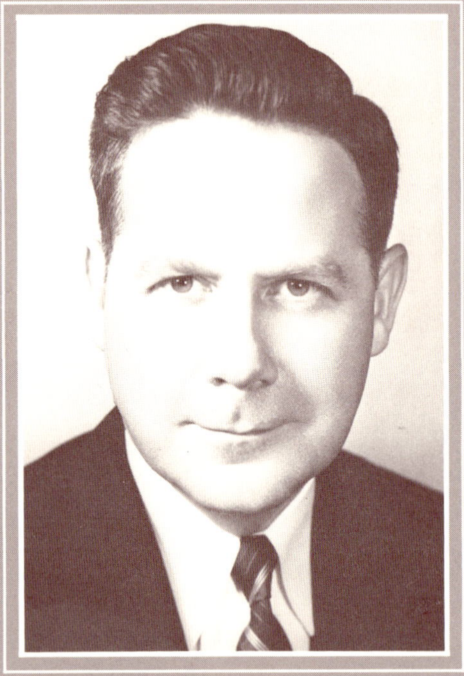

GROVER C. BOWLES

"Where we go from here will depend largely on our ability to continue to learn and . . . to change."

WHERE DO WE GO FROM HERE?

Thank you Mr. Macy, distinguished guests, fellow pharmacists, and friends. This is indeed a momentous occasion for me. I suppose that more nice things have been said about me in the last 30 minutes than in all the rest of my life put together. The praise has been over-generous but, even after discounting, is music to my ears. It is very pleasant to receive such compliments, especially in the presence of one's wife and boss. However, both of them know me so well, they are not likely to believe all that has been said.

To be named the 1962 recipient of the Harvey A. K. Whitney Lecture Award brought me a signal honor, one which I accept with a sense of humility and deep appreciation.

I am aware that this honor is not purely a personal accomplishment but reflects the influence and assistance of a host of friends and colleagues who, since early childhood, have kept me moving along a well-defined pharmaceutical path. Of these many people, the only one I shall attempt to single out is my wife, Mary, who gave up a promising career in hospital pharmacy to become associated with me on a permanent basis. While she has not written my speeches as some of you here tonight have inferred, she has played the role of a most astute critic. More important, through her efficient management of our household and family affairs, I have been able to devote more than a reasonable share of my energies to a rewarding and satisfying career.

Along with the honor that goes to the Whitney Award recipient goes the sobering responsibility of presenting a lecture, the subject of which is left to the recipient. So tonight, fully aware that nothing is more subject to the "Law of Diminishing Returns" than an afterdinner speech, I would like to talk with you in much the same manner that we would talk if you stopped by the hospital or our home for a visit. After an exchange of pleasantries and perhaps a brief review of current problems, I suspect our conversation would turn to the question of: "Where do we go from here?"

We are all familiar with the rapid growth of hospital pharmacy during the last two decades. Only 10 years ago, Alex Berman, the pharmacy historian, writing in the decennial issue of *The Bulletin*, had this to say about the development of hospital pharmacy:

> *One of the most dramatic and significant developments in the whole range of American pharmaceutical history has been the sudden emergence in recent years of a nationally organized and vigorous body of hospital pharmacy practitioners. Founded in 1942 as the American Society of Hospital Pharmacists, an affiliate of the APhA, this organization has in a brief span of 10 years become a potent force in American pharmacy.*

Yet progress in the decade just completed has been even more phenomenal than that described by Dr. Berman.

Fortunately, we have had more than our share of dedicated leaders like Harvey Whitney to see that hospital pharmacy obtained an enviable place within the profession and within hospitals. As a result, we have our own *Minimum Standard for Pharmacies in Hospitals* and the *Minimum Standard for Pharmacy Internships in Hospitals.* The growth of specialized courses in hospital pharmacy at the graduate and undergraduate levels has been stimulated in many colleges of pharmacy. We have our own literature. The *American Journal of Hospital Pharmacy* is second to no publication in the entire health field. The *American Hospital Formulary Service*, with its continuing flow of supplements, is another tangible contribution of the Society which stands on its own merit. The institutes on hospital pharmacy sponsored by the American and Catholic Hospital Associations have done much to improve standards of practice and to stimulate hospital pharmacists throughout the country to do a better job.

We have attracted a significant number of young people in hospital pharmacy. Preliminary results of the Audit of Pharmaceutical Service in Hospitals, as reported at our annual meeting last year, reveal that an unusually large percentage of the pharmacists practicing in hospitals today are young. One-third of all hospital pharmacists are less than 30, and over 50% are less than 40 years of age. However, the fact that more than 50% of all hospital pharmacists are under 40 years of age and have worked in hospitals for less than six years indicates that our specialty is not maturing as it should. Further, the fact that 40% of the chief pharmacists in the country are under 40 years of age and 33% have practiced in hospitals for less than six years is cause for concern.

Can hospital pharmacy as a specialty attain maturity when each year we experience a significant loss of leadership to other fields? We might ask ourselves why do so many hospital pharmacists of all ages leave to enter the community practice of pharmacy, to become hospital administrators, to join the pharmaceutical industry, to enter graduate programs leading to other fields, or to study medicine.

In editorializing on hospital pharmacy manpower needs, Don Francke points out that the Audit results show the replacement factor for hospital pharmacists to be 9.8%. This is approximately three times greater than the replacement factor for other branches of pharmacy. In spite of the rapid turnover, hospital pharmacy has been and I believe will continue to be the most rapidly growing and dynamic area of specialization within the profession. However, thinking leaders in pharmacy cannot afford to overlook the advantages to be gained by making long-term careers in hospital pharmacy more attractive.

I believe the following situations are largely responsible for the rapid turnover of pharmacists in hospitals. First, too many hospitals have failed to provide challenging opportunities for hospital pharmacists and, second, they have failed to pay hospital pharmacists sufficiently to compete with other areas in pharmacy for top level people. Third, pharmaceutical education has failed to prepare undergraduate students to recognize career opportunities in hospital pharmacy and, finally, too many pharmacists have failed to recognize that most of the opportunities in hospital pharmacy come disguised as hard work.

Hospitals that fail to provide a climate for professional growth in depth and breadth are not likely to attract and hold progressive pharmacists for very long. Providing a growth climate includes many factors. First is acceptance as a professional department head. Next is recognition of the needs for adequate physical facilities for the pharmacy, including a well-equipped laboratory so that pharmaceutical procedures can be carried out properly. Here I am not thinking so much about bulk compounding but rather adequate space and the equipment needed to provide those pharmaceuticals essential to high quality patient care that are not commercially available. Sufficient personnel is important too—not only to provide adequate service but to permit the pharmacist to have the time to work closely with the medical, nursing, and administrative staffs of the hospital and to take part in hospital committee activity.

To have a full and satisfying career, hospital pharmacists need to do some teaching and have the opportunity to further their own education. The pharmacist must also have time to participate in professional meetings and to attend institutes and refresher courses. He should be encouraged, preferably by financial assistance, to pursue academic studies. Highly necessary, and yet difficult to define, is freedom of movement. To me this means the freedom to operate the department, within the general policies of the hospital and in keeping with the standards of practice and ethics laid down by the profession. Finally, he needs the assignment of additional responsibilities, from time to time, to provide new challenges and to sharpen his managerial ability. Here, I would like to say that it is my good fortune to be affiliated with a hospital that offers all of these opportunities and more.

One of the more serious problems facing career hospital pharmacists today and in the immediate future is this matter of income or, more accurately, the lack of it. Hospital pharmacists, in common with other American citizens, have every right to get married, have families, go into debt, provide summer vacations for their families, and send their children to college. Many hospitals recognize these and similar desires for all their personnel and in recent years have done much to institute salary scales comparable to similar jobs in the community.

For the most part, salaries for staff pharmacists in hospitals have been elevated to compare favorably with other employed pharmacists. Hospitals that have failed to do this have simply failed to get their share of available pharmacists.

The pharmacist-in-charge has not always fared so well. In many cases, his salary too has been limited by the going rate paid to employed pharmacists in the community rather than being based on the income of those pharmacists with significant managerial responsibilities. This unfortunate situation has forced some career hospital pharmacists to accept part-time employment in community pharmacies and, in a significant number of cases, to seek full-time employment in other branches of the profession.

Hospitals must realize that to hold well-trained, mature pharmacists as department heads, they must pay them sufficiently well to enable the pharmacists to provide a standard of living for his family on a par with other successful professional people in the community.

The educational needs of the hospital pharmacist need reexamination and study. Today, undergraduate orientation courses are not uncommon, and almost one-half of the colleges of pharmacy now offer graduate work in the area of hospital pharmacy. Many of these programs are quite new and reflect the growing popularity of graduate study in all phases of pharmacy. I am inclined to think that we now have too many rather than too few graduate programs in our specialty. If this is true, it is our own fault since many of the programs resulted from the stimulation, clamor, and pressure from hospital pharmacists for the colleges to do something about graduate education in our area.

Without attempting to force all hospital pharmacy graduate students into the same mold, I would like to see fewer and stronger programs. Since the hospital pharmacist as a practitioner will be concerned primarily with drug therapy, it seems to me that it is important for him to be thoroughly grounded in the biological sciences. Advanced work in physical pharmacy, product formulation, and the like is necessary for background. However, primary emphasis should be placed on advanced work in pharmacology, biochemistry, and microbiology from a patient-oriented point of view. The college of pharmacy which is an integral part of a medical center complex is ideally situated to provide a strong graduate program in the area of hospital pharmacy.

By reducing the number of graduate programs in hospital pharmacy, sufficient students would be enrolled in each program to permit courses to be offered in the proper sequence. This would allow completion of the academic portion of the program in one calendar year. The second year would then be devoted to an internship which the student would spend with a qualified preceptor. The primary purposes of the internship would be to teach the intern managerial skills and to expose him to the day-to-day problems in the operation of a hospital pharmacy.

Since we have a solid core of well-trained hospital pharmacists, many of whom would welcome the opportunity to participate in preceptor programs, the problem of internship accreditation that has haunted us for the last decade would be partly solved. Certainly no internship program, regardless of the hospital, will be any better than the preceptor.

At the risk of being labeled well meaning but misguided, I would like to make a comment or two about the ultimate aim of the graduate programs in hospital pharmacy and the degree to be awarded. In the past, we seemed to have been confused. Some programs have offered professional degrees through the college of pharmacy while others have offered academic degrees through the graduate school of the university. Unfortunately, the confusion has not been limited to just the type of degree but also to the purpose of the program, and I think they go hand in hand. I can see only one purpose for graduate programs in hospital pharmacy and that is to train practitioners. Every phase of the program should be directed to this end, and the degree should be considered terminal. We are not training teachers or researchers or providing a steppingstone for a Ph.D. This does not mean that the occasional hospital pharmacy graduate student could not and should not alter his plans and elect to teach, become a full-time researcher, or go on for a Ph.D. It does mean, however, that as in the case of the M.D. who elects to earn a Ph.D. in pharmacology or physiology, it will be more costly to him in terms of time.

If graduate programs in hospital pharmacy are geared to producing practitioners, the degree should be one comparable to that awarded to others in the health profession who have completed six years of academic work plus a year of internship. Thus, it would appear that the Pharm. D. or Doctor of Pharmacy degree would be most suitable for the graduates of such a program.

I am impressed with the caliber of pharmacy students these days. They are intelligent, alert, and eager to learn. There is some evidence that the students are changing faster than the colleges. While studies indicate that 85 to 90% of the current graduates enter retail pharmacy, these studies cannot show the percentage of the current graduates that will practice in hospitals sometime during their career. However, it is generally accepted that approximately 30% of the legend drugs now flow through hospitals. Further, it is anticipated that hospital drug purchases may account for as much as 50% of the legend drugs that will be sold in 1975. This can mean only one thing: many more hospital pharmacists will be needed in the years ahead. It would appear that the colleges of pharmacy must alter their approach if their graduates are to be equipped adequately for the future. Strong orientation courses in hospital pharmacy at the undergraduate level should be offered and the lectures supplemented by required visits to hospitals in the community.

At the University of Tennessee, hospital pharmacy is a required course for seniors. As part of the laboratory exercise, the students in small groups spend three hours in each of four hospitals. An attempt is made to expose the student to what takes place in the hospital and give him some idea of what constitutes adequate pharmacy service.

Now in its third year, this program is too young to evaluate. However, the students have shown considerable interest, and we believe this experience will be of value to them in later years should they enter hospital practice on either a full- or part-time basis. It stands to reason that another by-product of this program will be the better understanding which will result between hospitals and the community pharmacists. Although no emphasis is placed on hospital pharmacy as a career, you will be interested to know that 20 students out of a senior class of 78 have indicated some interest in hospital pharmacy following graduation.

In the past, we have spent much time in proving that pharmaceutical service is essential in all hospitals regardless of size. For the most part, we recognize that many hospitals, particularly those of less than 75 beds, cannot afford the services of a full-time pharmacist and, if they could, pharmacists would not be available. While we have suggested that these hospitals should seek the services of a pharmacist in the community, we have not done all that we could in bringing about a working relationship between the small hospital and the community pharmacist. It is estimated that only 500 out of the approximately 4000 hospitals that do not have a pharmacist on their staff utilize the services of a community pharmacist.

Hospital pharmacists must provide the leadership necessary to bring the administrators of hospitals too small to require the services of a full-time pharmacist together with the community pharmacists interested in hospital affiliation. This program should also be expanded to include nursing homes. By assisting in the establishment of working relationships between small hospitals, nursing homes, and community pharmacists, hospital pharmacists will be fulfilling one of the major objectives of the ASHP and at the same time assisting the profession as a whole.

As Chairman of the House of Delegates of the American Pharmaceutical Association for the past two years, I have been exposed at close range to many of the problems confronting American pharmacy. We would be less than realistic if we fail to recognize that we do have many serious problems—problems that need the attention of every thinking pharmacist in the United States.

It has often been a source of considerable disappointment to me that hospital pharmacists have not taken a more active part in pharmacy affairs in their communities and throughout their state. Hospital pharmacists do have an obligation to the profession, and they should measure up to this obligation. We should certainly carry our own weight, and to do this we must know what is taking place in local, state, and national pharmaceutical affairs. I have no patience with hospital pharmacists who clamor for representation on state boards of pharmacy and public health committees and want to influence pharmaceutical affairs in their area when they make no effort to share in the solving of problems of total pharmacy.

No other group has the opportunity to contribute so much towards the professional survival of pharmacy as do the pharmacists practicing in hospitals. Medical practice is now centered around hospitals. The hospital is where the medical student is first exposed to the use of drugs. Experience, good or bad, with pharmacy service in the hospital as a student, intern, and resident will make lasting impressions which the physician will carry into private practice.

As good citizens, hospital pharmacists have obligations to take an active part in community affairs, service clubs, church activities, and the volunteer health agencies. The hospital pharmacist will find that in order to have a satisfying career, it is necessary for him to contribute to both his profession and his community.

This is an exciting time to be in hospital pharmacy. Many of the future breakthroughs in the medical sciences will be in the area of drug therapy. Throughout our lifetime, hospitals will continue to undergo dynamic growth in size and complexity. Where we go from here will depend largely on our ability to continue to learn and, more importantly, on our ability to change.

Already studies are going on in hospitals across the nation that will revolutionize the distribution of drugs and other pharmacy practices. The day of disposables is here. Within the next few years, almost all small volume injectibles will be dispensed in self-contained units with needles attached ready for administration. None of us here tonight would care to guess if strip packaging, unit dose dispensing, automation, and decentralized pharmacy services will win out over the highly centralized, efficient pharmacy equipped with a battery of electronic devices to transmit medication orders instantaneously to the doctor's handwriting.

One thing for sure, the role of the hospital pharmacist will become increasingly important and complex. However, even in the days ahead, the teachings of Harvey A. K. Whitney and his followers will remain valid. Tom Reamer, one of my preceptors, described Mr. Whitney as a man not satisfied with slow growth. Neither can the hospital pharmacist of today be satisfied with slow growth.

Where we go from here will not depend so much on unusual intellect or gifted vision but on our dedication to do those things we know should be done. The art of work and the realization that people, not organizations or machines, get things done will continue to be as important in the future as they have in the past.

Despite world tensions and the sometime seemingly insurmountable obstacles confronting our profession, I view the future optimistically and with enthusiasm. In the words of the poet Henry van Dyke:

This is my work, my blessing, not my doom.

At the time he received this award, Grover C. Bowles was the Director of Pharmacy Service at Baptist Memorial Hospital, Memphis, Tennessee.

1963

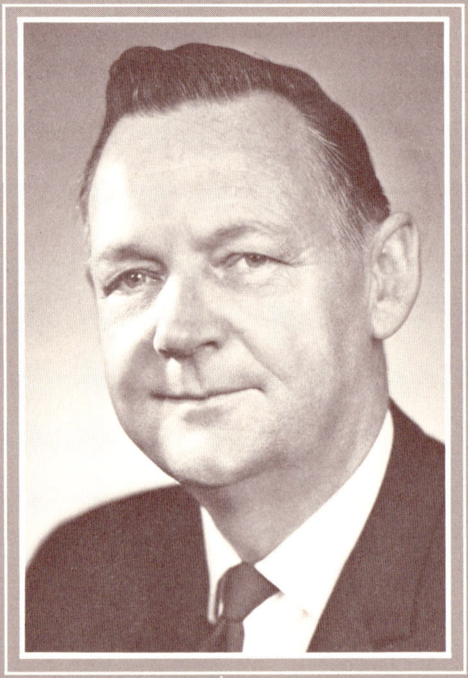

VERNON O. TRYGSTAD

"Even greater achievements and higher standards will be expected."

TO WHOM MUCH IS GIVEN

In St. Paul's Cathedral in London, a simple slab marks the tomb of its architect, Sir Christopher Wren. The inscription reads: "If you seek a memorial to this man, gaze about you." It was not my privilege to have known Harvey Whitney during his lifetime, but it would be hard to imagine hospital pharmacy today without his inspiration, his influence on the practice of pharmacy in hospitals, on the birth of our professional Society, and on the many leaders and practitioners in hospital pharmacy whose professional lives were touched by Harvey Whitney. "If you seek a Whitney memorial, gaze about you."

Some of those who preceded me in the honor you are bestowing tonight—in memory of Mr. Whitney—knew him well. It is heartwarming indeed to be included with those distinguished hospital pharmacists who previously have had the privilege of addressing you on this occasion.

I am deeply grateful to the Michigan Society of Hospital Pharmacists for selecting me for this honor and to the many hospital pharmacists and others throughout this nation who helped me to merit your recognition.

The title I have chosen is only half of the theme on which I have based this address: "To Whom Much Is Given." The rest of it is: "Much More Will Be Required."

As pharmacists, and more specifically as hospital pharmacists, what have we earned and been accorded? And because of these gains, how much more is required of us? Hospital pharmacists have earned professional recognition, the respect of co-professionals on the health care team, a *needed* status in the total hospital complex. You have the authority and responsibility for the management of a vital department within the hospital; for the professional selection, pharmaceutical evaluation, and proper dispensing of drugs. Your authority is a high trust. You have accepted and faithfully discharged a responsibility in the training and guidance of hospital pharmacists. For this accomplishment too, hospital pharmacy has been acclaimed; and because it has, even greater achievements and higher standards will be expected.

We often hear hospital pharmacy referred to as a vigorous, growing, young specialty. There can be no doubt of its vigor, of its growth, and that it is a specialty. But the historians tell us it really is not so *young*. Perhaps the first *institutional* pharmacy was practiced in the monasteries of the 13th or 14th century. Pharmacy in Egypt, Arabia, the Roman Empire, and other ancient civilizations antedates pharmacy in England, but there is a record of the employment of an apothecary in St. Bartholomew's Hospital in London in 1572. Interestingly and familiarly enough, one of the problems of that day was finding a means of reducing the cost of drugs.

In America, the first hospital pharmacist was Jonathan Roberts, who served as apothecary in the Philadelphia Hospital until 1755 when he was succeeded by John Morgan. Another somewhat familiar story—Mr. Roberts left for a better paying job, and Mr. Morgan later left to study medicine.

Hospital pharmacy in military and government hospitals has closely paralleled that of civilian hospitals. During the Revolutionary War, Andrew Craigie was appointed as the first Apothecary General in the "Army of the Patriots" under General George Washington. It was his duty, and that of the apothecaries under him, to procure and dispense medicines for the army hospitals. This was a position of high rank and prestige, which later appears to have declined until military pharmacy again began its upward movement in this generation, as did pharmacy in civilian hospitals. Among the first medical care institutions for war veterans were the National Homes for Disabled Volunteer Soldiers established following the Civil War period—eight of them from 1866 through the latter part of the 19th century—today remaining, with new buildings and facilities, as parts of modern Veterans Administration hospitals. Although little has been recorded about their first pharmacists, it is known that early in the establishment of Veterans Administration medical care facilities pharmacies were provided for and operated by qualified pharmacists. A "Chief Druggist" was provided for in these facilities in 1881. As in civilian and military hospitals, pharmacists in the Veterans Administration were classified in a "subprofessional" category until the "rebirth" of all of hospital pharmacy in the forties when they were given full professional status.

Pharmacy historian Alex Berman describes the "awakening" of hospital pharmacy in the twenties and its advance in the thirties in his discussion of the formative period of hospital pharmacy. You know well the events leading to the founding of the American Society of Hospital Pharmacists in the forties and of the leaders—their plans, hopes, disappointments, and successes. But to appreciate the advancement and development of hospital pharmacy practice as we know it today, I took a look back to see what hospital pharmacists were doing professionally in Harvey Whitney's time—what they were talking about and what was thought of them.

I still enjoy reading the weekly newspaper from my hometown in Minnesota, although the most familiar names, I find after these many years, are in the "Harkening Back" column—a column of news events from 25 years ago. I wondered what a "harkening back" column of hospital pharmacy would show. It wasn't hard to find out, because hospital pharmacists then, as now, were professional-minded, dedicated, and articulate individuals, though perhaps not at that time accorded the stature and professional prestige of our present-day practitioners. Thus, their writings in hospital literature were readily available and revealing.

In our "harkening back" column of 25 years ago, we would find articles on sterilizing medicinal substances, about making medications more palatable, a description of a plan for training pharmacy interns, of the conversion of two basement rooms of a hospital to a new pharmacy. One pharmacist-author wrote:

> *Cooperation between the pharmacist and the medical staff of the hospital is of vital importance*. . . and: *The pharmacist must be considered a vital part of the modern hospital and should be consulted by the different members of the staff when the occasion requires. Only in this way will the patient receive the utmost in medication and the hospital the ultimate in economy.*

Another said:

> *In addition to being a specialist, the pharmacist is a business and professional man. The administrator looks to him for help from a business standpoint, while the physicians and nurses look to him for professional help.*

A commentary on hospital pharmacy education urged the addition of courses in X-ray and clinical laboratory techniques to the pharmacy curriculum to increase the pharmacist's usefulness and employability, especially in smaller hospitals. With newer manufactured preparations available, pharmacists especially in tuberculosis, psychiatric, and smaller general hospitals would have *more spare time,* the writer said, and, furthermore, drugs were being supplemented by other forms of therapy such as light, heat, water, electricity, and exercise.

They *could not have known* at that time that we were on the brink of a breakthrough in drug therapy, which in the years immediately to follow would save and prolong the lives of thousands of tuberculosis patients, convert their hospital beds to other uses, and help to return many, many, previously hopeless mental patients to useful, meaningful lives in their communities; that would take the fear, the dread, and the tragedy out of many illnesses of only a generation ago. A breakthrough that would make drugs, and the pharmacies that dispense them, one of the most essential elements in all of hospital care. Hospital pharmacists were advised that the enterprising hospital pharmacist should be a member of the major hospital staff—attending conferences and participating in them; that he should be an important member of the nurses' training school staff and, even more important, he should be the director, in his own way, of a certain postgraduate instruction to the intern corps.

That is our "harkening back" column. Harkening back to the days in which Harvey Whitney practiced and wielded his influence on those who were to follow and bring even greater recognition to hospital pharmacy and to make it more useful. Hospital pharmacy, even then, was on the move—restless, emerging, and getting set for more progress within the 20 years to come than the most optimistic would have predicted. But there were no more than 1000 pharmacists practicing in hospitals at that time—we probably have closer to 6000 today—and they had not achieved the professional stature of today's highly regarded hospital pharmacists.

And now, two decades later, what are hospital pharmacists doing, what are they discussing, and what are their professional accomplishments? What is it that has elevated hospital pharmacists to this generation's position of professional prestige and recognition? Summed up, it probably would be education, hard work, dedication, service above self. But for more specific explanations, look at the program for this Annual Meeting. Note the subject material in the four annual institutes on hospital pharmacy, now sponsored by the ASHP. Look at the *Minimum Standard for Pharmacies in Hospitals*; look at the recommended standards for residencies in hospital pharmacy.

If a profession can be judged by its literature, look at the subject material in the *American Journal of Hospital Pharmacy*. I took note of a few from recent issues: "Allergenic Prescriptions"; "Adverse Drug Reactions"; "Clinical Testing of Drugs"; "Tests for Identification of Drugs"; "Incompatibilities of Parenteral Products"; "Refractometry in Quality Control"; "Pharmacy Staffing and Workloads"; "Detecting Medication Errors"—the latter a field, incidentally, in which hospital pharmacy has pioneered in cooperative efforts with other professions, an example of assuming responsibility with patient safety and well being as the sole objective. Most of these articles were written by hospital pharmacy practitioners. I know of no other field of pharmacy practice, other than in pure research, in which the contributions to the professional literature are so voluminous or useful.

Hospital pharmacists and pharmacy educators have been working together the past three years in constructive efforts to improve the education of pharmacists for hospital pharmacy practice. To assure this, the abilities required of hospital pharmacists have been analyzed and summarized. A look at these abilities—found in today's practicing hospital pharmacists—offers another clue to the reason for their position in the profession. You as a hospital pharmacist, if you head your department, must be a manager. Your responsibilities include program planning and integration with other hospital departments, interpretation of trends, budgeting, inventory control, personnel administration, and general administration of the pharmacy in a business-like way.

You have a thorough knowledge of drugs and their pharmacologic actions. You know the pharmaceutical properties of drugs and can judge their quality. You must be able to develop special product formulations and to manufacture in bulk quantities. You must understand and apply quality controls. The hospital pharmacist performs pharmaceutical research of an applied nature and develops new or improved products, and he participates in medical research. He teaches both pharmacy students and residents and pharmacy-related subjects to students and practitioners in other disciplines.

Hospital pharmacists also are looking to the future. Serious consideration is being given newer techniques and methods involving automation—not with misgivings and fear of change but with hope and expectation of even better things to come. They share with interest and enthusiasm the previews given us of the fast approaching future use in hospital pharmacy of automated data processing and other electronic aids. They know that the successful, progressive pharmacists of the future will be those who not only accept the changes made possible by newer methods but who find more ways of applying their knowledge and skills to improve ways of doing things more effectively and efficiently. Hospital pharmacy will not be the champion of the *status quo.* This is not unlike the acceptance of prefabricated pharmaceuticals, in contrast to the handmade ones of a few decades ago, which, while decreasing the demand for compounding services in some instances, has made drug therapy and pharmacy itself better, more efficient, and more accurate than ever before. And this change has by no means decreased the need for the education and knowledge of the pharmacist. On the contrary, he needs *more* knowledge, *more* education, to be applied in *more* useful ways now that less of his time is taken up with the technical chores of hand-fabricating medications.

Some pharmacists have concerned themselves a great deal recently with the "image" of pharmacy, with what the public thinks of our profession, of the way it is practiced, and what is thought of us as practitioners. Perhaps the truest of all "images" can be found in a mirror. It can only reflect what actually is there—no more, no less. It cannot flatter, and seldom can it misrepresent. A photograph, of course, also is an image and can be retouched to bring out the most favorable points in its subject. But the lasting impression is made by the subject itself—not by what the expert "retoucher" puts into the image. So it is with pharmacy. We may seek the advice of experts on how to put it in its best light, but the true image in the long run can only reflect what actually is there.

No public relations headlines are needed to establish the professional status of hospital pharmacy. No legislative acts or administrative decrees are needed to declare hospital pharmacy a profession. This you already have. Let us be sure in accepting this status, in accepting authority and responsibility, in accepting the respect of our associates and plaudits of the public, that we have actually earned them—and in return are providing even more in service and professional excellence.

I am convinced that one of the essential characteristics of pharmacy in our relation with the public is *genuineness.* Let the professional achievements of pharmacy practice be the *reason* for its existence, not merely one of its status symbols. If this is so, the "image" will take care of itself.

Much is said about the pharmacist in his role as an expert on drugs—as an authority on the pharmaceutical and therapeutic properties of drugs and their usage and dosage. Then let us *be* the "genuine" expert on drugs. Let us not be merely drug label readers or quoters of product package inserts. If we are to be experts on the properties of drugs, let us be experts in depth. If yours is the authority and responsibility for selecting the maker or source of supply for the drugs you dispense, accept that responsibility but be sure it is carried out well. If a physician prescribes a drug by a nonproprietary name without specifying a brand, he confers on you an authority and responsibility to apply your knowledge in selecting a product of the highest quality, effectiveness, and assured safety. This is a trust which hospital pharmacists strive for and are accorded more than in any other specialty of our profession. Guard it well.

Let us never go to the lawmakers for *economic* advantages under the guise of "protection" of the public health. If these are needed, let the reasons for them be *genuine.* Let us not jeopardize the elite, highly respected status of our Boards of Pharmacy by asking them to include "trade" control along with their vital responsibility for professional regulation. Pharmacy cannot afford to be found shallow and wanting in any of its claims when there is so much on the positive side to enhance its professional position. We live in a sophisticated society. It is true that pharmacists are university educated and that ours is a learned profession. But so are many others with whom we have daily associations—our patrons, colleagues, and the patients we serve—and many of them also belong to learned professions. No longer is the label of an educated person applied to a select few professionals in the community. We are not likely to convince many with exaggerated claims of professionalism if it is not a reality. But at the same time, our educated, sophisticated society, I am confident, is willing to accept, albeit take for granted, professional status wherever it *genuinely* exists.

I am convinced that long after the derogatory headlines have been forgotten, many more of our people are going to be grateful for the health-giving, lifesaving drugs developed by the scientists of pharmacy than were swayed by the economic charges during the tempest of the past two years in Washington.

I am convinced that long after the headlines are forgotten, more people are going to have reason to be grateful for the *effectiveness* of our food and drug laws and the way in which they have been enforced for the protection of the public than were frightened by the publicity and drama during this period of strengthening and improving them.

I recently read an editorial in a small town weekly newspaper praising the community pharmacy—the only one in town—and urging its support on the basis of the *need* for it in that community in time of sickness and for the town's other health care needs. This theme appealed to me particularly because I happen to have grown up in that pharmacy as a boy, but I believe this sentiment is typical of the feeling about pharmacies throughout this country, though not often expressed. I am convinced that long after the criticisms about prescription pricing and merchandising practices are forgotten, the good people of that community are going to be grateful for the assurance they get from having that pharmacy down on Main Street.

I am convinced that long after our current discussions of formulary systems, outpatient prescriptions, and the many other problems with which we now are concerned—long after these have been resolved—hospital patients and their physicians will be grateful for the hospital pharmacy and the hospital pharmacist in his essential role on the professional team.

One of the more serious responsibilities of hospital pharmacists, when they are given the opportunity, is the teaching and training of future practitioners. Professional training has been one of the responsibilities accepted by many pharmacists from the time our profession began. Probably it is because of its origin, because of tradition, and because few other centers of pharmacy practice were available that most preregistration internships have been served in community pharmacies. But is this still necessary, or adequate? More recently, we have seen the development of internships, now coming to be called residencies, in hospital pharmacy. Harvey Whitney was one of the early leaders in establishing hospital pharmacy internships. These are not intended primarily to qualify the intern for registration but rather to prepare him more thoroughly for the practice of pharmacy in hospitals. The American Society of Hospital Pharmacists has established high standards for hospital pharmacy internships (residencies), and a program for formal accreditation by the Society is now becoming a reality. Hospital pharmacy internships and residencies meeting ASHP standards offer exceptionally well-rounded training in professional pharmacy practice. In most states, this properly is accepted in fulfillment of the internship or "practical experience" requirement for registration.

In my view, another forward step in the training of *all* future practitioners of pharmacy would be the encouragement of a period of internship *in a hospital*, regardless of the type of practice the new graduate intends to go into after its completion. In this regard, perhaps we could draw an analogy with medicine. Internships in preparation for the practice of medicine are taken in hospitals. I am sure that many medical students and interns plan to practice in private offices or in group clinics. But regardless of this, the internship is taken in the hospital where the number of patients, the complexity of medical cases, and the variety of diseases provide the greatest opportunity for learning in the constant, concentrated, day-to-day treating of the sick and injured. Here the professional demands on the practitioner are the very greatest. The same could apply to pharmacy. What better training for the application of professional pharmacy *in any setting* than a period of internship furnishing pharmacy services all day, every day, to those sick enough to be hospitalized. In addition to its value as professional training, a period of internship in a hospital for *all* pharmacists would prepare them, as future community practitioners, for assuming a professional role in the hospitals and nursing homes of their communities, should the occasion arise.

The medical practice of most physicians is carried on both inside and outside the hospital. There is no reason why this dual area of service should not be followed by many pharmacists. Hospital pharmacists have long encouraged practitioners in community pharmacies to provide their services in hospitals in which there is not and perhaps, for economic reasons, cannot be a full-time hospital pharmacist. Some are doing this. But with the more than 3500 smaller hospitals in this country, and the number growing each year, without professional pharmacy services, there would appear to be little reason why a part of each day in the community hospital should not be a normal way of life for many community pharmacists.

In a special message to Congress this February, President Kennedy said:

Perhaps the most threatening breach in our health defenses is the shortage of trained health manpower.

He also said:

Although some progress has been made in meeting the backlog of need for chronic disease hospitals and nursing homes, it is estimated that less than one third of this need has been met and that an additional 500,000 beds for long term patients are required to meet today's demand.

If these facilities the President said we need are to be provided, and indications are that they will be, tremendous increases in drug dispensing will follow, and this is going to require pharmacy services. Where are the pharmacists coming from? Some, no doubt, will be full-time hospital pharmacists. But in many cases, the opportunity and the need for community pharmacists to provide their services will be there.

Pessimists in pharmacy have seen the times in which we live as the "beginning of the end" of pharmacy as a profession. Hospital pharmacy is proving this is not so—that we have just reached the "*end* of the beginning."

Why has hospital pharmacy so rapidly gained the professional position it now enjoys? Deno, Brodie, and Rowe in their book *The Profession of Pharmacy* explained it this way:

The combination of right times, right leaders, and right organizations has given hospital pharmacy an opportunity for rapid growth unequalled in any other branch of the profession.

I believe it also is because hospital pharmacists, under the forward thrust of modern medicine, were given a challenge to provide higher level professional services. You accepted and met that challenge, and in so doing earned your present enviable place on the health sciences team. You have made the most of your opportunities and, as the servant in the parable, having been given five talents, invested them wisely and returned 10; and the one given two returned four; not as the third servant, given one talent, hid it and returned only the one, for he had been afraid of losing the one he had. You had confidence in your capabilities and the courage of H. A. K. Whitney. The evidence of the achievements of hospital pharmacy and the challenge of even greater ones are all about you.

We have been given much.

But much more must be given in return.

At the time he received this award, Vernon O. Trygstad was the Director of Pharmacy Service at the Veterans Administration, Washington, D.C.

1964

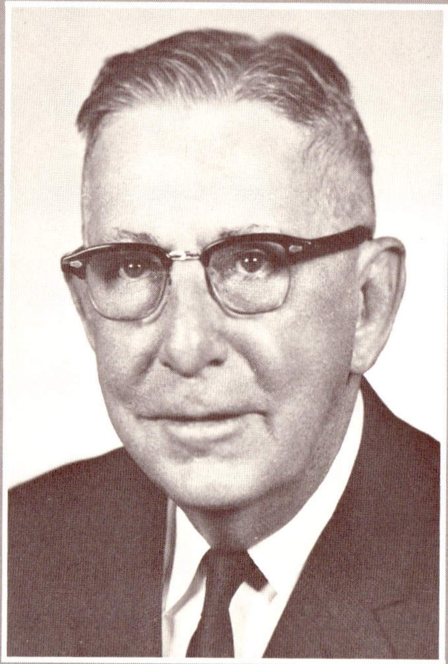

ALBERT P. LAUVE

"Success always seems to accompany professional satisfaction."

COMPATIBILITY OF PROFESSIONAL SUCCESS AND SATISFACTION

Reverend Sisters, honored guests, officers and members of the American Society of Hospital Pharmacists, fellow pharmacists, ladies, and gentlemen: To tell you that you have honored me today beyond my fondest expectations would be a grave understatement. To say that I cherish this honor above all others would be a gross misrepresentation of my true feelings this day. Accordingly, do not misinterpret my next remark as being false humility: I can assure you that our Society is composed of individuals so much more worthy of this award, and, incidentally, I recall this as my initial feeling and first impression at being notified of the award.

For just a moment, allow me the privilege of indulging in the satisfaction of examining the significance of this cherished award to me. First, it is awarded by a committee composed of past recipients of the award. Imagine, young pharmacists, imagine the hall of fame of hospital pharmacy that the individuals of this committee represent: the Franckes, the Bowles, the Flacks, the Fraziers, the Scotts; what glorious company to find yourself in.

Second, and possibly most important to me, is the fact that this award is given in honor of an old and cherished friend of mine, Harvey A. K. Whitney. Some of my fondest memories date back to the days when a vigorous, young pharmacist from Ann Arbor and I exchanged ideas on vague and unheard-of pharmacy practices, which we also disseminated in a one-sheet newsletter then called *The Bulletin*.

As you know, the recipient of the Harvey A. K. Whitney Lecture Award delivers a lecture which is intended to provide hospital pharmacists with a message or an idea which is meaningful and significant. This assignment was a much easier one to carry out several years ago, because today we have so many fine leaders in hospital pharmacy who, incidentally, never cease to amaze me with their vision and their ability to say things which stimulate other hospital pharmacists everywhere. Originality of thought was, therefore, somewhat of a stumbling block for me in preparing my remarks for this evening.

In somewhat of a reflective mood, I recall some of the events in my career in hospital pharmacy, and I quickly come to the conclusion that I am really quite a lucky man. "Why lucky?" you may ask. In a nutshell, I have been granted the things that have made a man's life enjoyable and rewarding: a loving family, a respected and honorable profession, and a feeling of success and accomplishment. All these are gifts that God has granted me. I am especially lucky because I have enjoyed professional satisfaction and the success of family and community life.

Consequently, it is extremely distressing for me to overhear a fledgling pharmacist remark, "Yes, Mr. Lauve, I'd like to practice professional pharmacy and utilize all my scientific training, but you cannot do that and be a success at the same time." In effect, he is saying that a pharmacist cannot enjoy professional satisfaction and be a success at the same time. How wrong he is, how narrow his vision, how misguided this unimaginative and unfortunate newcomer. To dissuade young pharmacists from the frustration, disillusion, and emptyness which oftentimes accompany material success alone, I usually preach a sermon which I entitle "The Compatibility of Professional Success and Satisfaction." It is really a simple sermon based on a simple doctrine. It goes like this: The past, the present, and the future success of pharmacy is dependent on the degree to which its practitioners utilize the unique characteristics which underlie and identify it. I refer specifically to the pharmacist's emphasis on the bulk formulation of pharmaceutical dosage forms, which may or may not be available from any other source. During recent years, I have had the feeling that I was preaching an outmoded doctrine—one contrary to the common opinion that manufacturing is a fast disappearing aspect of a pharmacist's activity. Recently, however, a statement in *Mirror to Hospital Pharmacy* renewed my confidence in this doctrine by stating:

> *The pharmacist who engages in manufacturing uses areas of scientific knowledge quite different from those used for dispensing and compounding. In fact, isn't it true that manufacturing and control are the only areas of professional practice which give the pharmacist an opportunity to use, to any significant extent, the large body of knowledge based on the physical sciences as applied particularly to pharmacy? If this is true, then must not hospital pharmacy chart a course which encourages manufacturing? This is an important question. A profession can't continue to be a profession unless a significant proportion of its practitioners utilize the knowledge and skill which underlie it.*

I have attempted to live by this doctrine in my professional life; and if I am judged a successful hospital pharmacist, then my success is a result of practicing the doctrine referred to. Looking back over the years, I can honestly say that were it not for this doctrine, Albert Lauve would not be here today. The desire and willingness to utilize formulation skills in the daily practice of our specialty have immeasurably contributed to providing us with the respect and admiration of the medical staffs of two institutions in which I have practiced. Furthermore, each time that I meet an old friend in medicine, we recall the challenge of developing together a drug formulation which many times was instrumental in successfully treating a patient. The product desired was usually brought to me in the form of an idea, incomplete and desperately in need of the skillful and creative development of a professional pharmacist.

Perhaps you would be interested in some of my earlier experiences which illustrate the close relationship of professional satisfaction and success.

My first experience with intravenous medication began in 1913 with the introduction of arsphenamine, commonly known as Salvarsan. This preparation was developed in 1910 by Ehrlich, after a long series of experiments, as a specific for syphilis. The preparation had to be freshly prepared. It was an acid salt and had to be neutralized before administration. Some of the doctors wanted to try this new specific for the treatment of syphilis, but there were no hospitals in the immediate vicinity where we could have access to an autoclave and distilled water—essential equipment for this kind of work. So we bought a small water still, an Arnold type of sterilizer, and a few Erlenmeyer flasks. We were ready for business. The arsphenamine was dissolved in 50 ml of sterile water and neutralized with 15% sodium hydroxide. No indicator was needed to determine the end point. The first drop of sodium hydroxide turned the arsphenamine very cloudy and we continued, drop by drop, until the solution turned to a golden yellow. The solution was then diluted to 250 ml with normal saline, taken to the doctor's office, and administered immediately. Crude as this method might seem, we administered over 200 doses without a single adverse reaction.

This is just one of countless numbers of examples that illustrate the dependence of professional success on our distinct and unique abilities. Even today, our department is called upon so much more to provide this essential aspect of our service.

The future holds even more success for the imaginative, creative, and astute hospital pharmacist. As in the past and as of present, this success will be firmly based on the foundation of the doctrine of formulation. We speak of unit dose dispensing, for example, and is it not true that the most challenging aspect of this contemporary concept lies in the compatibility and stability of medicaments in unique and possibly untried packaging materials? And who are the pioneers in this area? Hospital pharmacists with deep interest in formulation and control skills.

We speak of drug information centers as intimately a part of pharmacy service. Is it not true that a commonly posed question, but a difficult question to answer, involves the compatibility of injectable mixtures of medications? Again, the answer to the problem is based on the pharmacist's unique knowledge of the physical sciences as applied to pharmacy.

Young pharmacists, take heed. My years offer me the protection of experience, but they also offer me the fruits of observation and retrospect. Society recognizes the contributions our profession has made and continues to make. It wants more of the same. Do not be overly concerned or tempted to cast aside the enduring rewards of professional satisfaction for the temporary and fleeting pleasure of material rewards. A close examination of the professional lives and accomplishments of the past recipients of the Harvey A. K. Whitney Lecture Award dramatically reveals the remarkable way in which success always seems to accompany professional satisfaction—satisfaction which in itself can only be obtained from a practice based on professional uniqueness.

Heed the doctrine which has permitted one Albert Lauve to receive an honor which, again, exemplifies the compatibility of professional success and satisfaction.

At the time he received this award, Albert P. Lauve was the Chief Pharmacist at Mercy Hospital, New Orleans, Louisiana.

1965

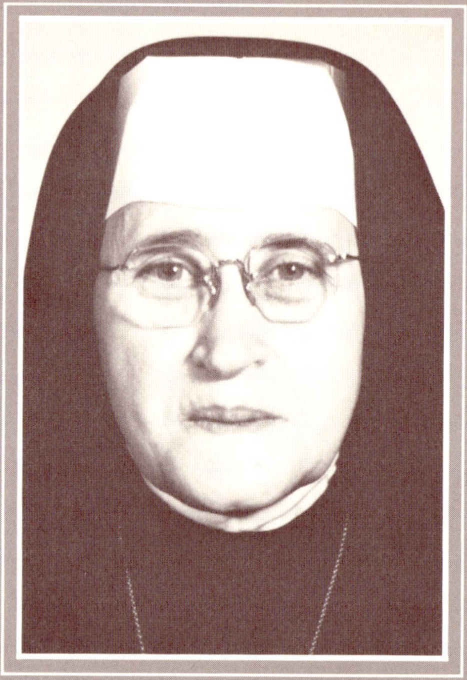

SISTER MARY BERENICE

"And so long live hospital pharmacy!"

QUO VADIS 20th CENTURY HOSPITAL PHARMACY?

It is a gratifying task to have this opportunity to review the Society's history from the vantage point of time and to trace in studied retrospect the touchstones of its stable progress, prudent adaptations, and provident changes.

The position and status of pharmacy in its relation to hospitals are significantly interesting and enlightening. At the turn of this century, hospitals bore the stigma of being "houses of death" rather than havens of cure and recovery. Accrediting bodies were nonexistent. Medical science was but in its infancy. Hospital pharmacy found itself in the company of a sapling profession.

The community pharmacist—or "druggist" of that day—provided relief for minor ills without a doctor's prescription since legal controls over medications were negligible. Prior to 1914, narcotics could be purchased over the counter with no ado. Possibly at this time the image of the community pharmacist fared somewhat better than that of the hospital. As the practice of medicine progressed and the uneventful recoveries of patients increased, the public's reaction towards hospitals took on a tone of confidence and the "house of death" image gave way to the "temple of hope." The very choice of the word "temple" presaged the growing respect which accompanied the discovery of successful new drugs and the introduction of Blue Cross and other insurance plans which militated towards the alleviation of financial stress. Doctors were regarded with unhesitating esteem, nurses and other personnel as "angels of mercy."

This utopian concept was dimmed by materialism and selfishness, and hospitals lost their enchantment in the emerging third image, which categorized them with such facilities as public schools, parks, and libraries or gave them placement with mere utilities such as gas, electricity, and water. Hospitalization was no longer recognized as a privilege but demanded as a right. Its services were price tagged, it knew the worries of litigations; and to the less dedicated and scarcely inspired, it became a place to work rather than one in which to serve. And yet despite these disappointing and disillusioning ramifications, the hospital continues to occupy a unique place in society, for in God's economy the foibles of human nature continue to be overshadowed by the dignity of man as the constant reflections of the divine in him mirror his changeless purpose in life and his intended majestic end.

Pharmacy was the first of the related medical professions to follow medicine in requiring registration by examination and the last to exact a hospital residency. All states except one require one year of practical experience for state board of pharmacy examination; this period often is loosely termed an internship but in most instances is wanting in caliber. (Mississippi requires only diploma registration for the practice of pharmacy.)

It is regrettable that most schools of pharmacy have lacked foresight in employing this formal educational associate to capacity, exhibiting a lamentable apathy in recognizing the urgency of upgrading the educational curriculum for hospital pharmacy in keeping with the steady advancement of its standards. We ask: "Is pharmacy now to assume the role of laggard where previously it merited the position of leader?" Colleges of pharmacy are not solely responsible for this plight. In general, hospitals must share the honest blame created by such diluting factors as unqualified personnel, insufficient knowledge, want of understanding, and lack of sympathetic rapport.

It gives me a warm happiness to point out, however, that St. Mary's Infirmary, St. Louis, Missouri, predecessor of the present St. Mary's Hospital and one of the 89 hospitals of the country and one of the two institutions in St. Louis, Missouri, approved in 1914 by the American College of Surgeons (now the Joint Commission on Accreditation of Hospitals), at that time enjoyed a stable superiority which has been transmitted to St. Mary's Hospital and the other hospitals administered by the Sisters of St. Mary. This unique position is due to the spirit and traditions of the Sisters of St. Mary but particularly to the faith, courage, and broad vision of Mother Mary Concordia, our fourth Superior General, whose reputation as a woman of God and a leading hospital administrator is surpassed only by her rich legacies to posterity. She, together with Sister Mary Irene, S.S.M., and the Reverend Alphonse M. Schwitalla, S.J., brought to birth collegiate programs in the various paramedical professions which hitherto enjoyed only a practical status. She opened St. Mary's Hospital to religious from every congregation in the United States and Canada and other interested persons for advanced education in the various hospital specialties. She also provided hospital facilities for the St. Louis University School of Medicine, thus enabling it to meet its vital accreditation requisite.

Startling developments in pharmacy practice were in the offing as World War I made history; and when physicians returned home, their battle-scarred achievements included the administration of glucose intravenously. This scientific advancement horizoned the necessity of the well-organized bulk compounding departments we know today. Dextrose and other preparations for parenteral use were not on the market; the market had to be created by the demand. Force of circumstances prompted the preparation of these solutions with materials and equipment that would not be acceptable today. Nevertheless, the hospitals engaged in this service then were among the best in the nation and were accredited by the American College of Surgeons, the only accrediting body for hospitals at that time.

It is interesting to note the changing patterns of practice from nearly total compounding with inadequate equipment to almost total purchasing, occasioned by the changing patterns of physicians' prescribing and of manufacturing firms' production. Hospital pharmacists, cognizant of the poor caliber of their working equipment, resorted to purchasing many products. A little later, as pilot-sized equipment became available, these same hospital pharmacists again took up their rightful prerogative of bulk compounding. The gap created by varying trends of the immediate past was again closing so that hospital pharmacists were once more in a position to fulfill their essential duties of service and education.

While it is conceded that many of our hospitals, especially the smaller ones, find it impractical to establish bulk compounding departments, still it is essential that these facilities be provided by teaching and research institutions to ground pharmacy students in the professional techniques involved in this vital area of service since frequently every hospital pharmacist must apply these techniques for small- or single-dose preparations. While colleges of pharmacy generally offer limited courses of this nature, not all offer curricula in manufacturing scoped to accommodate the specific needs of hospital pharmacy. Today, we find that more teaching hospitals are utilizing the services of product-development specialists, assay and control specialists, and research specialists to work with the medical staff in developing and testing new drug products and preparations for patients.

In the early part of the century, few drugs gave prolonged relief and fewer cured anything. Reactions resulting from drug therapy were generally unrecognized and, consequently, unheeded since the existing relationship between the action of drugs and the chemical composition and physiological properties of the body had not as yet been discovered, probed, and proved.

Standardization measures, communication media, and scientific advancement saw themselves personified in formal attire as the American Society of Hospital Pharmacists in 1942. Its initial 152 organizers were designated as charter members. In the following year, it gained 265 new adherents who well deserve to be designated informally as "near-charter" members, helping as they did to lay the arduous groundwork of the Society's foundation. Harvey A. K. Whitney was elected its first Chairman, a position comparable to today's President.

In Mr. Whitney's initial message, "Getting Out of the Cellar," he viewed the Society's members as pioneers who, "like the early settlers devoted themselves to hacking, scratching, and building pathways through unchartered areas of the hills and swamps, overgrowth, undergrowth and other imposing obstacles." All of these difficulties, he hastened to add, "should never be allowed to obscure the general direction we shall set toward the goal of professional respectability and secure a free way of living in the atmosphere of our chosen field of special endeavor." One can't help wishing that all hospital administrators and hospital pharmacists would have grasped the import of Mr. Whitney's provocative message and that our vineyard would be teeming with a happy abundance of qualified workers.

An understanding of the progress of the Society from its beginnings may be observed by reviewing the Society's publications, choice distillations all of the determination, courage, and convictions of hospital pharmacy pioneers whose luster shone in their simplicity, whose strength rested in their frail beginnings, whose wealth was their personal loyalty to the cause they served so well. In 1944, they passed a resolution stating: "the Finance Committee may without further action pass on all accounts or appropriations not exceeding $25.00." Our present annual budget of approximately one-half million dollars evidences how they envisioned the oak while planting the acorn! Certainly, it is a warm satisfaction to every member of the Society to know that this budget is being applied constantly in bringing increased services and educational opportunities to its more than 4000 members. You must be more than pleased with the services provided, services which dedicated and tireless workers have blessed into significant educational and professional profits for the advancement of pharmacy and its pharmacists.

Were Mr. Whitney to return to earth today to roam the ground of hospital pharmacy, I believe he would know neither surprise nor frustration. Rather, I think the milestones of advancement of pharmacy would delight his heart and transfuse him with renewed positive restlessness for the Society's continuing progress. Effortlessly, I think he would join forces with those "poets of the intellect" whose scientific research knows almost daily reward as the Lord of all creation blesses their tireless endeavors with miniature souvenirs of His omnipotence and omniscience. I like to think that this delicate courtesy of God is in recognition of His creatures' eagerness to fulfill His command to subdue the earth and bring all things under subjection.

God's benevolence towards mankind knows no respite, permitting Dr. John R. McGibony and like men of wisdom to dream on and on about miniaturization of modern facilities that will produce automatic bedside techniques for instant diagnosis; remote consultation through microcircuit television media; microwave cooking with floor vending machines; disposable or edible dishes; garbage disintegration; electric power through transmitters or small atomic energy units; walls and ceilings adapted to supply light; electronic prevention or removal of dust and dirt; blanket heating, cooling, and ventilating for entire communities rather than for individual units; entirely disposable linens; and transportation via moving corridors, sidewalks, and highways.

As the fantasy of these and other wonders give way to actuality, data processing eventually will score admittance throughout entire hospitals as pilot plants now apply themselves diligently to testing various systems and ascertaining economic modes of installation. Universities are teaching courses in electronics for application in hospital operations. A singularly facinating device, described in the January 1, 1964 issue of *Hospitals,* points to error prevention in the administration of drugs. For example, should a request for a wrong dose or an incorrectly named drug be inserted into the machine, the device will immediately type back "this is an incorrect dose" or "there is no such drug; please check with the physician." We know that the device can return only that information which has been stored in its memory. This information should be provided by the pharmacist. The inadequacy of my description should serve but to heighten your interest in scanning the entire article.

Pharmacywise, it is hoped that data processing will provide time for the pharmacist to function more fully in his professional capacity. Today, medications are being added to intravenous solutions during actual injection. It is essential that the person functioning in this capacity knows whether or not these drugs are chemically, physiologically, and pharmacologically compatible, for often they are not. Often, queries of just this nature are directed to the hospital pharmacy from various nursing divisions. The diminution of clerical duties should relieve the pharmacist to serve more adequately in his roles of consulting, teaching, and investigational research, especially in conjunction with the newly established drug information centers, and as the reporting center of the hospital for adverse drug reactions. This type of service is a new breakthrough towards progress—one that all hospital pharmacists should endeavor to establish. While it may seem that hospital pharmacists have practically always been the source of drug information, this new concept offers a far broader service and accommodating scope in its tremendous potential for better patient care. Data-processing equipment will be invaluable in this particular area, in fact almost indispensable as the program becomes fully developed.

This last-mentioned item has brought us to the very doorstep of the January 1965 issue of the *American Journal of Hospital Pharmacy* and the February 1965 issue of the *Journal of the American Pharmaceutical Association.* A soul-searching look of gratitude is directed to the past; a smile for work well done suffices for the present; a stable willingness of body, mind, and heart welcomes the future. And so long live hospital pharmacy! As we continue down the corridor of time and perform our life work in this field, let us be reminded that somehow we know that something of the awful sameness, kindness, and clearness of Providence will continue to shine through the reverses and successes that trample and temper as God seasons the raw matter of our efforts with His readying grace and halos seeming failures with divine unpredictability. Somehow, we know that often those who till most fervently and tirelessly reap but poorly. But smallness knows no entree in devoted, dedicated hearts. Garnered for posterity, the vintaged steadfastness of our pioneers has braved the chasmy gap of diffidence for those of us who often might falter still were it not for the timeless bridge which their love for mankind fashioned for all future hospital pharmacists worthy of the name.

In the convergence of human interests, as hospital pharmacy converges for us, no life is a purely private affair, and no one knows the numbers whom he has helped or hindered along life's road. Our actions as echoes ring down the valleys of other lives like voices of distant bells, quietly and impartially reaching to the most secluded, almost forgotten hamlets of men. Our lives sweep through those of others like the wind over the waters of the sea, whose waves reach even unto distant shores. Our acts of kindness, an encouraging word, our courage to fight for better patient care through quality pharmaceutical services are seen and heard or noted, imitated, and, in turn, pattern happiness in the lives of others, give proper direction to future hospital pharmacists and aid to the sick and injured in our communities.

Again, I thank each one of you! May God always bless you for your goodness and your kindness to others!

At the time she received this award, Sister Mary Berenice, S.S.M., was the Director of the Department of Pharmacy, St. Mary's Hospital, St. Louis, Missouri, and the Treasurer of the American Society of Hospital Pharmacists.

1966

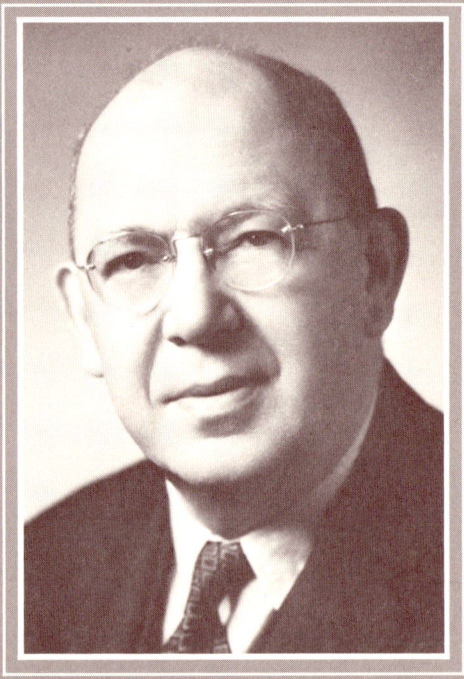

ROBERT P. FISCHELIS

(Speech is unavailable)

At the time he received this award, Robert P. Fischelis was the Dean of Ohio Northern University College of Pharmacy, Ada.

1967

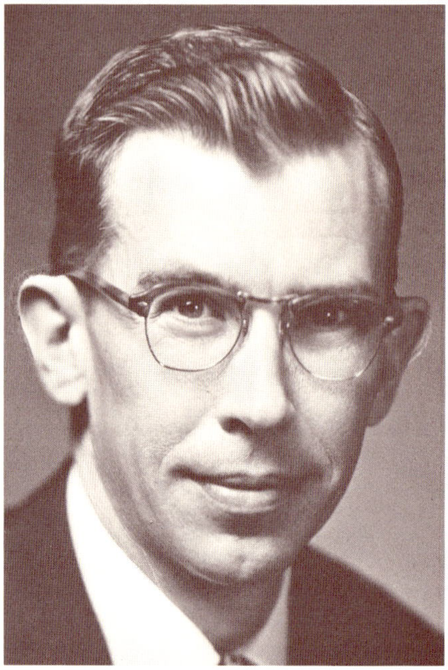

PAUL F. PARKER

"Pharmacy is in a rather remarkable position today to blaze a new trail."

DRUGS AND THE PEOPLE

American life is a continuous and unconscious revolution. . . America wants everybody to be happy, healthy, and useful; an idea regarded as wildly "radical" in some parts of the world. America works toward that ideal in every town, factory, school, and legislature until it changes the things that get in its way.

These words were used by James B. Reston, Washington Bureau Chief of the *New York Times*, to describe the bumper crop of legislation in the continuing American revolution.

Social change is all about us, and certainly health is one of the most significant of these changes. The people who provide health care no longer have the responsibility to the people for merely treating their diseases, mending their bodies, and immunizing their children but for maintaining their health from the cradle to the grave. While the American way of life in general is undergoing a social revolution, it appears that many of us in the health field still are unconscious of change. Those of us in pharmacy are more a part of this revolution than we may realize, because drugs are surely one of the most important components of health. To illustrate, let us divide the total concept of health care into any number of identifiable components such as medicine, surgery, dentistry, nursing, radiology, pathology, equipment, facilities, etc.—just as long as one component is drugs. Now, if we had to eliminate these components, one by one, when would drugs be eliminated? Surely, most people would list drugs as one of the last to go. But are pharmacy and drugs completely synonymous? Of course they are not. We must give credit to the scientists who discover and test drugs. We must recognize the very legitimate and important involvement of all our colleagues in the health field who concern themselves to varying degrees with drugs.

When we view pharmacy in the social revolution, perhaps we should ask ourselves: Does pharmacy adequately involve itself in the total concept of drugs, or do we limit our professional emphasis to the sciences of drug development and their physicochemical relationships or to drug distribution and control? Do we balance judgment concerning our business and scientific interests against the interests of patients and the public? Do we function effectively as members of the health team? Do we specialize sufficiently to make drugs as effective and efficient as they should be in relation to their relative importance in health care?

As I have thought about the subject of this lecture during the past several months, I began to develop some rather deep personal feelings about some of the issues confronting pharmacy today. I could not confine my thoughts to hospital pharmacy and the programs in which I am involved daily, but neither could I exclude these matters. I thought, too, about our drug industry—the kind, quality, and quantity of drugs which it makes available throughout the world. Most particularly, I also thought about the practitioners who comprise the major segment of our profession—the community pharmacists. Nor was I unaware of those in pharmacy who direct our associations, those who write and report as pharmaceutical journalists, and those who teach in our colleges of pharmacy.

I fully respect the fact that individuals in each segment of pharmacy see the issues of the day in a quite different perspective. For instance, when viewed as a business, representatives of industry have one kind of interest, the wholesaler another, the community pharmacist another, and the hospital pharmacist still another. When viewed as a science, the industry researcher would hold one view, the educator-researcher another, and the clinical researcher—to the extent that we have clinical scientists in pharmacy—still another. When pharmacy is viewed as a service to the public, even though we may have a different perspective because of our business involvement or the kind of work we do, it is my opinion that we must all consider the needs and views and interests of the public itself. Therefore, even though you may find it difficult to remain completely neutral about my remarks, my purpose is to direct your attention to some matters of public interest regarding drugs and to propose some basic principles for pharmacy to help us serve the public better.

When I speak of public opinion or the public attitude about drugs, I refer to the total American society—the informed as well as the uninformed. Recently, I read an article in one of the new drug journals which reported public opinion as represented by an interview with 121 housewives. I refer here to public opinion which might be represented by even one person who might be in a position to obtain public support for his viewpoint. The heart of the matter is, if the facts of any particular issue were known or understood, what would be the public reaction?

In my opinion, the most sensitive public concern about drugs is their cost. This issue is seen in many different ways by different segments of society. For instance, a legislator may start a congressional investigation of drug company profits or, indeed, explore the idea of placing the drug industry under public control. Still another may investigate drug advertising and promotion. Someone may ask whether it is really necessary to have thousands of detail men call on physicians, pharmacists, and others almost every day of the year. Many Americans may want to know whether the cost of drugs is covered or is not covered by his insurance or by Medicare. Other Americans may call for a drug prepayment system. And, too, if my next door neighbor made less money than I did, then he might think drugs cost too much because pharmacists made too much money.

I cannot, in good conscience, tell you that I believe drugs cost too much. But neither can I completely justify the cost of drugs. I have read most of the canned speeches that come across my desk from the Madison Avenue boys. Some of these people and, indeed, some of my professional associates believe that I should accept this material and present it before groups such as my local Rotary Club. The fact is the evidence about drug costs has just not been adequate to convince me that I should go out and explain to my fellow Americans why drugs cost what they do.

I believe that drug research is expensive; I believe we should have good production and distribution controls; I even believe we should use packaging systems, such as are represented by unit dose packaging, to extend controls to the point where the drug is administered to, or used by, the patient. All of these things make drugs expensive. I believe any expense is justifiable that assures better quality and control to the patient.

There are two areas of cost that I would question, and even here I hasten to add that I am not passing judgment. These are the cost of marketing, including advertising, promotion, and detailing on the one hand and the principle of markup for distribution on the other. I do not recall any data that have been made available concerning marketing costs. Nor do I know of any professional conferences or other efforts on the part of the profession that explored the subject. Can the profession face the public squarely and say the cost of marketing is essential? Undoubtedly, individual companies have determined that the present methods of marketing produce the highest volume of drug sales—but, again, does this mean that the public is best served?

The profession has, indeed, faced the issue of the markup principle by advocating the use of the professional fee. I believe the pharmacy practitioner will have made a monumental step in improving his public image when he fully accepts the professional fee concept and divorces his professional services from the cost of drugs.

We need to take a fresh new approach to the clinical evaluation of drugs. The 1962 Harris Amendments to the Food and Drug Act are a rather obvious example of the public getting what it wants and changing things that get in its way in order to do so. But the answer is not merely so simple as passing a law to require the government to make a judgment on whether a drug is safe and efficacious or whether it is not. Good judgment to determine drug safety and efficacy can be only as valid as the scientific and clinical information to make such a judgment. I refer here to the loose organizational arrangements that exist between preclinical research groups and clinical research groups for drugs. In the past, such research has been coordinated largely between the medical departments of drug companies and individual physicians. The new legislation has required so much red tape and paperwork that potential clinical scientists are not encouraged to do clinical research. The support for clinical research from industry is not as attractive now as it has been in the past, because so much other research monies are now available.

It is timely and appropriate for colleges of pharmacy and hospital pharmacy departments to create and develop drug research programs in the medical center environment. Is there any good reason why the interdisciplinary team approach to drug research, including the clinical component, cannot be applied in the academic and clinical environment as well as in the laboratories of the pharmaceutical companies? I believe some precedent already exists to do this to a limited degree but largely on an individual basis. I believe that an organized program of this type would attract good pharmaceutical scientists as well as good clinical investigators.

Physicians need help in conducting good clinical drug investigations. The subjective clinical judgment which only they can provide is essential, but subjective judgment must be framed in an appropriate research design (protocol) to provide adequate objectivity. The pharmaceutical scientist might well devote a major part of his research effort developing this protocol, making objective measurements, providing double-blind bases for the studies, and, in general, bringing scientific depth to clinical drug research. Such programs would serve as a training ground for the development of more scientists who are so badly needed in this field. But most importantly, it would produce scientific results to support our nationwide need for determining drug safety and efficacy.

For the past five years, I have directed a drug distribution program which produces drug usage data showing statistically how much of what drug was used and on whom. These data are relatively unsophisticated and, unfortunately, do not include why the drug was used. Even without computerization of these data, our physicians can easily see from the drug usage information that they overused certain drugs even though they themselves wrote the original orders for the drugs. We like to think that we have a good program to guide physicians in the rational selection of drugs, but, obviously, there are areas of drug use that give us concern. What would happen if all drug usage in the nation was reviewed objectively? Would such a review stand the test of public scrutiny? In other words, do we use the drugs we should use and not use the drugs we should not use?

For over 25 years, hospital pharmacists have championed the cause of Pharmacy and Therapeutics Committees. The basic purpose of this cause has been the development of a more rational drug therapy. Unfortunately, some of us have not fully understood the basic reason for Pharmacy and Therapeutics Committees and, as a result, have overemphasized standardization and economics. This is wrong, and I believe we should take prompt action to correct it. While standardization and cost reduction may result from good, rational drug therapy, they cannot and should not be the basic reasons for it.

Even though hospital pharmacists have steadfastly pursued this course for over 25 years, the results are not yet adequate. I can foresee no particular reason for physicians to play a more important role in drug therapy in the future than they have in the past. The only answer I see is for pharmacists to become more directly involved in drug therapy. This applies to patient care programs outside the hospital itself and into group medical practices, or what is sometimes referred to as the total concept of institutional health care from a social viewpoint. This means clinical pharmacy must become a fundamental component of pharmaceutical education. In retrospect, I believe we are already 25 years late in doing this, but even now we must first develop a clinical faculty and find a way to weed out some other segments of the pharmaceutical curriculum.

We must admit to ourselves that we have a long way to go to become clinically involved. But I have a real fear that clinical involvement will soon become such a popular idea in pharmacy that everybody will want to get into the act. As a result, we will use such terms as "drug consultant to the physician." Is that discreet? Wouldn't it be much more appropriate if a pharmacist had aided or assisted a physician in some meaningful way and the physician said he had consulted with the pharmacist? Someone might contend that he was clinically involved because he regularly went on rounds with the physician. I would only ask, "For what purposes, and what did he contribute?"

In the first place, we need to become comfortable and at home in the clinical areas with physicians and patients. Secondly, we need to understand the clinical jargon, particularly as it relates to drugs and specific patient conditions, laboratory or pathological studies, etc. This will not be easy. But the most difficult part of all will be for the pharmacist to make a meaningful contribution to drug therapy or drug use in general. To me, this means that the pharmacist will need to know more than anyone else about drugs in their application to patients.

The subject of clinical involvement of pharmacists is not to be taken lightly; and I say to pharmacy educators, hospital pharmacists, or any other pharmacist who may have reason to become involved clinically that the issue should be approached in full cooperation with physicians and with sufficient support to make it work.

By advocating that pharmacists assume a meaningful role in drug therapy, we are not saying that physicians are not doing a good job, nor are we saying that physicians must not have ultimate responsibility to prescribe drugs. Indeed, they must retain this responsibility. We are saying that drug therapy is sufficiently complicated that we must provide a drug emphasis that is consistent with the importance of drugs in the total concept of health care. Neither are we saying that drug distribution cannot or should not be a fundamental role of the pharmacist, but rather that his time and knowledge must be more effectively directed to the total concept of drug use.

If we are successful in introducing a clinical component to pharmaceutical education, there is little doubt in my mind that we will also introduce a variety of specialists in pharmaceutical practice, that drug detailing as we know it today will disappear, and that the team concept of health care with respect to drugs will start to become meaningful.

Still another aspect of drug selection that must be considered in the light of public interest is the inconsistency between the drugs physicians prescribe and payment for these drugs by welfare programs, Medicare, or other third-party payee plans.

It is obvious that the pharmacist must take a more responsible political role at the federal, state, and local levels in drug therapy and payment programs. As he does so, he will be faced immediately and squarely with some of the most puzzling questions of our time. He will need to apply a superior quality of judgment to balance the quality and selection of drugs on the one hand against the cost of drugs and maintenance of the free enterprise system in the drug business on the other.

Pharmacists in America have always had the basic elements of a monopoly on drugs. Not completely so, but at best they had a situation with which they could have drawn the string tighter or made it looser. By default or misjudgment, they allowed the latter to happen. With the advent of the principle of self-service and mass merchandising, we became more obsessed with the loss of business than with the principle of protecting the public against itself. As a result, we advertised drugs directly to the public, mass merchandised them in our drugstores, and placed ourselves in direct competition with the people who had a business advantage to gain from loosening our drug monopoly. Now we know that if this monopoly is ever to return drugs to the control of the pharmacist, it can do so only by justifying the control in terms of protecting public health. To justify this cause, it will not be adequate for you and me to simply say it is so.

There may be on the horizon a new hope and justification for more completely controlling drugs. I am told that each drug may have a rather standard metabolic path, rate of excretion, etc., but that when two or more drugs are taken or administered simultaneously, a new set of pharmacologic facts comes into existence with respect to each drug. Imagine what this would mean when some of our patients take 12 or 15 drugs simultaneously. Although we may now be approaching a time when it can be demonstrated scientifically that drugs need to be controlled, is it now also time to strengthen our professional position on this subject? In seeking its remedies, should the public listen to the television commercials or be guided by the advice of the checkout girl at the grocery store or the checkout girl at the drugstore? Maybe our educational curriculum should be more directed to a scientific understanding of these remedies and less concerned with methods of merchandising them.

We live in an informed society, and I can see no reason why it is not appropriate for my friends, neighbors, or relatives to know what drugs they are taking and what effect they are supposed to have. I would go further and ask why we should not have programs designed specifically to inform the public about drugs. As the situation exists today, any person with a reasonable amount of initiative could find almost any information about any drug if he would only take the time and effort to do so. Obviously, I am not speaking of the rare situation in which it would be in the patient's best interest to withhold drug identification. This could be overcome easily if it was understood that prescription containers would be labeled with the name of the drug unless the physician indicated otherwise. It is well understood that there would be better continuity if therapy and drugs could be more easily identified in case of an emergency. Now that the American Medical Association has officially taken a position on this subject, it is obvious that pharmacists are the principal deterrent to keeping the public informed. It appears to me that the real reason is that pharmacists think patients might shop for their prescription medication.

There is still another, less controversial, but more serious side to the subject of patient information about drugs. I refer here to the patient's understanding of how he should take his drugs, the emphasis of drugs in relation to disease, the factors of home environment that interfere with good therapy, and whether he even has his prescription dispensed. As an example, a physician on our staff once conducted a survey of patients to determine their degree of understanding about their illness and home care as they were being discharged from the hospital. To my chagrin, even though their drugs were labeled by name, there was less understanding about their drugs than any other aspect of their illness. I have since been able to interest the chairman of our Behavioral Science Department in doing a study of patient understanding and use of drugs.

I believe pharmacy can act responsibly to the public in all of these areas, but in order to do so, there must be a new philosophy and sense of direction among its practitioners. This brings me to the four principal points of my lecture. I believe these points, if applied, will make us sensitive to our responsibilities to society and, to some extent, capable of fulfilling them:

1. *Pharmacy should involve itself in the total concept of drugs in health care.* In other words, pharmacy should involve itself intimately and responsibly with every aspect of drugs—from their discovery to production, evaluation, and testing, to their being prescribed, distributed, administered, and used by patients.
2. *Pharmacists should be socially responsible individuals who are patient and drug oriented.* This point introduces two components to our philosophy which, in my opinion, are remarkably weak—"socially responsible" and "patient oriented."
3. *Pharmacists should function as integral members of the health team.* In this respect, we are not referring so much to personal acceptance as to meaningful contributions.
4. *Pharmacists should be encouraged to specialize functionally.* The emphasis should be to specialize in various areas of drug concern such as clinical pharmacology, biopharmaceuticals, clinical pharmacy, drug information, etc., rather than hospital pharmacy, community pharmacy, etc. Since environmental specialization is not based on a fundamental set of knowledge, a set of skills, or a quality of professional judgment, is it specialization at all?

Pharmacy is in a rather remarkable position today to blaze a new trail and take a leadership role in health professions because of the importance of drugs to health care and the social revolution in which we are involved. But there are problems of communicating this challenge throughout our profession. I am reminded of the story told by the dean of our Dental School about the Kentuckians who were squatted before the court house of a rural town. One turned to the other and drawled, "How's your wife?" The other removed his pipe and, after unhurried deliberation, responded, "Compared with what?" I would then hope to respond, "Compared to all other health professions, which is the way people see us." There are so many differences in our profession because of age, time of attending pharmacy school, business involvement, scientific background, environment of practice, etc., that it is difficult to see what common factor or focus of interest might lead the profession in one direction. I would hope that one focus might be "Drugs and the People."

At the time he received this award, Paul F. Parker was the Director of the Pharmacy Central Supply Department at University Hospital and an Assistant Professor at the College of Pharmacy, University of Kentucky, Lexington.

1968

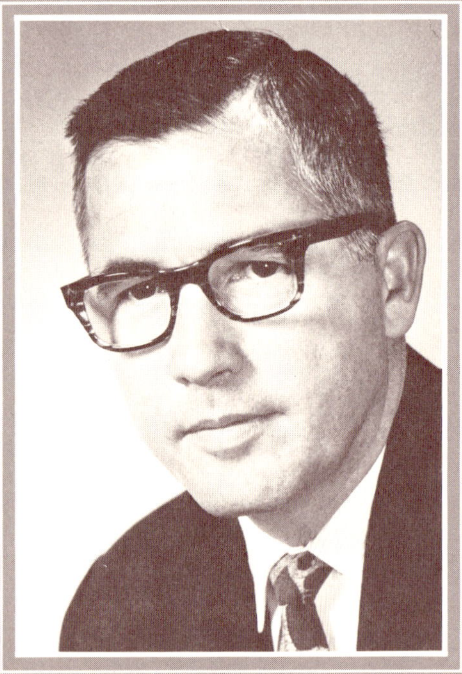

CLIFTON J. LATIOLAIS

"But perhaps this is the time . . . to assess our present position and to determine our future direction."

AS WE MOVE INTO HISTORY

"We must dream," said Thomas Jefferson, "of an aristocracy of achievement arising out of a democracy of opportunity." While Berman, the historian, described the trials and tribulations of hospital pharmacists during the awakening twenties and advancing thirties to gain national recognition in American pharmacy, it was this "democracy of opportunity" that provided the mechanism for the formation of the American Society of Hospital Pharmacists in 1942. Certainly, during its brief quarter century of existence, the ASHP has not attained an "aristocracy of achievement."

In fact, perhaps hospital pharmacy resides at a lower celestial level than its high priests would care to admit. Yet, it has amassed a wealth of accomplishments in American pharmacy amid a plethora of pharmaceutical organizations in existence at the time of its formation. While many of these organizations have inflicted what I call "organizational malnutrition" upon its members, perhaps the Society has made some of its members so-called "organizational fat cats." Such achievements have intrigued me to undertake this brief analysis of some underlying forces behind the Society's success, its present practices, and its future direction.

History tells us that organizations, societies, and cultures which made tremendous progress were goal oriented. Their peoples were committed, without reservation, to achieve these goals. However, to sustain the acid test of time, a goal-oriented society must be based on altruistic principles which foster the public good. While this must be its prime objective, it can, does, and must also serve individual human goals which society values so highly. If, on the other hand, individual goals are the prime objective and the public good is placed into secondary consideration, then that goal-oriented society shall fail. Two examples might suffice to illustrate the point, namely, the Al Capone organization and Hitler's Third Reich on the one hand and our American democracy on the other.

Capone was one of the underworld's most brilliant organizers. Unquestionably, the Al Capone empire was a well-structured "goal-oriented organization." In fact, he organized it in such a way that even his opposition contributed to his organization. Its members were quite dedicated to their goal, and they achieved it successfully. Fortunately, it failed to survive the test of time because its objective was against the public good. Likewise, Hitler's Third Reich was heavily goal oriented and it achieved its objective temporarily. Because it was not based on altruistic principles which foster the public good, it failed to withstand the test of time.

Our great nation was founded by a relatively small group of people highly motivated towards a common cause. They had a unity of purpose, an agreement of objectives towards the basic principle that "all men are created equal." They formed an altruistic goal-oriented society. The development of America as the greatest nation in the world attests to the power or strength of a goal-oriented society. Yet, amid all its strength, our nation strayed from its altruism by allowing the development of slavery, which was an opposite pursuit from its basic doctrines. Because of this, history shows that we have paid the price, from the Civil War to the Selma March, and we shall continue to pay that price until our people refocus their attention on the original altruistic goals the pilgrims incorporated into our Constitution.

Arnold Toynbee has documented the fact that 19 out of 21 civilizations have died from within and not from outside conquest. Something happened to their peoples; they no longer cared. Their demise occurred slowly, quietly, when no one was particularly aware of what was happening. I wonder how many organizations died the same way. I wonder how many pharmaceutical organizations have developed long-range fatal anemia, for a pharmaceutical organization is of no use unless it serves a great cause.

It has been stated that formation of the ASHP was one of the outstanding achievements in the history of American pharmacy. This statement is somewhat misleading for, in itself, formation of the Society was just another accomplishment—another organization. It was the adoption of a philosophy of service by those hospital pharmacists during the twenties and thirties which formed the basis for the development of a goal-oriented Society. Their unifying goal was the adoption of the philosophy that the purpose for the existence of pharmacy is to provide pharmaceutical services as an integral part of the total patient care concept in the interest, safety, and welfare of the public health. This purpose serves a great cause. Their "purpose" was placed above their "interests." Calvin Coolidge eloquently stated the difference between purpose and interest when he said:

No enterprise can exist for itself alone. It ministers to some great need, it performs some great service, not for itself but for others; or failing therein, it ceases to be profitable and ceases to exist.

In reading the early history of the ASHP, one cannot help but feel the verve, the vigor, the dedication, the enthusiasm, the unity of purpose among the membership towards the pursuit of a common goal. This was the force which propelled organized hospital pharmacists to make significant progress. For, as George Santayana so poignantly stated, "What we call the contagious force of an idea is the force of the people who have embraced it." Such is the characteristic of many newly formed organizations.

The question is, however: Does an organization move into history with this initial drive, motivated dedication, and contagious enthusiasm which are so essential to progress; or might it slowly change in character? As the ASHP develops, it may or it may not maintain this force. It may or it may not lose sight of its original goals. It may or it may not respond to the contemporary social forces in such a way as to continue along its chartered path. It may or it may not develop leadership to chart its course clearly through the troubled times ahead. It may or it may not depend on the few to do the job of many. It may or it may not lose its altruism for personal self-interests. It may or it may not develop an overly paternalistic attitude over its members. It may or it may not make the membership subservient to the organizational structure. It may or it may not develop pecuniary interests which can sidetrack its basic mission.

Whether it does these things or not will determine its future survival as an effective organization. Analyze these points to see whether they are, or are not, some vital causes of ineffective, nonproductive organizations similar to some of our pharmaceutical organizations which, at best, are running to catch up to the status quo.

We ought not ask ourselves: "What is the ASHP doing about these essential elements of an effective organization?" Rather, we should ask: "What are we doing about it?" After all, we, the membership, are the ASHP. While authority in the Church stems from God, authority in an organization stems from the membership. The ASHP should not be viewed merely as an organization housed in Washington. The ASHP is really an associative group of professional practitioners who have banded together to assist each other to pursue a common goal in the public interest.

An organization is not an end in itself. Rather, it is an instrument of society and fulfills itself by the contribution it makes to this outside environment. Likewise, the ASHP is an instrument of the membership and fulfills itself by the contribution it makes to society. After all, did we form the ASHP to resist the social changes demanded by our society? To maintain traditional practices which are not in the public interest? To get a few to do the work of many? To use the organizational strength to develop personal self-interests? To develop an organizational structure which makes the membership subservient to it? To elect individuals to represent local or geographical self-interests? To use organizational strength to promote protective legislation? To develop enough organizational prestige to make us aloof of the other essential segments of the profession? No, our Society was not founded on these principles; it never would have survived if it had been.

Yes, the ASHP has made great progesss—its founders left us a rich tradition and everything seems to be going well. But perhaps this is the time, the moment in history, to assess our present position and to determine our future direction. Let us not wait until greater problems develop. I say this because, as I attend meetings and talk with hospital pharmacists around the country, I see some evidence of certain grass-roots attitudes, as well as regional and national attitudes, which could be helpful or detrimental to the Society, depending on what we do with them. Some of these attitudes are, perhaps, a reflection of problems which a growing organization must go through. On the other hand, perhaps they are not.

Some have wondered about the trend in which the ASHP is moving. One cannot say categorically that this trend is good or bad. It is not so much the trends *per se* but subtle changes in the trends which are truly important events. These subtleties are major contributing factors which ultimately determine success or failure of an organization. These subtleties must be perceived; it is difficult to classify or quantify them. It is the responsibility of all of us—and particularly our leaders, our elected officers, and directors—to develop the ability to perceive these subtleties and to refocus the direction of these trends into proper perspective.

Our professional organization must provide a forum whereby all members have an opportunity to participate by contributing their ideas, to develop new concepts, to present their problems and their concerns, to express their views and philosophies about future directions of the profession, to obtain constructive advice and assistance, to develop programs collectively which cannot be accomplished individually, and to be positively responsive to the needs of its members. The organizational structure of a professional society should be fluid enough to flow with the mainstream thought of its members. Its structure should not stymie this mainstream thought. For as Frazier said, "the authority of ideas shall prevail."

If we were to be forthright, and we are, we would admit that we have lost some of that original verve, vigor, and dedication. Perhaps we have developed an organizational structure which has become less responsive to the needs of the membership. Perhaps we are asking the organization to do too many things for us, for this is the easy way out. Maybe we are using the organization to develop self-interests. Are we jockeying for a more prestigious position among other organizations within the profession? Perhaps we are developing unrealistic, grandiose plans, which might be good but which limit our resources to do the job which needs to be done today. We might be developing an organizational system which stifles initiative.

Self-criticism, even at its best, is most difficult. Yet, hospital pharmacy is on record for admission to self-criticism. The Audit of Pharmaceutical Service in Hospitals was an extensive exercise in self-criticism in order to improve our practices. I strongly recommend a similar audit on our national Society, the ASHP, as well as its affiliated chapters.

This "organizational audit" would involve an indepth self-appraisal of goals and objectives, practices and services, membership and staff, membership needs and capabilities, affiliated chapter activities and requirements, and overall strengths and weaknesses. It would identify the good, the bad, the excellent; thus, we could eliminate the bad, improve the good, and polish the excellent. Indeed, such an organizational audit could pave the way for unparalleled achievements within the sphere of organized American pharmacy. For it is the opinion of those outside our profession, not our own good opinion of ourselves, that will determine our status.

We must certainly assess our position in relation to the social forces of our times and to the grassroots attitudes of our members. We must continue to demand of our committees, our officers, our board, and our full-time staff the kind of leadership and motivation which will help attain our goals. As we initiate demands individually or collectively, locally or nationally, let us ask ourselves, "Is this an altruistically motivated program for the improvement of pharmaceutical services to the public, or is this a personal or organizational self-interest-motivated program?"

A solid foundation has been laid for the development of an elite corps of career-minded hospital pharmacists. The founders of our Society, Harvey A. K. Whitney and his colleagues, left us a rich, proud tradition, a dedication towards professional ideals, a challenge to the pursuit of excellence, a strong, effective goal-oriented organization with proven success, and a membership with the intestinal fortitude to submit to organizational self-appraisal for the common good.

With such a background, hospital pharmacy is but one step away from greatness—a mere attitude away from the Jeffersonian dream of an aristocracy of achievement. With a properly directed, goal-oriented Society, let us take that step, let us mold that attitude to achieve that dream, slowly yet methodically, practically yet idealistically, authoritatively yet softly. . . as we move into history.

At the time he received this award, Clifton J. Latiolais was the Director of Pharmacy at University Hospitals and an Associate Professor of Pharmacy at the College of Pharmacy, The Ohio State University, Columbus.

1969

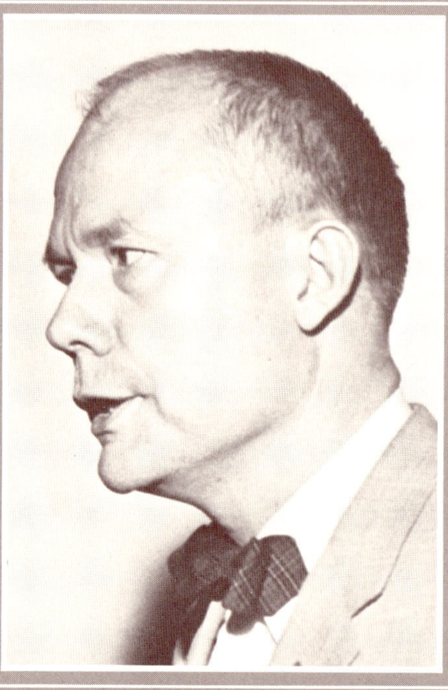

LEO F. GODLEY

"I would like to see practitioners who have been taught by other practitioners."

FORM AND SUBSTANCE

At the outset, I would like to declare myself a part of the establishment. I am a product of it. I helped to build it. I function in it, to some degree, on almost every level: I count, I pour, I teach, I consult, I study, I edit, I administer, I assay, I research, I inform, I gripe a lot, I praise a little, but, most of all, I administer.

And since I am a member, a product, and an architect of the establishment, I have the right to criticize and to suggest—and I criticize and suggest with pride because I love the establishment. I sometimes annoy myself and wish I were more like my administrator who always warns us that we should do something nice for somebody every day, even if it means leaving them alone. Consequently, I feel compelled tonight to comment on some areas of the establishment that concern me a great deal. How could I have deserved such an audience? Surely, from this pinnacle on which I tremble tonight, exquisitely conscious that I share it with those who have touched the "Golden Fleece" of accomplishment and possessed of this heady euphoria and this pounding heart that seem to be all mine, I am sensitive to these things because they are your concerns also.

Every now and again, I read that a colleague speaks of the "over-education" that the pharmacist must buy in the five-year curriculum; and the general trend of the reasoning usually concludes that to put the profession back on an even keel, we need to return to the four-year plan.

Now, this may be all right, but the arguments that I have heard don't appeal to me. I think we need some serious and honest thinking on education. And I am not certain that my idea of how the pharmacist should be educated is possible, at least not without some heroic shifting of long-established concepts and values.

Very simply, I would like to see practitioners who have been taught by other practitioners wherever possible; and further, I would like to see this practitioner in a working environment where his associates on the same staff are, generally, his equal in education and outlook.

I get so depressed at seeing the graduate with the fine mind—top man in the class, or very nearly—who loses the interest, initiative, and ability to apply the service of professional politeness to the dispensed product. I guess the product itself, or the volume of it, has loomed so big and bewildering that the "priceless ingredient" is dwarfed, consciously at first, because it is hard to come by. Then, as hundreds of product dispensings go through the practitioner's hands, the necessity to know no more than a token of information about it becomes easy to accept. This elusive "priceless ingredient"—now called "clinical involvement" because it embraces, as it should, the whole transaction: the pharmacist, the product, and the patient—becomes lost in a miasma of social graces and pseudoprofessional scramble.

This kind of outcome is unfortunate; and if that's the way it has to be, I guess it doesn't matter if we have only a four-year curriculum. But the five- or six-year man has a little more maturity and, hopefully, his decline into professional ugliness would become more painful.

So what does all of this mean? Does the pharmacist decline in professional integrity because he has too much to do, or because the job is not professionally interesting, or because he wasn't educated in the most effective way, with the most effective curriculum, by the most effective instructors?

The truth of the matter is that it's probably a combination of all of these forces. Let's consider some of these things and superimpose them on the so-called "changing image" of the pharmacist. I suppose I need to speak primarily of the institutional pharmacist because that's what I am and that, also, is what Mr. Whitney was.

So we have a new image—or we hope we have in this strange wonderful trivalent combination of pharmacist–product–patient. Image is important if it's good. It makes us happier and healthier; and if we're happier and healthier, we should be wealthier; and if we're wealthier, we can buy a new image. So what will it be next? Are we going to be physicians? I don't quite know, but I do have some ideas about what we need now.

Benjamin Franklin said, "By failing to prepare we are preparing to fail." And a few weeks ago the president of my alma mater said: "We never learn anything from people who agree with us. It is in the act of conflict-of-ideas that learning takes place, and this we must not forget."

If we apply these philosophies to education and get the curriculum really cleaned up, I think we will have achieved a giant step. It needed cleaning up in 1939, and now, 30 years later, it still needs cleaning, and of many of the same things. Cannot educators and clinicians and industrialists get together? Shouldn't clinicians be involved in education in a meaningful way? If the clinician isn't qualified to educate, neither is the educator for very obvious kettle and pot reasons. I say that in the direct application of the professional curriculum, the educator and the clinician must often be one and the same. As long as the clinician remains a "cut below" the instructor, neither can support, in deed and word, the mandate of the profession. Ironically, the educator cannot advance himself until the practitioner is advanced.

There is still the old duplication in chemistry, and calculations, and pharmacognosy, and operations, in the professional school and in the school of arts and sciences. We must have the preclinical sciences at least as advanced as the physician, and these must include human anatomy, human physiology, human pathology, and therapeutics. These disciplines must be a part of the professional degree—not graduate study.

These are the curriculum changes the practitioner needs for responsibility and respectability today, not tomorrow. I have thought about it a great deal—so much, in fact, that I might call myself an authority on curriculum "thinking."

I cannot appreciate the graduate programs in hospital pharmacy where this preclinical background hasn't been satisfied and such ancillary niceties as data processing and personnel management and the like are piled on top of this inadequacy.

The clinician can "pick up" these ancillary disciplines "on the job." It's not quite so easy to study anatomy and pathology on the job when he needs them to perform in a clinical climate.

I know that this kind of curriculum treatment is coming out of some few colleges even now; but there are many areas yet that have not reacted to the demonstrated need of the practitioner with clinical responsibility.

Also of great importance to the practitioner is the ability to use and appreciate the periodical literature. I am appalled at the inexperience in this area of most graduates who come through my practice. It should be a graduation requirement that at least two subjects be researched, in depth, in the library, with reports properly prepared and presented; and every professional course should require regular periodical literature assignments. It is unfortunate when this skill has to be acquired after graduation, for this is very difficult, especially if the graduate skips a residency and goes directly into professional practice. Often it's a thing that the practitioner never has time to acquire, mainly, I think, because he hasn't been schooled to appreciate this need in his practice.

Another important point on education that bothers me a great deal is that, to my knowledge, the professional curriculum of most schools does not provide instruction in the dispensing of sterile prescriptions. We were taught how to count and pour, but the preparation of prescriptions for our sickest patients must be learned on the job or taught by the nurse. Most pharmacists are ashamed, and appropriately so, to tell the nurse that they don't know how to compound an injectable prescription.

I would like to mention a disturbing kind of situation that we seem to perpetuate among hospital pharmacists—the relegation of the staff practitioner to some kind of second-rate status. The real glory boys in our ranks are the administrators, the drug information pharmacists, the educators, and even the purchasers. I know that we stress the status symbol of being a chief too much, for it seems that the holder of a residency certificate considers himself something of a failure if he isn't able to find a director's job at graduation time.

Yesterday's staff pharmacists must be today's clinical pharmacists. The specialty activities generated by specialty pharmacists on a pharmacy staff should, in my opinion, be directed through the staff practitioner to the patient, the nurse, and the physician. These staff pharmacists must represent the best blood in the profession—not men who couldn't quite make it in administration, or the assay laboratory, or the library—but practitioners who are specialists in clinical practice!

I must not forget that I cannot dignify my own office until I dignify the practitioners on my staff as clinical specialists. These practitioners must be competent in the library and the clinical laboratory; they must school their personalities into a compatible and acceptable pattern, for the ability to relate to other people and the possession of professional competency are equal criteria for patient care.

I would like to talk now about some ideas and impressions that I have on clinical experience. As I discuss with my colleagues over the country the evolving concept of clinical practice, I note the great awareness of the excitingly gratifying experiences of administering pharmacy services on the patient areas. It is very obvious that the pharmacist's "in vitro" knowledge has become functional in its "in vivo" fulfillment.

Pharmacists in clinical areas are applying their services now, on a consultative basis, in regular visits to patients with the physician or the nurse, to discuss and suggest in matters relating to the drug therapy programming. Pharmacists answer emergency calls to the bedside along with other professionals. Pharmacists are performing patient interviews for drug history information, as well as correlating the biochemistry of the patient's therapeutic program with laboratory and other diagnostic procedures that the physician has ordered for the patient. And while these relatively new thoughts and ideas and procedures are emanating more frequently from teaching medical centers, they very surely and certainly are being studied and practiced in community and government institutions as pharmacy clinicians learn to extend the humanness of their art.

As I mentioned earlier, in talking about these trends with other practitioners in other hospitals as well as in my own beginning experiences, I notice that the pharmacist very quickly relates his disadvantage in the doctor–nurse confrontation on the nursing areas to his bedside inexperience. I think we have demonstrated that this experience cannot be effectively achieved by "observing and visiting." Comfort at the bedside appears to come gracefully to those who have been deliberately taught patient care responsibility.

We are thinking very seriously of introducing an exercise into our residency program in which the pharmacist will be taught this patient care responsibility. Our thinking now is that the pharmacist will be assigned to a specially selected nurse. This nurse must be in sympathetic agreement with the pharmacist's educational need; and the pharmacist will work with this clinical nursing practitioner during her shift of duty—40 hours a week—caring for her assignment of patients.

The plan is that the pharmacist will give medications, including injections and suppositories. He will apply the treatments and administer the tender love and care under the direction of this clinical preceptor. This patient assignment will include 10 or 12 patients, and the pharmacist will be concerned with this same group of patients from admission to dismissal. During his experience of administering treatments and medicines and care, he will also be observing patient responses to drugs and how these responses are affected in a variety of physiological systems by a myriad of pathological, psychological, and environmental parameters.

The pharmacist will be required to carry out the patient care procedures alone when his instructor considers him competent, and he will have ample opportunity to discuss his patients with the nurse and the attending physician. As each of his patients is dismissed, the pharmacist will be required to document his experience with the patient, the nurse, and the physician. This documentation will include a detailed discussion and rationalization of the therapeutic and treatment programming. We think these exercises will demonstrate the value of this experience to the pharmacist in his clinical function.

At our hospital, nursing care is administered on the "total care" plan. Each staff nurse is given a patient assignment, and she manages the entire spectrum of care of the patients assigned to her. We feel this approach to patient management is especially compatible with the educational need of the pharmacist.

We think that six weeks of this concentrated experience in exploring the mystery of patient care will give our pharmacy residents the kind of maturity that they need to function effectively as pharmacists on patient areas in the hospital. We have no interest or desire to create a nurse-pharmacist. We simply feel that it is our responsibility to give the pharmacist an experience base for his comfortable and effective function with the nurse and the physician at the bedside. If we can increase the pharmacist's usefulness and confidence in an association in which he belongs, we will have achieved our need. We have not effectively satisfied this need in the past by putting the pharmacist through patient area observation exercises.

When I look at the prospectus of this program and realize what I project into it, it seems unforgivable that we have overlooked this approach to establishing clinical sensitivity in our practitioners.

If our clinical image is important for our productive professional future, an integrated compulsory performance at the bedside will give maturity and substance to an image that often, now, has only shadow or form.

Surely then, with an appropriate curriculum administered wherever possible by practitioners, with an effective residency strengthened with clinical experience, and with an adequate laboratory in which to serve mankind, we can feel the stir in the "womb of time" of a progeny of practitioners with purpose, compassion, and humility. And I say to you that the greatest of these things are purpose, compassion, and humility.

At the time he received this award, Leo F. Godley was the Director of the Department of Pharmacy and Central Sterile Supply at Harris Hospital, Fort Worth, Texas.

1970

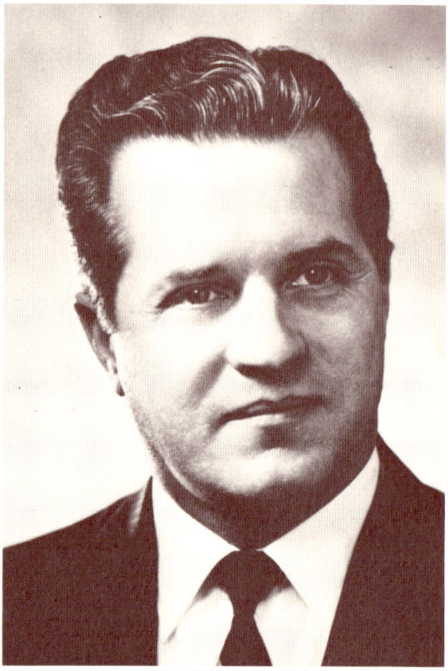

JOSEPH A. ODDIS

"To strive continually for commitment and involvement is essential in our pursuit of excellence."

COMMITMENT AND INVOLVEMENT

If the decade of the sixties is to go down in history for its positive accomplishments—in spite of such blots as violence in our streets and the assassinations of three great Americans—the resounding voice and influence of the consumer is one notable observation. We, as citizens and consumers, have finally come out of our shell of complacency. We are demanding quality and safety in all aspects of our life, and our government must not fail to respond to our cry. Americans are demanding quality and safety in our air and water, in our household appliances, in our President's nominees to the Supreme Court of the United States, in our drugs, in our total health care. This quest for excellence has affected all professions, business enterprises, and organizations which collectively comprise American society—from giant corporations which manufacture automobiles or drugs that are sometimes less than safe, to professionals who provide health care which is often less than optimum.

In this new era of consumerism, it is easy to strike wildly. The hippie philosophy appears to be that nothing is worth saving, that it is better to destroy our social structure completely and start again from scratch. This element is adept at identifying what is wrong but almost totally inept at offering remedies. Despite the problems and injustices in our contemporary society, I believe there is much good that needs to be preserved. As responsible citizens and professionals, we need to retain what is good in all aspects of our lives, including the delivery of health care and the practice of pharmacy, and rebuild only what is bad. This constructive approach must not be allowed to give way to destruction of our very principles and foundations.

Among the many problems of contemporary America—problems that require immediate attention through a constructive approach—is that of providing adequate health care. Our health resources are being strained beyond their limit. Among the factors exerting pressure on our health resources are population growth, the changing age structure of the population, better education, urbanization, and the long overdue realization that good health care is a right of all citizens, including the poor and the aged. Still, perhaps more progress has been made in the health sciences in the past decade than during the entire half-century preceding it. This progress, in large measure, can be attributed to the increased willingness and obligation of our government of the people to respond to the health care needs of all citizens. We are in the midst of a new era of the consumer, and his bill of rights is irrevocable. There is no turning back.

Along with government, health practitioners and, through them, their associations and organizations deserve credit for their role in improving the quality, scope, and availability of health care. Unfortunately, some have lagged behind and have only adjusted their blinders in a futile attempt to preserve the status quo. Among organizations in the health field, our own American Pharmaceutical Association and American Society of Hospital Pharmacists need not take a back seat to any in terms of aggressiveness, progressiveness, and social as well as professional commitment.

I believe we are well prepared for the decade ahead. Early in this decade, it will be necessary for this nation to enunciate a basic policy of health goals at all levels and to delineate the mechanisms which will be required to support this policy. Pharmacy must participate, and it must do so with the realization that no single element of the profession nor, indeed, any single member of the profession has a monopoly on ideas. Working together, I am confident that we can demonstrate the commitment and involvement that will be required. In participating in the development of a policy for health care, pharmacy must make a place for its students and its youth; they have amply demonstrated that they have the commitment, but we must now provide more opportunity for meaningful involvement.

In considering some of the possible causes and effects of a national health policy, one observation stands out. Despite the continuing need for total, integrated delivery of health care, such care will be largely institution based—not necessarily within four walls but emanating from behind the walls and extending into the community. Further, it is already evident that total health care is shifting towards large institutions, and this pattern will probably continue for reasons of efficiency and economy. The small hospital, despite its importance and continued need, will care for proportionately fewer and fewer patients as a system continues to develop. One social force that is accelerating the trend towards institution-based health care is the migration of the independent, solo health practitioner, along with his affluent patients, to suburbia, leaving the inner city and rural America deficient in the availability of health care services. This deficiency will never be solved on a solo practice basis—some form of institutional or group practice is the only answer. In short, health care will revolve more and more around the institutional setting regardless of the number of pharmacists who will be considered institutional practitioners as opposed to community practitioners.

Other observations with specific reference to pharmacy will influence our national health policy:

1. In his attempt to restrain the spiraling costs of quality health care, the consumer, through our federal government which has repeatedly examined practices of the pharmaceutical industry, will focus more and more attention on archaic methods of dispensing prescription drugs to patients. The big question is whether pharmacists will meet the challenge or whether the consumer, through his government, will force the issue.
2. Related to this, it is widely accepted that many of the routine, traditional dispensing and administrative functions performed by pharmacists can be performed more efficiently, more economically, and more safely by machines or technicians. Thus, by judicious use of automation and technicians, under the control and supervision of pharmacists, pharmacists will continue to expand their professional responsibilities in the area of drug information, clinical practice, and other emerging functions. More and more supportive personnel will be employed in hospital pharmacies. Not only will technicians dispense, manufacture, and package, but other professionals—chemists, systems experts, business managers, and others—will find a place in the hospital pharmacy of the future, particularly as total health care continues to shift to larger institutions. The hospital pharmacist will serve as scientist-administrator-director rather than dispenser.
3. By teaching students about drugs in real life, i.e., in the hospital, schools of pharmacy will educate every student so that he will be able to practice in any environment he chooses. This means that all schools will have a clinical facility as a laboratory and a clinical faculty composed primarily of experienced hospital pharmacists. The professional Doctor of Pharmacy degree will be standard for those who plan to become practitioners.
4. Externship or internship for pharmacy students will either become unnecessary in this clinical environment or, if it is retained, it will be fulfilled primarily in the hospital. Licensure will be based on a stringent standardized national examination which will enable the graduate to practice his profession anywhere in the United States.
5. As pharmacy continues to shift emphasis to the patient as well as the product and as the body of knowledge of the physician becomes increasingly specialized, the pharmacist will be accepted as the drug expert on the health team and he will exert a profound influence on the prescribing of drugs, particularly in hospitals. This will happen in spite of parochial interests and the reluctance of some health professionals to change the status quo.

6. As the consumer continues to insist that the government increases its regulatory powers and as the effects of formulation of drug products on their efficacy become better understood, differences among brands of a drug will become a minor consideration in the future practice of medicine and pharmacy. The physician, pharmacist, and patient will have reasonably complete assurance that any drug product available for use will perform in the expected manner and with brand-to-brand consistency of effectiveness. Thus, the pharmacist will become less concerned about *whose* drug product will be used and more concerned about *which* drug the patient needs. This reinforces the belief that he will markedly influence prescribing habits.

It is abundantly clear that the practice of pharmacy must better adapt to contemporary needs. Pharmacy, individually and collectively, must rise to the occasion, and organized pharmacy must lead the way. In light of the developments taking place around us, some basic questions require answers:

Can a coordinated organizational system for American pharmacy evolve which has as its basic objective the interest of the public in matters relating to clinical pharmacy and drug use control?

Can this coordinated organizational system be so designed as to be truly representative of, and responsive to, practitioners in different settings who perform a variety of specialized functions?

Is it possible that there should be more emphasis on unity of purpose and cooperative organization—on unison as well as on "one voice" for pharmacy?

Past Whitney recipient Latiolais, in his lecture two years ago, called for an "organizational audit" of the ASHP and its affiliated chapters. Such an audit, he stated, "would involve an indepth self-appraisal of goals and objectives, practices and services, membership and staff, membership needs and capabilities, affiliated chapter activities and requirements, and overall strengths and weaknesses." Mr. Latiolais continued: "Indeed, such an organizational audit could pave the way for unparalleled achievement within the sphere of organized American pharmacy." I concur that an organizational audit is called for. Further, I believe that such an audit should be applied to organized American pharmacy as a whole.

In an editorial in the July 1962 issue of the *American Journal of Hospital Pharmacy* entitled "The American Hospital Pharmacy Movement—Episode or Event?", Dr. Don E. Francke stated:

A movement is a connected and long series of events leading toward a goal. In contrast, an episode happens and comes to an end; it is an independent action that stands alone. A review of the records shows that the hospital pharmacy movement is a series of interrelated, planned events which continuously generates new events.

Dr. Francke then continued by separating the events of the American hospital pharmacy movement into four rather distinct phases. A decade has passed since the beginning of the fourth phase. In view of the developments and influences we have pondered, perhaps it can be said that we are now entering the fifth phase of the American hospital pharmacy movement, a phase which may be identified with the new challenges which face us. Throughout all phases, we have witnessed a commitment and involvement on the part of members of the American Society of Hospital Pharmacists unparalleled in the history of the profession. Today, more than ever before, we are being asked to dedicate ourselves to a life of commitment to and involvement in the things that face us daily in our homes, our profession, our government, and in a host of activities relating to our existence on earth.

To strive continually for commitment and involvement is essential in our pursuit of excellence. But in this pursuit, we must keep in mind always the warning of John W. Gardner who, as President of the Carnegie Foundation, wrote:

A society that has reached the heights of excellence may already be caught in the rigidities that will bring it down. An institution may hold itself to the highest standards and yet already be entombed in the complacency that will eventually spell its decline.

This is a danger to which we must ever be alert.

And so, as we enter the decade of the seventies, almost three decades removed from the founding of the Society and two decades since the establishment of the Harvey A. K. Whitney Lecture Award, we are challenged with a resolve for greater commitment and involvement not in terms of self-interest but, in a larger and more meaningful sense, in terms of public welfare.

The Society can be thankful for its achievements in a brief span of 28 years. These achievements can be attributed to a number of factors. We have been successful because of our involvement in professional activities both at the national and local levels. We have been successful through constructive confrontation by facing issues when they have been clearly identified and a reasonable and rational course of action has been outlined. We have been successful because we have established realistic goals and objectives and have worked to achieve them. We have been successful because of our receptive attitude to change in the public interest. We have been successful because we know the value of introspection—of constantly looking at ourselves and our Society to ensure that our programs and objectives are sound and in keeping with contemporary needs. Finally, we have been successful because we have been unafraid of hard work and are willing to give without waiting to receive.

All of this can be summarized succinctly, I believe, by a quote from the Society's *Statement on Goals for Hospital Pharmacy*:

> *History shows that groups which unite with a purpose, which give a selfless service for the greater good, which make plans and keep driving forward, which set immediate objectives yet maintain a degree of flexibility, which prepare themselves for the future—are those which make tremendous progress.*

At the time he received this award, Joseph A. Oddis was the Executive Secretary of the American Society of Hospital Pharmacists, Washington, D.C.

1971

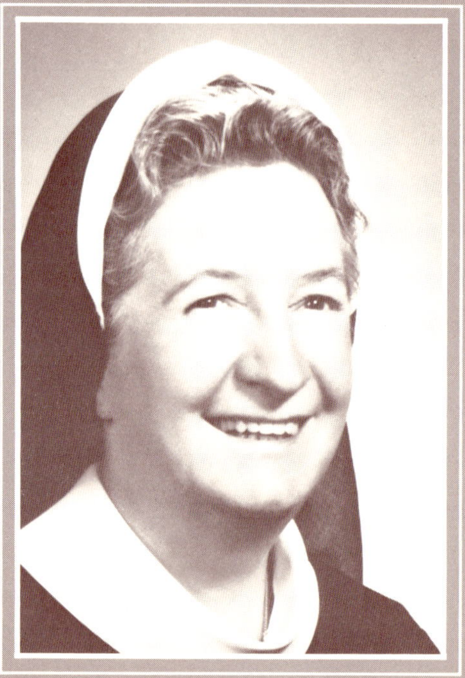

SISTER M. GONZALES

"Patient contact. . . .reveals an added dimension to our previously established services."

AN ADDED DIMENSION

It is the best of times, it is the worst of times, it is the age of wisdom, it is the age of foolishness, it is the epoch of belief, it is the epoch of incredibility, it is the season of Light, it is the season of Darkness, it is the spring of hope, it is the winter of despair, we have everything before us, we have nothing before us.

So wrote Charles Dickens in 1859 in the opening paragraph of his immortal classic *A Tale of Two Cities.* These words can appropriately be applied to the present state of pharmacy and, particularly, pharmacy as it is practiced in hospitals today. Only we, the practitioners, can assure by our personal contributions that positive statements from the above quotation become reality. We have within our reach. . . the best of times. . . the age of wisdom. . . the spring of hope.

Today, one major concern is the patient–pharmacist relationship. We are moving from a service of things to a service of people, service to and with others—the patient, nurse, physician, as well as specialized services to our fellow pharmacists. Sufficient studies have now demonstrated what should long have been an obvious fact—many pharmacists have been overeducated to do "count and pour" jobs. Admittedly, "count and pour" is an oversimplification of the traditional pharmacy service, but we have been educated to do more. And that "more" is a service that is needed! Our experiences with drug information services demonstrated also that it was not enough for us to sit and wait for the physician to ask us questions. Somehow, we had to find a way to be on hand to assist and offer information before we were asked to do so. Incorporating the pharmacist into the team in a more realistic way seemed to be the answer.

The evolution from the "pharmacist-in-the-pharmacy" to the "pharmacist-in-the-patient-care areas" has been a torturous one. Full potential is far from being achieved, but we are working on it; and almost each day, new doors are opened as this concept grows and the needs we fulfill are recognized. Another example of this challenging aspect of pharmacy is seen when a pharmacist interviews the patient.

Let me briefly describe what I envision comprises a patient interview, because it is this type of patient contact that reveals *an added dimension* to our previously established services. We have what is called the initial interview, at which time the pharmacist chats with the patient in an effort to learn as much as he can about the patient's medication regimen and habits.

This first contact with the patient is used to obtain as much detailed information as possible concerning the patient's use of prescription and nonprescription medications. The interview often uncovers situations which are clinically important to the patient and to his physician such as the patient who is not taking his medication as prescribed, or the patient who has simply stopped taking prescribed medications, or the patient who has experienced allergic or adverse effects. Occasionally, we find that the reason the patient is in the hospital is drug related.

The information obtained in the interview must be communicated to the patient's physician. This is done in a variety of ways, perhaps the most effective being the documentation of the medication history in the patient's chart as a permanent part of his record.

Interim visits with the patient throughout his hospital stay offer us the opportunity to participate in the assessment of the patient's response to therapy. It also provides the patient with one more indication that "this hospital is concerned about me!"

Discharge interviews are of considerable value to many patients. The likelihood that a patient will follow his prescribed regimen is directly proportional to his understanding of the purpose of the therapy. For many patients, this is a paramount consideration. It presents a challenge to the pharmacist to discuss and explain the therapy in terms the patient can understand and to give a reasonable and balanced discussion of potential side effects to which the patient should be alerted.

Frightening things emerge when a patient "tells all" to a pharmacist. And how can we expect our patients to know that some of the nonprescription medications they have been taking could alter their wellbeing? The lay person today learns his pharmacology from the television commercials and his physiology in the pages of *Readers' Digest.* And these popular founts of wisdom seldom relate the side effects of the miracles they promote. Further, the often harried physician is not geared to indepth exploring of his patient's medication sprees. Yet, somehow, the patient willingly relates to a pharmacist a detailed history of all of the medicine he has been taking. And haven't we all had nurses present us with brown paper bags of drugs that patients have brought with them to the hospital?

So it is a new era, and understandably so. Medication regimens resulting from potent, often specific, drugs are complex. And the patient-oriented pharmacist cooperating with a pharmacist-conscious physician or nurse can together achieve a high level of service. As we study this type of service, it seems we have been a missing factor for too long—or may I use an already overused phrase and say: the hospital pharmacist was needed to "put it all together."

To prepare our pharmacist to serve in this new role, all manner of changes have been made. Universities have established new departments; schedules have been rearranged to permit students to work in clinics, to make patient medication rounds, and to attend grand medical conferences. The recent literature is replete with examples of what I am saying. However, there would seem to be one area about all of this that is slighted and about which much more needs to be said—the importance of the *manner* in which pharmacists approach the ill patient. Do we detect a dangerous gap here? Not all of us are equally equipped to daily confront the ill, any more than all physicians are so blessed. It takes a certain type of individual to effectively work with sick people. Some are gifted with personalities that lend well to daily contact with the sick, others we must train. And we would be unrealistic if we said all pharmacists can, or even desire to, serve in this capacity.

We are in a period of great medical achievement—a time in which much medical gadgetry is used. Many practice in the impressive, stainless steel and glass glare of the modern hospital. But, unfortunately, on close inspection it would seem that in these monoliths of modern medical madness, everything and everybody come before the patient. In following my trend of thought here this evening, I would not have you think I am in any way degrading these spectacular, computerized, scientific advances that we now have for our use. I am not!

What I am saying is let us take all that is good today and yet not dehumanize the patient. The emotional side of the sick must never be overlooked. I personally wanted to use this forum this evening to focus on this aspect of hospital pharmacy service. We hospital pharmacists have within our grasp a powerful means of helping to mend this gap in today's hospitals and health programs. It could be our timely contributions to add to—not subtract from—the care of the sick patient just by our manner of approach and our personal philosophy of the uniqueness of each patient. Would that we will grow daily in this specialty of helping the sick, but remember—we must always help them one by one!

Health-maintenance organization programs dominate the political scene today. Such political crusading can only result in a greater number of health programs and increased numbers of people applying for health care. Our national leaders are well advised to give to these health plans their most careful attention. In our own situation, three primary care stations and a Care-mobile that operates from Mercy Hospital in Pittsburgh have revealed alarming statistics of a large population of chronically and acutely ill people who have never had any medical treatment or ever been seen by a physician—this in a midtown ghetto that is surrounded by six large hospitals. Our health care systems are demanding to be revised. But, here again, the patient can easily be only one more statistic in such systems and personal, individual care can be overlooked.

President Nixon recently made a revealing remark that was reported in the *U.S. News & World Report* of January 11, 1971. He had just been given a clean bill of health after his annual physical checkup. Mr. Nixon said, "I've seldom been sick in my life. But I know the main thing that patients need is not for someone to talk about their illness but to have someone smile at them." With a President that thinks like this, perhaps there is hope that in the legislating of new health programs, there will be heart as well as help.

Physician-teachers from Hippocrates to Osler have lengthy writings on the importance of good physician–patient contacts. Osler has said somewhere, and I will paraphrase him to make it apply to pharmacists, that "no matter how vast is your knowledge of pharmacology or how experienced you may be in recognizing the drug–laboratory test interferences or the drug–drug interactions, it is of little value if you do not approach the patient with real concern and interest. If a patient senses your haste or your impatience with his rambling accounts, you will leave him depressed, rejected, and you will have done nothing to his mental attitude which is so important to the healing process." I hope Osler forgives the liberties I have taken with his words, but all of his writings, as well as those of many of his present-day counterparts, stress the invaluable contributions that can be made by a warmhearted attitude towards patients.

So it is just because of our increased contact with patients, physicians, and nurses—but mostly patients—that we need to rethink the importance of our personal contributions. We are no longer handling bottles and things but people. And people, not things, engender problems; people need help, appreciate care, and recognize love. Yes, love at its purest and most unselfish, most precious best. And love is something more than a word surrounded by flowers painted on the side of a Volkswagen bus. The opposite of love, you know, is not hate but indifference. And no one can inflict a greater hurt than an indifferent, thoughtless person. The ill patient, alone for many hours, uncertain of the outcome of his illness, is a prey to indifference the likes of which a busy, healthy individual would not notice.

Not only does the individual sick person view his world differently from the healthy, but there are numerous factors that influence him other than his illness. The young and not-so-young can profit by an occasional meditation on the trauma produced by illness. Illness causes fears, frustrations, and impatience in most. Pain elicits a variety of reactions often determined by the patient's cultural or ethnic background. The transition from health to a recognized, accepted illness is bound to be a period of anxiety and apprehension. An educated, successful businessman's reaction is often similar to that of a newly caged lion, while the grandmotherly little lady may use her illness to attract all the attention and pity she can capture. Her moanings and groanings are often (not always) a means of milking every drop of sympathy she can get from relatives and strangers alike. It is to complex, emotionally distraught individuals such as these that we are sending our pharmacists. Have we honestly prepared them adequately for this pivotal role?

It would seem that hospital pharmacy and hospital pharmacists experience a recurring cycle of metamorphosis. At our first seminars and early conventions, the live topic was bulk compounding and we went home feeling richer if we had gathered some new formulas. Later we were euphoric with success when we had compiled our first hospital formulary. Then came the hassle of generic dispensing and proper labeling with the proven necessity of having good controls and control numbers. And remember when having a walk-in refrigerator was a mark of prestige? Honestly, I may not have fallen into this temptation to reminisce if the familiar faces of long-time friends were not in front of me. But I think we do admit that although the Pharmacy and Therapeutics Committee brought us closer to physicians, and inservice nursing programs as well as teaching pharmacology in schools of nursing opened doors in the nursing field, we still had, for the most part, only over-the-counter contact with our patients, usually on an outpatient basis.

To function as an integral part of the health team, to daily meet and talk with the ill, is a new challenge for us in these years of the shaking seventies! A challenge we need to acknowledge, define, meet, and accept.

There are some in our modern society who claim we live in an age of insensitivity. Perhaps we do, but I hope not. There should be no taboo on tenderness. It was Hippocrates who cautioned that our first rule should be "do no harm"; Dr. Francis Peabody simply says, "The secret of patient care is caring for the patient." Bishop Fulton J. Sheen amusingly reminds us that the best medical men should be equipped with a topnotch education, a sense of humor, and an incision! Of all the various aspects of our service in the past, perhaps our present trend to supply this most important link between patient and physician needs our best efforts and most cautious acceptance. If this is what we call clinical pharmacy, it is also a scientific art and a humanistic science. The art and science must be intermingled, symbiotic, and inseparable. Without the art, the skills, and the tenderness, there can be no data for the physician and only trauma to a patient. Without the science, there can be no reason for the art.

I had only one goal this evening and that was to call your attention to this new facet in the practice of pharmacy today. I hope I have done just that. And if I may be permitted to close with a prayer, I would have that prayer be this:

May we be mindful of the fact that our Creator, who has placed us here on earth to do a work, touches the world mainly through the ministration of human services. We labor in an atmosphere where frequently good must battle evil, where some must suffer and die. May it be our happy task to ease the ways of all those for whom we care. May we be brought to the realization that true happiness is found in the knowledge that a job assigned to us here and at this point in time has been a job well done.

At the time she received this award, Sister M. Gonzales, R.S.M., was the Director of Pharmacy and Central Service at Mercy Hospital, Pittsburgh, Pennsylvania.

1972

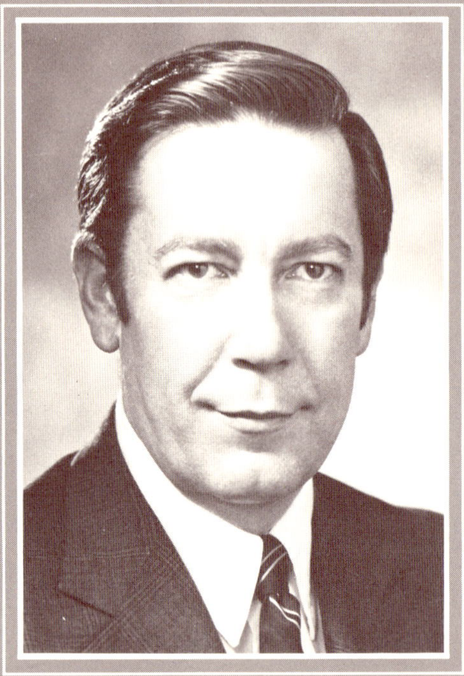

WILLIAM M. HELLER

"It is only on maturing that most of us realize that we can contribute more."

ON MATURING

On Maturing. Isn't that an impressive title for a talk! Doesn't it sound profound? I hoped it would. But actually it's an idiot title, picked at a time when I didn't know what I wanted to talk about, picked as so nonindicative that I could develop any number of subjects and wiggle them around to fit.

For instance, it is only on maturing that most of us realize that we can contribute more and even carry our own pet ideas further if we have a good team, help our teammates join their ideas to ours, and then give them the freedom and wherewithal and finally the credit due them in pursuing those ideas with far more talent and time than we have at our own command. The satisfaction that we know as youngsters when we accomplish some new thing for the first time gives way, on maturing, to a greater joy in seeing the team win a big one, with individual members fulfilling their functions far more expertly than we could ever hope to.

I've been a lucky fellow all my career because of the teammates I've had, and I accept this Award tonight only as a token of recognition to them.

When I started at Arkansas in 1955, I was the one and only pharmacist in a one-room pharmacy that served a 200-bed hospital with 60,000 outpatient visits per year—and didn't even have a typewriter or a file of yesterday's prescriptions. Into that mess came Louise Pope, who had learned from Leo Godley what a hospital pharmacy could do. Harold Hamilton joined us and, with his experience in retail pharmacy, started a teaching program that students recognized was relevant. Carl Brooks integrated our staff before Little Rock became a worldwide symbol.

A fellow named George Provost called from Watertown, New York, and was persuaded that Arkansas was indeed the Land of Opportunity, as the state slogan went. It didn't seem like that a couple years later when a big budget cut knocked off one-third of the beds in our new hospital. But just at that time a little sideline operation we had been working on for the ASHP was put on the market, and we suddenly realized that the *American Hospital Formulary Service* was going to need a full-time writer if we were going to keep it up to date as promised. We let George do it.

Not being too proud to take Yankee money in the absence of any prospects at home, we submitted a grant proposal to NIH to do a unit dose dispensing demonstration project. This was turned down in 1959. On my innocent inquiry as to why such an obviously good idea was rejected, I received a detailed explanation that was incomprehensible to me. With this rejection slip in hand, I met a big fellow who was finishing his residency at Florida under Warren McConnell. He was the first hospital pharmacist I'd known who had taken graduate work in the social sciences with the intention of making a career in research. His name was Ken Barker, and he interpreted that rejection slip for me. Said my proposal had been turned down for every reason in the social science research books except bad grammar and the idea itself.

Now Ken had listed himself in the ASHP's Personnel Placement Service as being willing to go anywhere except the South (which the Placement Service stated positively as a willingness to work in the North, East, or West), so I told him Arkansas was really the Southwest, just like Texas, and besides where else would anyone let him investigate medication errors and take drugs off the nursing units and supply only single doses. So he decided discretion was the better part of geography and took over a budget slot we had called Pharmacist in Charge of Central Sterile Supply and Infant Formula Room. Some two years and $80,000 worth of altered payroll slots, scrounged supplies, and unpaid overtime later, Ken had not one but two significant grants: one from the Hartford Foundation for a full-scale study of medication errors in a nonuniversity hospital and the second a Public Health Service grant for an experimental hospital medication system featuring automated data-processing control of medication orders and unit dose dispensing. These studies formed the scientific basis, I believe, for the sweeping changes in hospital medication systems and pharmacy practice of the last few years.

I shall ever be grateful to Arkansas for the opportunity we had there. At other universities, top faculty members would have been already immersed in their own research and not available to join the multidisciplinary research team that Ken put together. And few hospitals would be willing to suffer the disruption of having all its medical, surgical, and pediatric beds shifted to an experimental medication system where observers were popping in and out or constantly trailing people around, Teletypes clacked away in the still of the night as well as the pandemonium of the day, and a 10,000-square-foot pharmacy was created by relocating several entire departments in a domino-like effect that ended up with the dean of medicine giving up the only classroom he had in the hospital.

Unfortunately, Arkansas couldn't afford to maintain the new system after the experiment ended, and the 27 pharmacists we had there at one time scattered to the four winds. The hospital administrator left; the directress of nursing left; the project director left; I left; but Bert Kossler, who had joined us as our primary medication administration observer, stayed on and became chief pharmacist.

I ended up on the ASHP staff. So did George Downs, and May Douglas, and Ray Jang, and Brenda Martinez (which meant that Domingo was close by); and if we counted George Provost as an Arkansas alumnus, we were about even with the Duquesne crowd on the staff. This was a delightful two years. To a hospital pharmacist, accustomed to contesting for financial and territorial rights with the many other professions and vocations required to operate a modern hospital, it was a real pleasure to work where the entire staff shares a common background and works towards common goals.

Joe Oddis never did replace me when I left the staff. I was hesitant to ask him whether it was because I was irreplaceable or expendable—I rather suspected the latter since Mary Jo Reilly was doing a masterful job with the *Formulary Service*, May Douglas was all wrapped up in *DPIF* tape, and, early on, Dwight Tousignaut had been hornswoggled into taking on the editorship of *International Pharmaceutical Abstracts*.

Well, I've dropped names all over the place and doubtless have left out some that I should have mentioned, but these are the people who have every right to feel that they have earned a piece of the 1972 Whitney Award too—they and my family which, with varying degrees of resignation over the years, has allowed me to do "my thing."

Lloyd Miller said my recruiting courtship for the USP continued for over 10 years, and I'm sure he has had pangs of doubt both before and since retirement that he should ever have been so persistent. Sometimes hospital pharmacists still ask me why I left hospital pharmacy. I don't consider that I have. The basis on which I was hired by the USP Board of Trustees is a very simple analogy familiar to every hospital pharmacist: I said the USP ought to be the Pharmacy and Therapeutics Committee of the country.

To help make these changes in direction of the USP organization, three hospital pharmacists have joined me on the staff: Ken Barker again, Ray Jang again, and, just to show that new blood is acceptable, Robert Henry. We have great hopes for this unique organization, not the least of which is to select the drugs for the federal formulary when and if one is legislated into being.

But that's another story.

Tonight I want to make just one point. I want to impress upon you as vividly as I can a perspective on the role of the pharmacist that is even more clear to me after three years on the USP staff. The story I am about to tell is true, as far as I know. You all lived through it last year. This story was reconstructed in stirring detail by Wallace Werble and the editors of *Drug Research Reports*, "The Blue Sheet," in the May 26, 1971, issue. It is with Mr. Werble's kind permission that I am able to plagiarize in such abundant fashion. And I chance these extensive quotations because "The Blue Sheet" costs $200 a year and it's just possible that some hospital pharmacies don't subscribe.

This has to do with the septicemia epidemic that was linked to Abbott parenterals.

The Abbott investigation was a classic epidemiologic detective story, involving at one point around 100 people on the staff of the National Center for Disease Control (CDC) in Atlanta. The action took place there and in half a dozen hospitals around the country.

CDC has an annual budget of $48 million, about as much as the combined advertising budgets for Anacin and Alka-Seltzer. The CDC staff consists of both career Public Health Service officers and bright young men fresh from medical and graduate schools, doing a two-year stint in lieu of military service. Among them was Dennis Maki, a 31-year-old University of Wisconsin M.D., who completed his tour last June and is now a resident at Massachusetts General Hospital. Dr. Maki was one of the key figures in the Abbott affair.

On November 1, 1970, Dr. Maki lectured to the sophomore students of the Medical College of Virginia on hospital-caused (nosocomial) infections. After the talk, he was called aside by one of the MCV professors who told him about several septicemia cases at the hospital during the past summer. These had been investigated by Dr. Richard Duma, a young assistant professor of medicine. The study showed that 24 of 69 Abbott intravenous sets were contaminated with microorganisms. These contaminants were thought to have been introduced at the level of the screw cap through breaks in sterile handling techniques by the hospital staff. Dr. Duma was preparing a paper on his findings for the *New England Journal of Medicine.*

Dr. Duma and his coauthors, one another M.D. and one a Ph.D. microbiologist, were the first in a long while to point out that IVs can serve as a vehicle of contamination. An article describing a similar problem was published in *The Lancet* in 1953. Although numerous articles had been published in more recent years implicating indwelling catheters in infections, no one had looked up at the bottle hanging above.

Maki decided to find out whether other hospitals were having similar problems and whether, as MCV concluded, Abbott sets were more subject to contamination. Disguised questionnaires were sent to the 70 hospitals that regularly reported to the CDC's Hospital Infections Section.

Abbott users reported a seemingly higher incidence of primary bacteremias, but the difference was not statistically significant. That seemed to be the end of that.

A call from the University of Virginia Hospital in Charlottesville on December 1 revived interest, however. Four of the five patients in the coronary care unit had developed septicemias during the past week. CDC normally expects five to 10 bacteremias per 1000 admissions.

Maki and a microbiologist from the CDC went to the University of Virginia and cultured the bottles then hanging. One-fourth of 72 hanging bottles were contaminated, mostly with low numbers of organisms. Two were heavily infected with members of the *Erwinia* group and *Enterobacter cloacae*, the same organisms cultured earlier from the coronary care bacteremia patients.

Erwinia is usually thought of as a plant pathogen, and hospital bacteriologists do not normally look for it. Furthermore, it tends to get lost in the usual mix of microbial contaminants cultured. But because *Erwinia* is such an unlikely contaminant, the CDC investigators turned it to their advantage and used it as a microbiological indicator.

Abbott officials meeting with the University of Virginia staff maintained there was nothing wrong with their products. Contamination resulted from sloppy hospital practices, they said. Lab studies at CDC showed that all freshly opened Abbott bottles were sterile, supporting Abbott's claims.

That was also the expectation of Dr. Carl Bruch, one of FDA's most consumer-oriented scientists and a man who has served enthusiastically on USP advisory panels. He was not unduly excited on reading a draft of Duma's report. Dr. Bruch had long been concerned with the sloppiness of aseptic techniques in hospitals. Only two months before, he had quashed a similar report of reputedly contaminated spinal tap trays, showing that there was nothing wrong with the trays and that the contaminators were the dirty-fingered hospital investigators themselves.

But other hospitals began reporting troubles with Abbott solutions. A former CDC man who had become chief of infectious diseases at Orange County Hospital, Irvine, California, called to report an outbreak of septicemias. *E. cloacae* was one of the infectious organisms.

During a routine inspection of IV systems at St. Anthony's Hospital in Denver, hospital bacteriologists discovered contamination with *E. cloacae.* Half the hospitals in the nation used Abbott parenterals, and the likelihood of three of them having the same problem was only one in eight. Furthermore, lab technicians at CDC headquarters found *Erwinia* in clinical isolates sent from St. Anthony's.

Maki and a CDC microbiologist studied and cultured the parenterals for five days at an Atlanta hospital using Baxter solutions. All new Baxter bottles were sterile, but 9% of the hanging bottles were contaminated. Significantly, however, the contaminants were neither *Erwinia* nor *E. cloacae.*

According to the textbooks, microbes just cannot live in dextrose solutions which lack organic nitrogen. Maki and a CDC bacteriologist cultured about 100 strains of hospital microbes in dextrose; 96 strains failed to live, but two that did were *E. cloacae* and *Erwinia.*

On January 26, the chief of infectious diseases at Detroit's Henry Ford Hospital reported an outbreak of septicemias. By then, Orange

County Hospital had linked its septicemias with Abbott systems and had isolated *Erwinia*, the indicator.

Maki, a CDC microbiologist, and a fourth-year medical student spending an elective semester at CDC conducted a prospective study at the University of Virginia Hospital, comparing Abbott solutions with Cutter. They found that 2.5 times as many hanging Abbott units were contaminated. In eight of the Abbott systems, they isolated *E. cloacae* and *Erwinia*. One Cutter system may have had the same microbes. In the eight Abbott bottles, contamination was heavy, although patients being infused from them had not been diagnosed as clinically ill from those organisms.

Maki and his coworkers checked everything. They took cultures from tables, sheets, and walls. They talked to nurses to find out what hand lotions, soaps, lipsticks, cosmetics, and deodorants they used. They also cultured nurses' hands, discovering that 25% intermittently had *E. cloacae* and *Erwinia* on them, but none was a permanent carrier.

Fresh bottles and sets were cultured but gave only negative results. Finally, they disassembled a bottle cap aseptically, dropped it into broth, and got growth. University of Virginia microbiologists repeatedly got positive cultures from caps, and this discovery was confirmed under ideal conditions at the CDC's own laboratories in Atlanta.

FDA found that Abbott had made a change in the cap liner material the previous September.

CDC staffers, convinced that the Abbott cap was the villain, worked double shifts, seven days a week, for three weeks. They discovered they could release bacteria into Abbott fluids just by opening the bottles and closing them again in 25% of the instances in which cap liners were contaminated. Further testing showed that bacteria could also be released into the system just by banging the caps, a standard procedure of nurses dealing with the hard-to-open bottles.

Additional reports of trouble with Abbott solutions came from New York Hospital and from St. Joseph's Hospital in Ann Arbor, Michigan. St. Joseph's was the first hospital participating in CDC's regular nosocomial reporting system to come into the picture.

Abbott insisted that it could not be held responsible for contamination that was introduced when caps were banged. The firm had never made sterility claims for its cap liners.

CDC tested the Abbott production process, showing that organisms could enter the bottle system without opening or tapping the bottle cap. The whole bottle, not just the cap liner, could be contaminated by organisms in the water used in the firm's cooling procedures. When the bottles came out of the autoclave and were placed in water to cool, fluorescent dyes placed in the cooling bath were sucked right up into the bottles.

Almost a year after Duma started his work and four and a half months after CDC became involved, enough evidence had accumulated that FDA could force a recall of Abbott solutions. An unknown number of patients had died. Henry Ford Hospital reported eight, and the press nearly wrecked Ford. The *Detroit News* said, cynically, "It is unlikely that any of the eight patients will have septicemia listed as the immediate cause of death."

I haven't had time to develop the full flavor, as "The Blue Sheet" did, but I think that's a fascinating story—a medical detective story. Sometimes we are told equally fascinating detective stories by manufacturers who have been successful in developing a new product that they happen onto almost by chance. But this story deals with practice, with the places we all have been working—our nation's hospitals.

And when you think about it, it's the most damning indictment of pharmacy ever written.

The basic premise of having a pharmacist in the hospital is to make sure that the patient is protected from bad drugs. Physicians and nurses will make sure that patients get drugs, but only the pharmacist undergoes a long educational program, largely at public expense, to learn the components of drug product quality.

What happened here? What happened in American hospitals in 1970 and 1971? Had pharmacists developed quality assurance programs to insure that hospitals *obtained* drugs of suitable quality? Even more importantly, since the manufacturers, the compendia, and the FDA were working towards that end, had the pharmacists established quality control programs to assure that drug products were *handled safely* after entering the hospital?

They had not.

Nowhere in that "Blue Sheet" story is a pharmacist mentioned.

And the result of this abdication of responsibility for drug product quality?

Instead of a program of detecting defective drug products through routine in vitro control procedures, pharmacists left detection of defective products to physicians, whose only test method is death—death, or if they are suspicious soon enough, exacerbated illness of the patient at best.

What kind of a quality control system is that? Why should our patients have to get sicker, even die, in order to show that the drugs we have given them are defective?

The American people are desperately concerned about product quality. They want protection from defective automobiles, hazardous toys, flammable fabrics. They want quality built into a nickel candy bar. Why should we assume they aren't willing to pay for the quality control necessary to protect them from the very drugs they are hoping will make them well?

And would it cost that much more, really? In a study published in the Society's *Journal* in January 1972, Ken Barker reported that almost half—47%—of the time of the pharmacists observed in five hospitals for one week was accounted for by personal pursuits or just plain idleness. This is a sunk cost; the patient is already paying these salaries. Somehow, some way, we have to reach these pharmacists with the message of what it is they are there to do.

But I'm sure I'm like most preachers. Those sinners of omission are not in my congregation tonight. The members of this congregation and your fellow pharmacists back home work hard all day long. There never are enough hours in the day to get all your work caught up. I know. I've been there myself. We are the sinners of commission. We waste our time and our patients' money, not by failing to work conscientiously and hard, but by failing to work at the things that really matter.

How many hours of your day, of your pharmacists' day, are devoted to opening up the manufacturers' drug product packages and destroying the assurance of quality that was built into those packages through the manufacturers' own quality control programs, through the thousands of volunteer manhours devoted to the compendia in establishing quality specifications, through the millions of dollars you and your fellow taxpayers pour into the FDA compliance activities? The elaborate system we have developed to bring the world's highest quality drug products to our practitioners is compromised, and perhaps totally destroyed, as we repackage—repackage a drug product of unknown composition and unknown stability when outside the container in which it was tested—repackage it into a container providing an unknown degree of protection. And for what purpose? For financial control! We assume that the patient is willing to pay for our pharmacists' time in assuring that all the charges are properly placed—as a by-product of the act of subdividing larger packages, he won't be charged for doses he doesn't get. But do you really think he would opt for *financial* control over *quality* control if *he* could direct those manhours of pharmacists' time?

Meetings of the various sections of the Pharmaceutical Manufacturers Association are usually held in such watering places as the Greenbrier, Boca Raton, etc., but traditionally the Quality Control Section has one meeting each year in Washington so the USP, NF, and FDA people can attend inexpensively.

One of my friends in the control department of a major manufacturer, who shall remain nameless for obvious reasons, shared a coffee-break with me at the meeting last month. I told him how useful and important I thought it was that they had one of their meetings each year where the compendial and regulatory people could come. "Why not," he said, "you and I and the FDA are all in the same business: protecting the public from my company's products."

I commend that attitude to you as hospital pharmacists.

We are hearing much this week about our responsibilities in selecting and purchasing quality drug products. Certainly, that is a basic responsibility of hospital pharmacists. But just as basic is the pharmacist's responsibility for maintaining that quality after the product enters the hospital medication system.

Your national P&T Committee, the USP, is dedicated to helping you in that responsibility. For decades, USP has trended towards standards and tests that can be applied practically only at the manufacturer and regulatory levels. We have no intention of deemphasizing that aspect of USP responsibility, but we do intend to try harder to introduce special procedures which practitioners can apply. The USP is not alone in this concern. The FDA has just awarded USP a $100,000 contract to coordinate a broad-scale approach of all the professional, scientific, and regulatory groups involved with large volume parenteral solutions. ASHP will be represented on this coordinating committee. Individual pharmacists are already involved with other health team workers on USP's own Advisory Panel on Hospital Practices. As Robert Henry says, we aim to assure the quality of IV solutions from the manufacturer to the needle point.

To get a broad perspective on hospital pharmacist's problems and to make them more aware of drug quality, we have been proud to participate with the ASHP and the FDA in a pilot study of a Drug Product Defect Reporting Program during the past year. The phenomenal interest of hospital pharmacists in this program prompted *Quality Control Reports*, Mr. Werble's "Gold Sheet," to state that "from the standpoint of the taxpayer, this is probably the lowest-cost nationwide government reporting program in existence." And just last month, the Deputy Director of the FDA Bureau of Drugs, Dr. J. Richard Crout, said in a speech that the ASHP–USP–FDA Drug Product Defect Reporting Program was one of four major surveillance procedures used by FDA, the others being inplant inspections, premarketing batch certification, and industrywide testing of all brands of specific drug products in the FDA's new automated testing center. Dr. Crout said "that the return rate in terms of useful information per dollar spent is greater in our pharmacist-oriented drug defect reporting system than in any other voluntary reporting program we have in the Bureau of Drugs." Furthermore, FDA was willing to put its stamp of approval on this approach of extending quality control to the practitioner level by giving USP a $68,000 contract just last week, enabling us to offer this reporting system on a pilot basis to community pharmacists and to nurses.

When I talk about quality control, quality assurance, in the hospital, I'm not talking just about some laboratory next to that drug storeroom called "the pharmacy" down there in the basement.

Hospital pharmacists have escaped from the basement. The whole hospital is "the pharmacy." The entire hospital medication system has become the pharmacist's responsibility. He has become patient oriented. Patient oriented, but—never forget—drug based. Nurses and physicians and physician's assistants are patient oriented too, and all have a part in the hospital medication system. But only the pharmacist is educated in drug product quality—how drug dosage forms are put together and what takes them apart. Your patients have only you to depend on for assuming the responsibility of providing them that quality assurance.

Back in the innocent days when I was graduated from grade school (grammar school, the city slickers called it), even some of the boys had autograph books. One of my classmates, Bob Gaither, asked me to write something in his. I remember envying Bob two things: he could make beautiful bulges with his biceps and I was just a skinny runt, and his dad had built a shower in their basement. Not many homes in Brighton, Illinois, had running water inside the house, let alone a shower—except when it rained. But Bob's father had built one in. Mr. Gaither was an electrician and handy with tools, but I had never thought of him as an intellectual. I don't know what I wrote in Bob's book, but I don't think I'll ever forget what his dad wrote there on the first page:

With maturity comes responsibility.

I think it's time for us to go home and grow up to assume responsibilities that really count—responsibility for hospital medication systems and community drug dispensing systems that protect our patients from our drugs.

At the time he received this award, William M. Heller was the Executive Director of The United States Pharmacopeial Convention, Inc., Rockville, Maryland.

1973

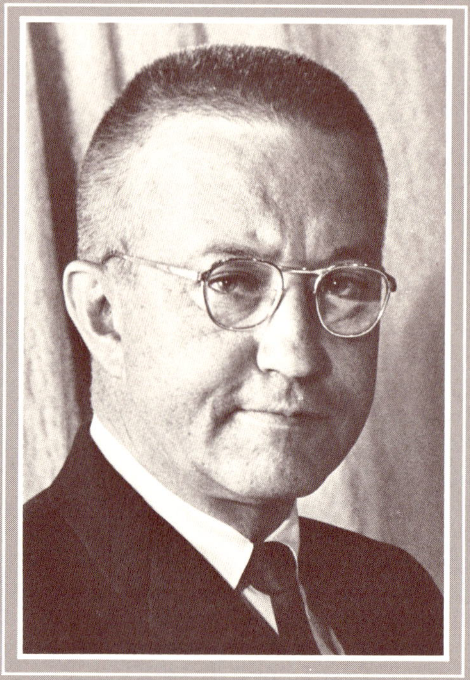

GEORGE L. PHILLIPS

"Uncle Harvey, as he was affectionately called. . ."

UNCLE HARVEY

Joe Oddis was first to both notify and congratulate me on having been named the recipient of the Harvey A. K. Whitney Lecture Award for 1973. In the same conversation, he advised me to start thinking about the title of my address. It occurred to me that I might be the last of Whitney's residents to receive this Award and that I am also one of the dwindling number of people linked to the times and life of Uncle Harvey, as he was affectionately called by coworkers and students. Therefore, I shall try to tell you why we are here to honor this man tonight.

A couple of days after Joe's call, Walter Frazier called to offer me his good wishes. I told him of my intention to tell the Whitney story and advised that I would be visiting Cincinnati to obtain information from Harvey A. K. Whitney II. Walter then invited my wife and me to stay at his home while we were in Cincinnati. Walter telephoned again on the evening of Wednesday, April 18, to firm up the date of our visit. Three days later, on Saturday, Harvey II called to relate the tragic news of Walter's death while working in the garden of his church. Thus, one week after last hearing from Walter, we were sorrowfully attending his funeral on Wednesday, April 25, 1973. Needless to say, this started off my historical search on a very sad note as Walter and I had been close friends since his postgraduate training days at Michigan nearly 30 years ago.

In 1958, when Walter Frazier received this same Award in Los Angeles, he said:

> *To be the recipient of an honor such as the Harvey A. K. Whitney Award causes one to reflect on his indebtedness to those who have been responsible for this recognition. This Award provides the opportunity for me to transmit the honor to my colleagues, to those who have generously given me ideas to use and who have inspired me to use them, and who have given me the insight to understand the true meaning of pharmacy and the vast possibilities for a full and pleasant professional life in the practice of hospital pharmacy.*

This nicely sums up the way I feel about many people, including:

1. Harvey A. K. Whitney I, my preceptor and first boss after my father.

2. Don E. Francke, my copreceptor and teacher, who stimulated me to write and teach and yet allowed me great latitude helping him to run the ship.
3. John Zugich, who started in residency with me and later went into hospital administration and became one of my closest friends and good fishing partner.
4. Joe Oddis, who guided me through three years as President and Board member of the ASHP.
5. Vern Thudium, who was my strong right arm as Associate Director of Pharmacy at Michigan.
6. The hundreds of pharmacy students and residents at Michigan who always tried to give as much as they received.
7. And saving the best for last, my dear wife Maggie, who literally keeps body and soul together. She was born under the sign of Virgo and, true to her sign, is neat and orderly and helps to rescue me from my own sea of disorganization.

Adrian, seat of Lenawee County, is a small college town in southeastern Michigan about 35 miles southwest of Ann Arbor. It is called the Maple City of Michigan because of the fine old trees that shade its quiet streets. It was here that Arthur and Emma Whitney lived during the 1890s and where Arthur served as fire chief. On the cool, crisp fall day of November 7, 1894, Harvey Whitney I was born to Arthur and Emma Whitney at home, as was the custom in those days. Dr. Allan, a friend of the family, was the attending physician. Harvey was the first-born child to be followed by brother Arthur two years later and four years later by a sister, Gladys. Arthur is still living in Adrian, and Gladys lives in Fort Lauderdale, Florida.

His natal day was also nearly his final one. Harvey often told the possibly apocryphal story his father, Arthur, had told to him. His birth had been difficult as Harvey was a bouncing 12-pound baby with an unusually large head. The nurse who was caring for Mrs. Whitney thought he would not be normal and should be allowed to die. She had relegated young Harvey to a basket behind the coal stove. It was there that his father found him that afternoon when he returned from work. He gently reshaped the baby's head and fontanelles and literally breathed life back into the little fellow. The excellent job Arthur did is evident; Harvey was a handsome boy and possessed a movie star visage in his twenties. The nurse was fired immediately.

The baby was christened Harvey Allan Whitney. Allan was chosen to honor the attending physician. The "K" was to come later.

Whitney's early education was in the Adrian schools, and he graduated from Adrian High School in 1912. During eighth grade and high school, he worked part time in the hometown drugstore. In 1913, he went to Toledo to work for the Rupp & Bowman Drug Co.

However, in 1916, he was attracted by the large salaries being paid by the automotive industry, and he took a job in the drafting division of Dodge Brothers in Detroit.

As World War I enveloped the world, Whitney served in the U.S. Army Medical Corps. After an honorable discharge, he entered the College of Pharmacy of the University of Michigan and received his Ph.C. degree in 1923. John G. Searle of Searle Laboratories was a member of his class, as was Dean Emeritus Troy Daniels of the University of California School of Pharmacy. Dean Daniels remembers Whitney as:

> *a gifted, conservative young man who was always well dressed and neat in appearance. He made friends readily and communicated easily but not excessively. He was a good student and demonstrated a well-organized mind. His notes taken from lectures were unusually well done. I recall especially his notebook and drawings in pharmacognosy as a work of art and Harvey received special mention for their excellence.*

At the 50th anniversary celebration of the founding of Rho Chi in Ann Arbor on May 19, 1972, Dean Daniels also revealed the key role played by Harvey Whitney in the founding of Rho Chi. Dean Daniels said that, to the best of his knowledge, Whitney was solely responsible for selecting the name Rho Chi and for the design of the octagonal key emblematic of that society. John Searle recalled pleasant memories and pleasant relations with Harvey as a member of the pharmacy class of 1923 of the University of Michigan.

The year 1923 was important to Uncle Harvey for another reason: he married Hildreth Katherine Wheeler, whom he often affectionately referred to as "the blond." I am most indebted to Mrs. Whitney Hewitt for many facts and pictures used here tonight. For example, Mrs. Hewitt also relates that the story of Harvey's birth came out when she found a crocheted baby bonnet large enough for a football player among his possessions. She now lives in Boca Raton, Florida, and is married to Al Hewitt.

Harvey was appointed to the pharmacy staff of University Hospital in Ann Arbor in 1925 and was named Chief Pharmacist there in 1927, succeeding Perry Briggs. The stage was now set for Whitney's major contributions to hospital pharmacy and pharmacy as a whole during the two decades from 1925 to 1945.

Of the many people I contacted who knew Whitney, most felt that his greatest contribution was as an inspiring leader. This was apparent in Dean Daniels' remarks concerning Harvey's activity in Rho Chi, and later in molding and developing a small group of hospital pharmacy practitioners into a subsection of the APhA and finally in August 1942 into the ASHP at the APhA convention in Denver.

One key to his success as a leader was his well-developed ability to communicate as a writer and a conversationalist. As an example of this, Leo Godley said:

> *I remember that he wrote me once, and I believe that I still have the letter. I still see it. The letter had great style and a great personal message. It made me feel that I had been chosen for something special. And I suppose that is what I think his greatest professional contribution was. He made us feel and know that we were involved in a specialty that was worthy of respect and preservation and development, and he compelled many to strive for this respectability and development through service and research. The electricity in the aura of his national influence was obviously the catalyst that influenced our professional effort. I really did not know Harvey on a personal basis. I always felt that I did and faked it.*

Whitney served as the first President of the ASHP from 1942 to 1943, as Vice President of the APhA from 1940 to 1941, and as President of the Michigan Board of Pharmacy in 1937 and 1938. Geraldine Stockert remembers him best from the APhA meeting in Detroit in 1941, one year prior to the official formation of the ASHP, when she was vice chairman of the group that preceded the ASHP. She said, "He was so sure the future of pharmacy was in hospitals and aware of the need to get the young pharmacy school graduates coming out of the colleges into hospitals and further build the profession."

Evlyn Gray Scott remembers Whitney's ability to see the potential of the young people around him and how he worked with them to see that they received a firm foundation in the profession.

Sister Mary John remembers Whitney as a friendly, compassionate man dedicated to hospital pharmacy, the education of hospital pharmacists, and the reduction of hospital costs through efficient pharmacy services.

Sister Mary Berenice remembers Whitney from the APhA convention of 1937 where he, Dean Spease, and Dean Muldoon all took special interest in the sisters attending the convention, made them feel welcome, and introduced them to the other APhA members.

Don Clarke sums up his leadership qualities with this thought: "Harvey functioned as a rallying point for his peers and, as such, generated in them a like spirit. This served to elevate many people out of a defeatist attitude to one of creativity and progressiveness."

To keep the ASHP alive in its early days and to allow for free interchange of information among its members, Whitney and Leo Mossman founded *The Bulletin of the ASHP* in 1943. Mr. Mossman is still practicing as Director of Pharmacy at Holzer Hospital in Gallipolis, Ohio, and last month reminded me that the ASHP has come a long way since May 1943 when the total membership was about 120. After writing *The Bulletin*, Whitney would go to the Addressograph platemaking section of the University of Michigan Hospital and personally make the mailing plates for the members. As you know, *The Bulletin of the ASHP* became the *American Journal of Hospital Pharmacy* in

January 1958. Thank goodness Editor Provost doesn't now have to make the mailing plates by hand.

Whitney is credited with establishing the first hospital pharmacy internship program, now known as a residency program, at the University of Michigan Hospital in 1927. This was 10 years before the first combined internship program would be offered by Spease at Western Reserve and 20 years before the second and third programs would be offered in Baltimore and Philadelphia.

Dr. Warren McConnell, a Whitney resident of the early 1940s, thinks this may have been his most noteworthy contribution:

> *What made the greatest impression on me was his recognition of the need for the well-trained hospital pharmacist to have a good understanding of the clinical aspects of hospital pharmacy practice. He insisted that his pharmacy residents attend clinical staff conferences, grand rounds and autopsies and that an intimate professional relationship be established between the pharmacy and medical staffs.*

McConnell also recalls the night he was on call as a resident and inadvertently left the pharmacy door unlocked after taking care of a late evening call. The next morning, he found the following note from Uncle Harvey in his mailbox.

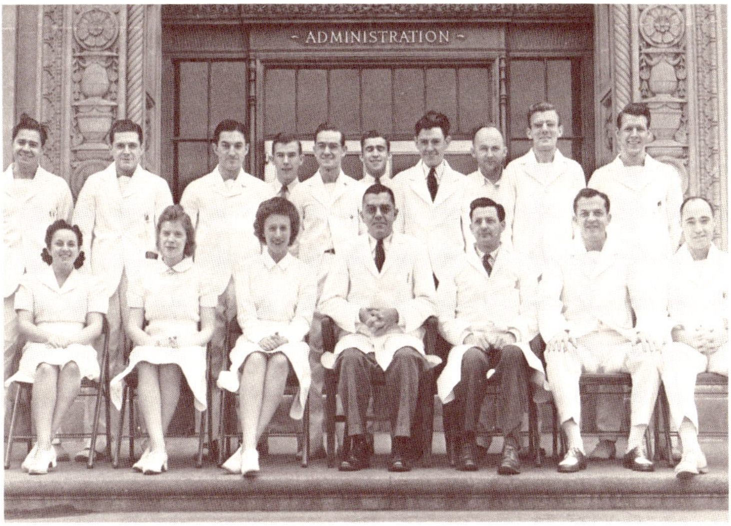

University of Michigan Hospital Pharmacy Staff, 1940–1941. Harvey A. K. Whitney I is seated at the center of the first row.

Flash Confidential:

Last night (11:27 p.m.) ye olde profit (sic) while engaged in "whether snifting" had occasion to consult the barometer in the "club headquarters." To his utmost astonishment the entrance way MCV *was left unguarded, open if you must know. This is a most reprehensible situation, one, in fact, that has been known to lead to a "terminal" situation.*

Signed: The Whipcracker

McConnell was so impressed that he still has the note and sent me a Xerox copy.

Don Creagan, a former Whitney resident with Mac and me and now with Squibb and known to many of you, recalls the following story of how Harvey I trained Harvey II, then known as Kim. Kim wanted to earn money as a boy by selling Sunday papers at a downtown Ann Arbor street corner on Saturday nights and Sunday mornings. Harvey was opposed because he could foresee problems in tieing up every Saturday night and Sunday morning, but he relented under persistent coaxing and agreed with the stipulation that once a thing like this is undertaken, it requires a discipline and a sense of responsibility to stick with it, rain or shine, no matter what temptation would arise to be absent every now and then. Everything went well until one night Mrs. Whitney thought Kim should eat supper. In order to reinforce the idea that it was important to "man the stand" without fail, Harvey, acting the part of a good father, took over to relieve Kim while he ate supper. Along came two U. of M. nurses out of uniform and, not sure that Whitney had recognized them, they went by looking a little embarrassed and sheepish. It was reported to Harvey later that they had felt so sorry for him, they didn't want him to know he had been seen. They thought it terrible that the chief pharmacist at a big place like the University of Michigan was paid so little that he had to moonlight by selling papers.

Muriel Creagan, Don's wife and a University of Michigan Nursing School graduate, is quoted as follows:

All the student nurses adored Uncle Harvey, who taught us materia medica. In that era, student nurses thought they were on the bottom rung in the hierarchy ladder because to them it seemed that no one listened and everyone put us down. Everyone except one Uncle Harvey, who remembered all our names and taught with a kind, gentle and understanding manner, always with a sense of humor.

My first remembrance of Whitney was when he lectured to our pharmacy class of 1939 and told us impressibly about hospital pharmacy and showed us the facilities at the hospital. Four members of my class became Whitney residents, proving how well he convinced us of the merits of hospital pharmacy practice.

Dave Hamilton, a Whitney resident of the late 1930s, remembers Whitney as a great organizer. The program of internship he installed in Ann Arbor was a masterpiece of organization. To quote Dave: "On the rotating principle of duties, a young pharmacist learned more about hospital pharmacy in one year than he could learn in four years of studies." Dave also remembers the drug card file that Whitney's secretary kept up to date for him on his desk. A physician would call the pharmacy for information about a drug, and Whitney would discuss current events while he was fingering through his drug information file until he found the card he wanted. Then he would offer the information requested. I am sure the physicians thought that Whitney had a photographic mind or a great storehouse of knowledge.

As you can see, Whitney was deeply involved in teaching pharmacy residents, nursing students, pharmacy students, and the medical staff of University Hospital.

In the day-to-day job of running the hospital pharmacy, Harvey also excelled. On April 4, 1928, Whitney was requested by the hospital director, Dr. Harley Haynes, to submit a written report of pharmacy needs for the next two years. Along with the usual requests for more space and personnel, he requested an autoclave, a hot air sterilizer, a steam bath, and a tablet machine. The closing paragraph in Whitney's letter to the director is especially typical:

> *Because these needs are regarded as necessary for the maximum interest and welfare of the care of patients, and because they are held as accessories to the efficiency of the pharmacy, they are not presented as debatable. In the event some reason must be attached to each request, I shall be glad to furnish this added information.*

In the early 1930s, 40 years ago, Whitney had already accomplished the following:

1. Distributed a printed formulary of available drugs which had been approved by the Pharmacy and Therapeutics Committee. He never stocked more than one brand of each chemical entity and had full permission of the medical staff to use professional judgment in brand selection. This formulary was later revised by Francke and became, still later, the basis for the *American Hospital Formulary Service* of today.
2. Published pharmacy drug bulletins for the nursing and medical staffs.
3. Prepackaged drugs in convenient dispensing sizes, coded and dated.
4. Manufactured many sterile products before they were marketed commercially, including allergenics and intravenous and surgical fluids. In the bulk sterile fluid manufacturing process, he, in conjunction with the U.S. Bottlers Company, devised a new mixing, filtering, and filling unit of corrosion-resistant stainless steel.

5. Prepared a wide variety of ointments and washable bases especially tailored to suit the needs of a large dermatology service.

Remember that he was doing all these things 40 to 50 years ago, several decades before they became accepted norms of practice.

Another of Harvey's good traits was his great willingness, almost an obsession, to share his knowledge with his fellow pharmacists. This was very apparent in the early issues of *The Bulletin of the ASHP.* Gerry Stockert says that he always had the answer when she would send him a "What do I do now?" letter.

Marjorie Zugich, pharmacist-secretary to Whitney, recalls his tolerance to the practical jokes of his residents, such as when a live goldfish would appear in a sealed "sterile" liter of intravenous water or when his Fatima cigarettes, which were stored in the pharmacy refrigerator, would be borrowed by a young resident until payday.

Uncle Harvey would frequently outdo us on the humorous side, as when he became the "flaming spot wizard" walking along the hospital corridors followed by a flame of ethyl chloride burning on the floor behind him. This he sprayed from a pressurized bottle of that local anesthetic which was concealed in his hand.

Tom Reamer cherishes his memory of Whitney during the Whitney Award banquet of 1957 in New York City. Tom was toastmaster; Sister Mary John, the Award recipient, was seated on one side of him and Harvey on the other. All evening long, Harvey kept telling Tom funny stories that made it difficult for him to keep his mind on toastmastering. That was the last Award dinner and ASHP meeting that Whitney attended, as he died in December of that year.

At the first Whitney Award banquet in 1950 in Detroit, when Arthur Purdum was the recipient, Harvey was asked to say a few words. He remarked that these honors usually come after one is dead. He quipped, "I may be diseased but not deceased as far as I know."

In May 1944, Harvey left the University of Michigan Hospital to again respond to his country's wartime needs. This time he went to Richland, Washington, to head the pharmacy department at the Hanford Nuclear Engineering Plant. One year later, he joined Ortho Products in Linden, New Jersey, as Director of Pharmaceutical Research.

The final decade of his life (1947–1957) was spent mostly in community practice, with one exception when he was Director of Pharmacy at Detroit General Hospital. During his last three years, he practiced at Middle Park Pharmacy near Detroit. Here, as usual, his patients felt that he was most understanding of their problems and always ready to help.

On December 2, 1957, Harvey came to the University of Michigan Hospital for the last time. There, on December 5, he was operated on for an abdominal aneurysm and he died 10 days later on December 15, 1957 at 4:40 p.m. following postoperative complications. I recall that my wife Maggie and I visited him at the hospital the night before the operation and that, as we were leaving and saying goodnight, Harvey laughingly said we should say goodbye as he fully realized the risk involved. Unfortunately, he was correct. His funeral was held on December 18, 1957, at the Muehlig Chapel in Ann Arbor, and he lies buried in Washtenaw Memorial Park on the north side of Ann Arbor. Pallbearers at his funeral were his close friend and hospital administrator, Dr. Albert Kerlikowske; a fellow pharmacist and state pharmacy board member, Jerry Totzka; and four of his former pharmacy residents, Don Francke, Don Creagan, John Zugich, and George Phillips.

Hildreth Whitney Hewitt admits that Harvey's first love was pharmacy. She is quick to add that his second love, his family, was never neglected. He was a fine husband and father. He was never too busy to help with the children; although he used a firm hand, he never failed to explain to them in detail any problems that might arise.

When Harvey II was born, Harvey I decided to name him Harvey Allan Kim Whitney II and legally to add Kim to his own name. Uncle Harvey was a great admirer of Rudyard Kipling, and Kim comes from the title of Kipling's best known novel whose principal character was Kimball O'Hara.

Quite possibly, the influence of Kipling's *Kim*, and certainly his poem *If*, helped Whitney set the pattern for his own life style. The dominant themes of *Kim* are tolerance, love, loyalty, respect, and self-realization. The dominant theme of *If* is that life is what we make it. Uncle Harvey's career and accomplishments are proof that he was able to follow Kipling's sage maxims successfully:

If you can talk with crowds and keep your virtue,
Or walk with Kings—nor lose the common touch,
If neither foes nor loving friends can hurt you,
If all men count with you, but none too much;
If you can fill the unforgiving minute,
With sixty seconds worth of distance run,
Yours is the earth and everything that's in it,
And—which is more—you'll be a Man, my son!

At the time he received this award, George L. Phillips was a hospital pharmacy consultant. He retired in 1972 as the Director of Pharmacy Service at the University of Michigan Hospital, Ann Arbor.

1974

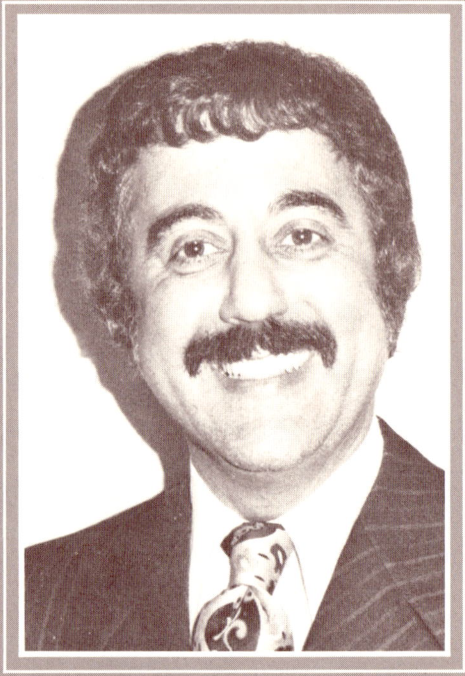

LOUIS P. JEFFREY

"Our interest is a commitment to our involvement in a profession in which we choose to serve."

A PERSONAL OPINION FOR PROFESSIONAL REFLECTION

This is a unique occasion for me, the members of my family, and the literally hundreds of pharmacists, residents, and students who have served the profession with me for more than two decades. I hope that each of you will permit me, as the 25th recipient of this distinguished award, to acknowledge and express my sincere appreciation to some friends to whom I am deeply indebted.

In the criteria for the selection of the recipient, it states that the receiver should have "made significant contributions to hospital pharmacy in the form of sustained exemplary service." The implication of this requirement cannot be met unless the recipient is supported by an outstanding group of colleagues who share with him their knowledge, their strong commitment to service, and their dedication to excellence in performance. Few of my peers have been as fortunate as I in being the beneficiary of so many talented pharmacists who by their performance have qualified me to meet the high standards of this award.

Thus, I would like to ask all those pharmacists who are here this evening, and who are responsible in part by their very hard work, to please stand and share at least for a moment this great honor which belongs to all of us!

It is not easy to devote a significant portion of one's life to his profession without compromising his personal time and family responsibilities. After many years of involvement and the hundreds of meetings which I have attended, I'd like to have you meet my parents, Mr. and Mrs. Samuel F. Jeffrey, who for the first time ever have attended a pharmaceutical affair of any kind; and my wife, Dorothy, and my children, Paul, Anne, and Michele, for they all have made a contribution of personal sacrifice on this road to achievement!

I also wish to acknowledge in silent tribute the many people with whom I have shared professional organizational experiences. While I would like to personally recognize them, they know who they are, and they too are the recipients of my deepest appreciation on this occasion.

This evening gives me an opportunity to share with you a personal opinion about the status of some of our current professional problems. While each of us is concerned as a hospital pharmacist, our interest is a commitment to our involvement in a profession in which we choose to serve. And this is as it should be. But it is imperative, more so now than ever before, that we view our role with a broader perspective. The issues confronting the profession are complex and transcend locus of practice. They allow no tolerance for parochial positions.

Hospital pharmacy has produced many leaders for our profession. In addition, our specialty has been a pioneer, from an organizational and practice viewpoint, in developing and establishing new concepts for pharmacy. The growth and progress of the American Society of Hospital Pharmacists are a reflection of the contributions and dedication of its members and staff. For hospital pharmacists to maintain their leadership role in the profession, they must take the initiative to transcend organizational boundaries and become involved in the equitable resolution of issues that relate to all pharmacists.

One of the conglomerate issues that currently influences all aspects of the profession relates to continuing education and professional competence. If an objective and unbiased analysis were made by a group of experts outside of our profession, I imagine that they would conclude that we have managed to complicate a desirable objective to the point where it becomes almost undesirable.

It is disappointing that some organizations at the national and state levels have acted precipitously in this area. There is little disagreement that continuing education is a lifelong process. To amplify this philosophy further, there are those who have concluded that continuing education should be mandated as a requirement for relicensure. While the objectives of continuing education may be essential for the profession, it seems to me that there are groups who have acted prematurely and, in some instances, in a self-serving manner.

The issue becomes even more of an imbroglio as national professional organizations and state regulatory agencies espouse and promote provincial organizational interests, rather than addressing themselves to the basic issues and objectives as they relate to the needs of the individual practitioner. It is unfortunate that the practicing pharmacist is facing the possibility of becoming a pawn on the chessboard of his own profession at the same time he is emerging as a bishop or a knight on the larger chessboard of the health care delivery system.

I believe that many of us here do accept the recommendations of the National Advisory Commission on Allied Health Manpower which state:

Professional societies and state governments should explore the possibilities of periodic relicensing of physicians and other health professionals. Relicensure should be granted either upon certification of acceptable performance in continuing education programs, or on the basis of challenge examinations in the practitioner's specialty.

The Commission's recommendation provides the profession with the opportunity to select one or the other proposal or, if desirable, to combine the two. It is interesting to note that boards of pharmacy and state pharmaceutical associations have now shed their rusty armor and have moved into the arena of continuing education. It is not difficult to misinterpret the rationale for their action. The reasons seem obvious enough to create disagreement within the profession and suspicion of the objectives of those organizations which previously had little if any interest in this matter.

Traditionally, the educational portion of our profession—undergraduate, graduate, and postgraduate—has been the province of the colleges of pharmacy and our national professional organizations. The latter, for years, have provided the programs and opportunities to meet the personal and practice requirements of the responsible pharmacist. It seems to me that the "new kids on the block" do a disservice to their brothers who recognized an inherent need for the profession long ago and made this service available to members and nonmembers. I find it very difficult from a personal viewpoint to support mandatory continuing education for pharmacy. Once again, members of the profession are utilizing the legislative process to resolve a basic moral obligation of some pharmacists. By following that path, we are in a sense making a public admission that the profession cannot regulate one of its principal concerns. Unless those involved assume a more statesman-like posture, the problem will take too long to resolve. All pharmacists must assist in the adjudication of this issue, because we simply have no time to waste.

It is difficult to discuss continuing education unless one is going to relate it to the reason for its existence: professional competence.

The need for the maintenance of a desirable level of competence on the part of the pharmacist was once of only cursory public concern. Now, however, it is becoming a matter of public demand and has become a professional dilemma. In order to achieve a satisfactory level of competence, we must first have a standard by which to measure competence. It is almost ludicrous to mandate continuing pharmaceutical educational programs and to try to increase the knowledge or intelligence of the practitioner when we don't know where he is or where we want him to be. I am in agreement with the philosophy expressed by Dr. Edmund D. Pellegrino:

Continuing education is the only guarantee of continuing competence and the ultimate protection for the patient of the quality of care he receives. It is too important to be left as an individual responsibility.

While the traditionally voluntary system of maintaining competence may now need to be changed, I am convinced that moving too swiftly and without sufficient forethought into this complex arena and trying to change it overnight is illogical, irrational, and ill-conceived.

As many of you know, I had a brief and enjoyable experience with the pharmaceutical industry. When we had a problem, we would meet as a group and form a plan of action. Perhaps what we need here in addressing ourselves to competence is a suggestion with regard to a plan for the profession. I shall use this forum as an opportunity to express my personal opinion for your professional reflection. I believe we need:

1. A clearly defined, professionally acceptable definition of a pharmacist;
2. A "Pharmacist Standard for Professional Competence," which has the approval and support of all components of the profession; and,
3. A nationally representative, professionally inclusive body that has the authority to create, develop, and approve continuing educational programs for pharmacists. It would have the additional responsibility to develop and implement a system to insure the profession and the public of the competence of all licensed pharmacists.

It would seem highly desirable for our leaders to agree to an immediate cessation of all divergent activities in this area until we receive the report of the profession's Task Force on Continuing Competence in Pharmacy. We must take a more rational approach to the problem before we proceed any further in the decisionmaking process. Fact-finding involves common sense, which is the application of truth derived from everyday practice. We should use this process, now! Waiting for tomorrow will further delay the resolution of this vital issue.

I wish to share with you a personal opinion concerning the report of the Commission on Goals of the ASHP. As you recall, the Commission presented its preliminary report at the 1973 Annual Meeting. The report was received with mixed and, in some cases, strong reaction from a significant number of members of our Society and several prominent members of the American Pharmaceutical Association. The controversial issue in the proposed document seems to relate to the desire of the Commission on Goals to broaden the base of the Society from hospitals to all pharmacists practicing in "organized health care settings."

The relatively mild negative reaction on the part of other national pharmaceutical organizations to the content of this as yet unofficial report may represent the "calm before the storm." The tacit implication in the Commission's report concerns the likelihood that adoption of the report may move the Society into areas of the profession which are currently within the territorial boundaries of other pharmaceutical organizations. The reaction is understandable. The justification is one basis of disagreement.

Up to late 1972, the Society had been identified as a specialty organization affiliated with our national professional association. This is no longer true. Even under the currently approved objectives and recently broadened definition of active membership, the American Society of Hospital Pharmacists is changing. During its relatively short organizational lifetime, the Society has grown into a prominent position in national professional and political affairs. This is not surprising, for this dynamic organization is composed primarily of dedicated, aggressive, often brilliant, young pharmacists who have moved prominently into the mainstream of the health care delivery system because of their practice environment.

The concern that I have relates to a realistic possibility. For the purpose of illustration, let us assume that the Board of Directors and the membership of the Society approve the Commission's recommendations and then translate them into new constitutional objectives for the American Society of Hospital Pharmacists. This would put the Society in a formidable position to become an even stronger pharmaceutical organization in this country. This is not beyond the scope of reality. The Society has a long list of successes into new ventures, services, and enterprises. It has developed its expertise in our health care system from the prominent position and the power base structure of the hospital and affiliated medical colleges. Thus, the American Society of Hospital Pharmacists, or whatever new name it may be called, would carve out a major role in the national pharmaceutical political and professional arena.

While the mainstream of the pharmaceutical component of our health care delivery system has a solid base in the 45,000 community pharmacies in this country, the 7000 hospitals and their 100 affiliated medical colleges occupy a strong leadership position in that same system and form the pinnacle of the pyramid. Added to this picture is the realistic need of our colleges of pharmacy to become more closely affiliated with hospitals in their area so that they may serve as an environment for clinical pharmacy education and training. To make one additional point, there will be an increased need for hospital pharmacies to support and absorb the increasing number of students seeking to comply with the current internship requirements. All these factors support the contention that the Society has become more influential in the affairs of pharmacy practice, health care legislation and regulations, student education and training, and a host of other areas.

In summary, an expanded set of objectives for the American Society of Hospital Pharmacists, in my personal opinion, will serve as the basis for another of the Society's successful ventures. If this prediction does materialize, my great concern is that functions and areas of interest will overlap with the three major national organizations representing pharmacy. For years we have had difficulty in getting our associations to agree and work together in concert. History has documented the failure of most troikas, except in the Christian dogma of the Holy Trinity. If my personal opinion becomes the basis for an organizational dilemma, it would certainly deserve your professional reflection.

In closing, I want to express my indebtedness to the American Society of Hospital Pharmacists and its members for giving me the opportunity to serve in so many ways for so many years. It is difficult on this occasion not to acknowledge the inspiration and influence that the Society has had on my professional career. Perhaps the words of the British statesman John Russell express my personal feelings better than I could:

To stand still today is to die. An organization must be bold, imaginative and alive to the unexplored. There must be a compliance for service, dedication to excellence and a zest for adventure. An organization which combines quality with the zeal of an evangelist will survive and thrive.

My commitment of service to the Society has always been stimulated by these descriptive words of Lord Russell.

And to all of you kind and thoughtful friends who are here to share this wonderful experience with me this evening, I wish to leave you with the philosophy of a personal credo which I borrowed from the poet Edwin Markham:

There is a destiny that makes us brothers
None goes his way alone
All that we send into the lives of others
Comes back into our own.

Tonight, you leave me with a heavy heart. I shall always be grateful!

At the time he received this award, Louis P. Jeffrey was the Director of Pharmacy Services at the Rhode Island Hospital, Providence, and Clinical Professor of Pharmacy and Chairman of the Clinical Pharmacy Advisory Committee at the University of Rhode Island, Kingston.

1975

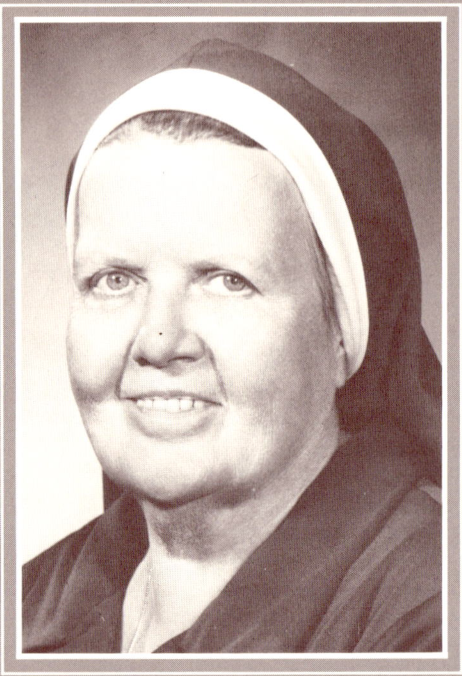

SISTER MARY FLORENTINE

"My enthusiasm for hospital pharmacy has been all pervasive."

ENTHUSIASMS

The mountain climber who, after the long, arduous, sometimes dangerous climb, rests exultant on the peak surveys the twisting path behind him with exhilaration, a sense of pride tempered by humility. He has been carried over obstacles along the way by enthusiasm for the climb, as well as the attainment of the pinnacle. As I stand here tonight upon what must surely be the pinnacle of a long professional climb, my feelings can best be expressed in these few lines, written many years ago by a friend of mine:

Now for a little hour let me stand
Here where the Past meets Future, face to face,
Let me lay one reluctant hand
Upon the years I see the Past embrace,
The while the other reaches valiantly
Out to unveil the Future's mystery.

Monday, January 13, 1975, began much like many other Mondays, with the exception of that "just before an examination feeling" that something dire was about to happen which has presaged many great events, both good and bad, in my life. The Irish call it "fey," I believe, so perhaps it is traceable to my maternal Irish heritage. In any case, the feeling persisted until late afternoon when the phone rang and Joe Oddis announced that I had been voted this year's recipient of the Whitney Award! Quickly bringing me back to earth was the dictum that the title of my address be forthcoming within the next couple of days! After much soul searching and brain wracking, I selected "Enthusiasms," the hallmark of hospital pharmacy, as my title and theme. Over the years, I've enjoyed a few pet enthusiastic projects which have finally come to universal adoption. This evening I would like to recount a few of these enthusiasms and then start what I hope will be a great ground swell for my most recent interest.

First, there was the enthusiasm for pharmacy engendered by accompanying my father who, on his day off, went to visit another pharmacy. It was further nurtured by a stubborn desire to become a pharmacist in face of equally obstinate opposition from that same father. Since first taking over as a very inexperienced hospital pharmacist, my enthusiasm for hospital pharmacy has been all pervasive; subsequent interests have been just by-products. That enthusiasm has encompassed even the day-to-day performance of merely routine professional functions. When performed for the love of the neighbor seen in outpatient clinics, even these can be soul satisfying indeed. Someone once said there were no small tasks, merely small persons doing them. Yet even small persons can make of these multiple small actions a mighty force for good. The phenomenal growth of hospital pharmacy and its impact on the entire field are evident proof of this.

This enthusiasm for pharmacy focused on hospital practice after my being literally plunged into it by stepping into a hospital position vacated by the death of the incumbent. Not the blunders, the long hours, nor the hard work interfered with the convictions, soon arrived at, that this was truly pharmacy and that pharmacy is service. In those early days, hospital pharmacists had only a section at the annual meetings of the American Pharmaceutical Association and of hospital associations in which to discuss their special problems and exchange ideas. The enthusiasm of the pioneer leaders was spread by state groups, the first institutes, and the generous sharing of ideas that characterized the beginnings of the Society. Few of us who sat with our feet in wet sawdust at the Princeton Inn that hot July in 1948 went away unmoved by Dr. Carl Walters' description of the "green seawater" technique of preparing hypodermic injections! For me, it was the beginning of a continuing enthusiasm for the preparation of sterile products—injections and ophthalmics as well.

Evolution is a slow process, and the progress from hypodermic tablets to disposable cartridges has taken several decades. Equally gradual has been the passage from the one-or-more ounce bottle of ophthalmic drops to today's sterile units. Yet a chance conversation with one of our ophthalmologists about preparing a "chain of sausages," each containing but a few drops, sparked in me an enthusiasm that could not be dampened by machines that failed to seal, tubes that spouted their contents unexpectedly or dried out because of water seepage through the walls! Bill Heller, remembering a disastrous demonstration at the Institute in Chicago I'm sure, suggested that I bring to this assembly a little tube which he remembered as the first unit dose eye drop. Enthusiasm and persistence have finally paid off, and today industry furnishes tubes that really work.

There have been other related enthusiasms as well, but why try to enumerate? Once, after I showed the director of trade relations for one of the large pharmaceutical companies through our department, he remarked: "You're very keen on your job, aren't you?" At the moment I was pleased that it seemed so obvious. As time passed and I reflected more deeply on his remark, I wondered whether I might have been too keen on the immediate job to see clearly the wider potential of service. The emphasis today, however, on clinical pharmacy as service has had unprecedented acceptance. A field of practice spawned in the hospital, the concept has spread to other branches of pharmacy.

The connotation of "clinical" has a certain detachment and sterility of approach that made my initial enthusiasm for clinical pharmacy something less than wholehearted. Nor was this apathetic view stimulated when senior pharmacy students, after a semester's exposure, declared themselves "clinical pharmacists." Further reflection produced evidence to convince me that this was just a new label on a time-honored method of practice in hospitals. For, after all, patient-oriented service had always been the goal; now it could be achieved on a wider scale. So much so, in fact, that warnings are being issued that we are training too many clinical pharmacists.

Today, in the leading medical centers and hospitals across the country, clinical pharmacy is the accepted standard of practice. Here, this one-to-one, patient-oriented service gives patients the advantage of rational drug therapy. Patients entering these hospitals (as well as any hospital which has a clinical service) have pharmacists taking the patient's drug history, which can be used by the physician as well as the nurse to improve patient care. Possible drug interactions, known sensitivities, favorite home remedies are pointed out. A pharmacist counsels the patient on the proper use of his medications. The patient improves, is discharged, and this service is abruptly terminated. And what of the more than 22 million of the population who are over 65 and are not hospitalized? In an editorial in the October 1973 *American Journal of Hospital Pharmacy*, George Provost spoke of the "advancement of rational, patient-oriented drug therapy," which would be provided in organized health care settings rather than hospitals.

By whatever term we choose to call it, we are moving inexorably in the direction of more government interest in, and control of, the delivery of health care and the regulation of hospital pharmacy along with the other health professions. We have read articles and heard leaders warn that change was inevitable. What direction that change takes can be influenced by the profession itself if we all turn our enthusiasm and innovative thinking towards a more subjective approach to our service. The February 1975 issue of *Pharmacy Times* quotes Julius E. Stolfi, M.D., associate editor of the *New York State Medical Journal*, who defines humane, humanism, and ethics and then asks, "Join us, please, in our prayerful hope for a return of humanism in all phases of the practice of medicine in the New Year." Our toastmaster, Grover Bowles, commented in his Remington address that students are not being adequately prepared in the humanities. To reinforce further the need for the trend towards wider scope for our clinical approach, one of our enthusiastic young leaders, Dr. Tom Mattei, asks:

What could we possibly accomplish if we freed ourselves from our frozen concept of pharmacy practice? The common denominator of our involvement must be the chronically ill patients' need for medication and their need to know how to use these medications properly.

This "need to know," the continuing thirst for knowledge that is man's inheritance from his first parents, takes many guises. It is present equally in the clinic mother who doesn't know whether she should remove the tinfoil from her child's suppository and the senior citizen who wonders how, when a number of pills of various sizes and colors are swallowed, each knows which part of the body to go to. The answer in each situation seems so obvious as to border on the ridiculous; yet it is of serious import to the questioner. So, for the moment, we become teachers and sharpen our communication skills to assure patient compliance. But even more, we must have concern for these questioners. Clinical pharmacy then will be enriched with an added dimension of communication and concern. Instead of being completely objective, it becomes more subjective and we become listeners instead of preachers. Speaking of U Thant's abilities as a listener, Robert Mueller said that "man can learn so much by simply opening himself to others, by lowering the barriers of his self-sufficiency and infallibility."

Concern, then, must be our watchword for the future. Concern is something more than routine and mechanical procedure. It is a gift of service, a gift of ourselves. Such service will be a natural outgrowth of present outpatient services flowing into neighborhood health centers, and there will be innovative preventive care as well as newer educational efforts. Currently, a large percentage of persons over 65 who are confined to nursing homes, extended care facilities, and long-term facilities are receiving pharmaceutical services from community practitioners. Here problems of overuse, underuse, and interactions of drugs are under surveillance. But what of the remaining 95% of this population? They, more often than not, live our their days in loneliness in apartments or rooms. They, too, are the patients on long-term drug therapy to whom the multiplicity of drugs is confusing. Time plays strange tricks with the memory. Was that dosage taken—and when it should have been? We know from studies performed that noncompliance with dosage schedules is widespread among patients attending our outpatient clinics. I do not recall seeing any compilation of statistics on the ages of the nonperformers, but I can venture a guess. So this is my latest enthusiasm, a greater concern for the older, sometimes confused, and often lonely segment of our population.

The Society has conceived, nurtured, and brought to fulfillment so many innovative methods in the past. It has such a wealth of eager, enthusiastic, and imaginative talent that a multitude of plans could be operable in short order. Perhaps a presentation of two simple, yet workable, schemes may stimulate many here this evening to think along similar lines.

The first plan involved a hospital where physicians maintained their offices and where the physicians' answering service was also hospital based. Here the hospital administrator became involved after noting the frequency with which recently discharged geriatric patients were readmitted in a badly deteriorated condition. Consultation with patients and physicians confirmed the fact that needed medications had been omitted or overdosed, primarily because these patients just could not remember whether or not they had followed the prescribed dosage regime. "How silly," we are inclined to say. Yet how often have the best of you forgotten whether or not you had taken a routine drug dosage? And you are young, knowledgeable, alert. What then of the old, confused, debilitated?

In this hospital, the administrator arranged with the answering service of physicians caring for these patients to call each patient daily to check on them and remind them to take their medicine. A patient load of six to 10 patients for each operator was maintained from a card file listing medications and times, as well as a neighbor's phone number. This latter information proved useful in one particular case where no answer was received and the neighbor's timely intervention was instrumental in obtaining prompt emergency assistance. Not only was the system helpful to the patients, by acting as a surrogate person who cared, but it also relieved the physician of many nuisance calls and acted as a liaison between patient and doctor. Think how much our services could expand by the use of volunteers to reach out to these patients who are waiting to hear a friendly voice, to know someone cares.

Your program tells you that I am a gadgeteer. With this in mind, the next plan is for a gadget, or a method, or any convenient way of reminding the patient to take medicine at appointed times. It would also serve as a check to assure that indeed they have been taken as ordered. Which one of us has not, in the middle of engrossing duties, paused to wonder whether or not he has really taken an appointed dose?

My interest in, and enthusiasm for, this phase of patient compliance was stimulated when visiting a really spry octagenarian, seemingly alert and responsible, who complained about inability to follow a rather complicated multiple medication regimen. The solution came in the form of a plastic container with days of the week listed across the top and a series of pockets below with times under each one. On the side opposite the designated times were the names of the drugs. All that had to be done, then, was fill the pockets once a week. An interested friend, neighbor, or relative could perform this service from well-marked prescription containers. A glance at the full and empty pockets will reveal at once compliance or noncompliance. Cards such as those designed to be filled and used as hypnotic records might easily be converted for use in such cases. In any event, I am sure there are many ingenious minds here that could devise a much better system. Think of the potential!

Finally, I would like to enlist you all in efforts to promote research into the pharmacological effects of drugs in older patients. As clinical pharmacists practicing in hospitals where great numbers of the patients seen in the outpatient services are in the over-65 group, you are the ones to see the drug-induced toxicity caused by diminished renal capacity, slower metabolism, or the lessened response caused by failure to take the drug. Where multiple-drug therapy is an additional factor, the potential for interactions and toxicities increases sharply. Or add to this conglomeration the doses of the leading products for the world's ills pushed on television. Is there any wonder that this potential for drug interactions runs so high? Pharmacy at large has begun a response to the needs of the patient in long-term care facilities. But what of the enormous population, mentioned previously, living out their lives in one room, lonely, often unwanted, who need a concerned, generous gift of our very special service. George Griffenhagen, in his editorial in the January 1975 *Journal of the American Pharmaceutical Association*, states:

Yes, we have come a long way in providing pharmaceutical service to patients in long-term care facilities but the results cited in recent studies lead to the unavoidable conclusion that we still have a considerable distance to travel.

Let us be on the road at once.

It would be inappropriate for me to close without thanking all those friends that I have met along the road who have helped me over the rough spots and have made this heady moment possible. So I thank God for the accident of having been born, as I've so often phrased it, "in a drugstore." My thanks are due to those farsighted teachers who insisted, while I was gobbling every science course possible, that I not become "one sided" and who fostered in me an abiding interest in the arts and literature. My deep gratitude, as well, must be tendered to the many great practitioners who have been an inspiration to me as well as faithful friends over the years. Nor should I neglect the scores of students who spent time in our department and always kept me "on my toes." I would be remiss indeed to neglect all those of the Society's headquarters staff without whose painstaking efforts this evening would not have been the perfect reunion and enrichment that have delighted us. Finally, let me thank all of you who have shared this glorious evening with me and close with these lines from the friend quoted earlier:

Ah soft the grey veiled Past now turns away;
Down darkening paths that greet her victory

She carries even this exultant day
Off to tear-misted hills of memory.

At the time she received this award, Sister Mary Florentine, C.S.C., was the Chief Pharmacist of the Infirmary at St. Mary's Convent, Notre Dame, Indiana.

1976

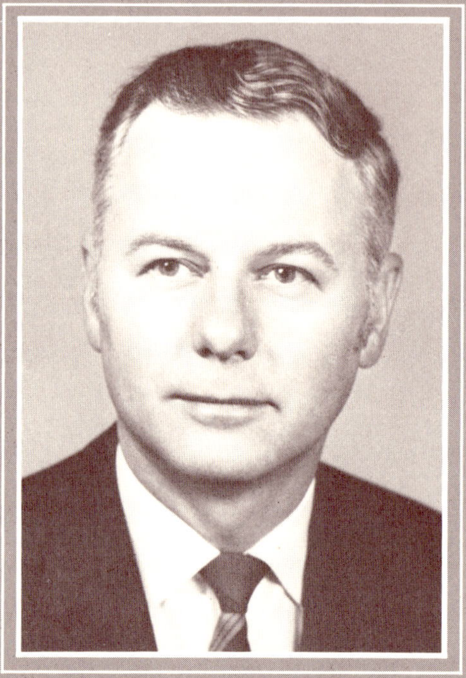

R. DAVID ANDERSON

"Hospital pharmacists have manifested a dedication to the career concept."

THE PERIL OF DEPROFESSIONALIZATION

The following thesis has a twofold purpose. First, I will repeat the often ignored warning that American pharmacy is in great peril of being deprofessionalized, that forces both external and internal, deliberate and unknowing, are intent upon reducing pharmacy to a technical vocation. Second, it is my belief that hospital pharmacy practice offers the best hope we have of reversing this trend and creating an environment in which pharmacy will be able to restore the respect which the public and other health professionals once had for this honored profession.

I fully realize that the breast beating, cynicism, and self-criticism which are to follow will be strongly offensive to some and that I will be taken severely to task for my disloyalty to the profession. However, few people can claim greater love for his chosen career than I have for pharmacy. My presence here tonight offers some evidence that I have worked diligently for the advancement of pharmacy. That is a path which I expect to follow for the rest of my life, and this is but the first step into tomorrow rather than the last labored step of today or yesterday. My effort here is to direct attention to some concerns that I feel must be dealt with if we are to achieve our destiny.

Five of the distinguishing attributes of a profession are: (1) a systematic body of knowledge or theory, (2) authority recognized by clients, (3) broad community sanction of this authority, (4) a regulative code of ethics, and (5) a professional culture sustained by professional associations.[1]

Many believe that pharmacy does possess these characteristics. Practitioners, educators, pharmaceutical scientists, and those who author the literature that sustains the body of knowledge upon which our work is based use the term freely. Some social scientists, however, consider our use of the "professional" designation as inaccurate. They point out that pharmacy fails to meet the criteria established for the ideal type profession. Indeed, we see references to pharmacy as a "marginal profession," a "limited profession," a "semiprofession," a "quasiprofession," a "peripheral profession," and an "incomplete profession."

Many of the intellectuals in pharmacy are strained to acknowledge professional status for the pharmacist. Numerous studies and commentaries depict the pharmacist as being in a class closer to technician than professional. Knapp[2] and his colleagues have studied the pharmacist's performance, and they have concluded that professional ability eludes the pharmacist. As drug advisors to physicians and the public, we fail to demonstrate good communication and consultation skills. Knapp's devastating evaluation, which I am grieved to accept, lumps me together with all those "who utterly failed the tasks presented to them—failed to the point of exposing their patients to the unnecessary risk of possible death. . . because of the overwhelming nature of the incorrect responses and the severity of the consequences of the pharmacist's actions."

George Provost[3] has observed that pharmacy is promising more professionalism than it is able to provide, while Robert Fischelis[4] noted that the public has lost faith in pharmacists as guardians of the public health and that pharmacists themselves are not sufficiently interested to perform functions they were trained and licensed to do. More recently, the Chief Justice of the U.S. Supreme Court proclaimed in a formal opinion that the pharmacist, when dispensing a prescription, is no more professional than the "clerk who sells law books."[5]

The public ranks pharmacists low on the scale of professionalism. The Dichter report[6] stated that pharmacists have lost contact with their patients. Forty-one percent of their respondents indicated that they never consult a pharmacist on medical or drug questions. Drug advice was obtained most frequently from friends and neighbors. Pharmacists were mentioned last, after physicians and the media, as sources of health information. The public is unable to identify the pharmacist as a professional.

Physicians and other health professionals have shown an alarming indifference to pharmacy. We are seldom called upon for more than simple advice concerning cost, available dosage forms, and brainless comparisons. In spite of frantic efforts by both community and hospital pharmacists to become useful sources of drug information, the services that have evolved are utilized infrequently and are of questionable usefulness in many instances. In those cases where pharmacists have gained a reputation as drug information specialists, they are rarely compensated for this knowledge, and there is little incentive to develop these abilities. A bound collection of official package inserts, supported by the pharmaceutical industry, and the detailman continue to serve as the physician's primary sources of drug information. The Study Commission on Pharmacy observed, "The least frequently used source of information (for the physician) is consultation with a pharmacist."[7]

The government and others who control our health care system demonstrate a remarkable disdain for the relevance of the pharmacist in all areas where drugs are being used. We are seldom called upon for advice, and we find ourselves cast in the role of storekeeper-conveyor-assessor of drugs rather than an authority on the use of drugs. We are more frequently considered extravagant, unessential purveyors of drugs who are overpaid and overtrained for the work we are required to do. Much of our time is spent in idle, nonproductive tasks requiring a low order of technical skill, which could be more economically provided by supportive personnel.

Pharmacists appear to have lost faith in themselves and have become resigned to a second-class role in the health care scene, knowing little and producing less that is absolutely essential to the safe, effective use of drugs. Regrettably, surveys have shown that some students in our colleges of pharmacy also appear to view their chosen career more as a business than a science or profession.[8] They look forward to years of frustration and lack of fulfillment for they know that their productive years will offer few opportunities to effectively use the training they have obtained. They cringe at the bleak outlook of prostituting themselves to the "commercialized jungles" where their extensive knowledge gained in a rigorous college education is soon adulterated by concerns for wine, auto parts, garden tools, and building supplies. They find little encouragement in the independent pharmacies which attempt to compete with the giant chains on their own terms only to vanish into that ever deepening vortex of merchandising and business conflict.

Those who select a career in pharmacy as an outlet for charitable service to fellow man soon find the path blocked and pockmarked by the practical economics of business and the moneymaking ethic. We are paid not for our knowledge and service but for the products we dispense. In short, we find that high ideals of professionalism are soon diluted by managers who thumb their noses at standards of excellence, acknowledge no sense of community responsibility, and resist application of special intellectual techniques and abilities which are unprofitable.

The above and many other citations can be provided which indicate that pharmacy is in great peril of being deprofessionalized in the eyes of those it serves as well as those who practice it. In the community, it is indulged by longstanding legal protection. It suffers from a decreasing emphasis on knowledge. It has foresaken much of its service orientation and sense of obligation to the sick and injured of society. In some settings, its status has deteriorated badly.

The true profession identifies early in its existence a sense of mission. It recognizes that it and it alone has the opportunity to develop and deliver those essential services on which the community depends for its very existence. In the case of pharmacy, it should rest in a devotion to patients and the acquisition of the knowledge, skills, and judgments that will assure optimum use and safety of drugs that are required in the treatment of illness. In my view, pharmacy is losing its sense of mission and thereby courts deprofessionalization.

Regrettably, most of those who use pharmacy to advance their own aims and many pharmacists have as their mission the accumulation of wealth. Once taken up, that goal obscures every value the professional holds dear: standards of excellence are eased to accommodate profit potentials, the sense of responsibility to community and profession is undermined, rules of conduct are relaxed, efforts by management to ease entry into its educational system become apparent, and its social standing begins to deteriorate.

Greenwood[1] has stated that the chief difference between a professional and a nonprofessional occupation lies in the element of superior skill which is supported by an organized, internally consistent body of knowledge. As we have already pointed out, the responses of pharmacists to the most elementary drug-related questions have soiled the name and reputation of pharmacy. Many of us are incapable of communicating in simple medical terminology. We demonstrate no superior skill, and the knowledge we attempt to manifest can be found largely between the covers of a pricing catalog.

The professional commits himself to a lifelong effort of study and contemplation. He requires no outside pressure to force him to study and develop an insight into the use of drugs. But pharmacy is struggling with the question of mandatory continuing education to coerce so-called professionals to become professionals. The typical pharmacist does little to elevate his level of competence. Very few commit themselves to serious study. Few pharmacists develop their own personal professional libraries. Those which are visible in most drugstores consist of the legally mandated USP and NF and a few free magazines that feature a small amount of pharmaceutical information sandwiched between advice on the latest deals in kitchenware and pantyhose. A few outdated textbooks on galenical pharmacy and inorganic pharmaceutical chemistry and, occasionally, a journal published by one of the state or national associations make up the bulk of the literature that is readily available. Little, if any, is permanently bound to provide quick access to needed information. Many hospital pharmacists, however, have recognized the need for comprehensive drug information services and have developed programs which meet the needs of a diverse clientele.

Those pharmacists who are not in constant face-to-face contact with physicians, nurses, and, particularly, patients where they are being treated and who are unable to see exactly how drugs work, what they do to people, and how they affect particular organ systems are destined to know little more than a myriad of unorganized details. No matter how vast the details known about drug products, the pharmacist who is unable to organize that knowledge into abstract principles, combine it with information gained from observation of the patient, and then interpret the relationships which exist between drug and patient will find that the element of skill which permits approval as a professional is missing.

We are destitute of experts in pharmacy. The plaintive cry is often heard that the pharmacist is the expert on drugs. Who can identify them? Where are they? We devote our lives to dealing with drugs, but we are satisfied to know so little about so many drugs. Few of us can claim to be expert in a single drug. Our failure to master the available information on drugs leads the public and other health professionals to reject us as advisors and colleagues.

A basic need of every profession is to control the manner in which its practitioners are recruited, nurtured, and secured to the ideals and mission of the profession. Pharmacy's practice component is losing its control over the breeding of pharmacists; unfortunately, hospital pharmacy has never exerted any effective control at the undergraduate level. Entry into the profession is largely regulated by the colleges of pharmacy, though they frequently plead for assistance from alumni and practitioners. Students are selected primarily on the basis of grades and the ability to meet demanding curriculum requirements. Little, if any, attention is given to identifying and rejecting those who would violate professional ideals and morality.

An insidious bureaucracy seeks to influence admissions and regulate the number of students. Capitation grants are dangled like a carrot before a dumb ass to increase the number of students, qualified or no. Research funds may suddenly dry up or the availability of other subsidies may be placed in jeopardy if the school refuses to lower its standards to a level of uniform mediocrity. A monolithic community pharmacy orientation continues to dominate the curricula of many of our schools. Faced with demands from every segment of the profession to increase curricular offerings to match the needs of special interest groups, the colleges frequently spawn a potpourri of courses which utterly fail to equip the student for a life of professional accountability.

Greenwood[1] declared that one of the distinguishing characteristics of a profession is the professional culture sustained by formal professional associations. Pharmacy has few peers when it comes to the number and variety of associations which vie for precious time, talent, and money. At every level of our society, city, county, state, and national organizations plead for allegiances, exhort us to get on the bandwagon, fight and bleed for dear old pharmacy. While many are of questionable usefulness, they offer common interests and goals around which some pharmacists will rally. They prevent isolation and loneliness by making available a forum for the expression of ideas, exchange of experiences, fellowship and contact with others having similar needs and views.

We hear constant calls for occupational and organizational unity. The premise is advanced that the ASHP has become too strong and powerful, that it duplicates the work of others, that the energies of its members are being wasted by devoting themselves to patients rather than the weightier matters of politics and the maintenance of a viable economic base for the independent practitioner of pharmacy.

Our leaders are criticized for harboring parochial attitudes. We are condemned for our failure to cleanse ourselves of provincial feelings and for speaking out on issues of common concern to our members. Hostile criticism is heaped upon us for our continued thrust towards improved standards for the profession. When we come together in free association to discuss common problems and attempt to define new areas of practice in which we can serve our patients more effectively, we are accused of developing pompous attitudes.

Strauss[9] points out that professionalism:

> *. . . complicates the task of developing teamwork between occupations. Each profession tends to develop a parochial, specialized point of view. As a result, jurisdictional disputes become more common, and the overall organization starts to break down into a number of semiautonomous departments.*

American hospital pharmacy has followed this predictable course and has rapidly developed an autonomous relationship with other segments of the profession. While exhibiting an earnest desire to cooperate in solving mutual problems, the Society and its members have rejected restrictions on our thought, activity, and political agitation.

Patient care, patient safety, and the public welfare have been our first considerations. If we demonstrate solidarity and single mindedness of purpose, it is because we share a common interest with many in a unique responsibility. This posture has created relationships with other pharmaceutical organizations that, at present, are free of serious conflict but characterized more by accommodation, avoidance, and competition.

We work under different circumstances. We work with a different type of people in different relationships in an attempt to meet the different requirements of a different patient or client. We work under a different form of bureaucratic management composed almost entirely of nonpharmacist administrators under the control of housewives, bankers, and farmers who sit on hospital boards of directors committed to altruistic service to the community. Regulatory authority imposed upon us by local, state, and national governments is vastly different from that which affects our compatriots in community practice.

We accept the description of the Millis Commission[7] as differentiated brethren, but we reject being categorized (by those who refuse to recognize these distinctions) as separated brethren to be shunned, avoided, and ignored. We will not go away; our organization will not go away. We will not be deprofessionalized by those who wish to recast us in a common mold whose shape is already flawed.

The prestige and dignity of a profession are largely determined by the trust and reliance placed in it by the public it serves. This confidence must be gained by strict adherence to a code of conduct; it is not willingly conferred by a constituency which is cheated, duped, and deceived. Failure to adhere to codes of ethics and conduct spawn laws, regulations, and interference by government—the people. Most pharmacists are law-abiding, ethical individuals, but we must recognize that pharmacy is one of the most rigidly controlled professions, which suggests that ethical imperatives are not as uniformly observed as we would like. There is ample historical evidence of gouging, rank substitution of inferior drugs, kickbacks, solicitation of premiums, fraud, and dishonesty to explain the necessity for many of the laws and regulations under which we function.

Marshall[10] defined a profession as an occupation in which *caveat emptor* cannot be allowed to prevail. Yet, we find in the recent scandalous revelations of the Senate Medicaid investigations that some pharmacists abused their clients and perverted their profession. Perhaps this disclosure will provide some relief from the stricken conscience we in hospital pharmacy experienced after similar practices were documented in some California hospitals. Who has brought charges against them? Have boards of pharmacy revoked or suspended licenses? Have local, state, and national associations censured them in any way or revoked their membership for such conduct? Indeed, have any of them called their ethics committees into session to investigate cases of misconduct against the public and professional standards? Are there, in fact, ethics committees to summon?

Hospital pharmacy, with a few exceptions, has generally escaped the slander associated with such dishonesty. But each of us can point to the acts of some who have violated the canons of human decency to take advantage of their fellow man. We have no code of ethics in hospital pharmacy. The Code of Ethics of the American Pharmaceutical Association is a document to which each of us should subscribe. Few of us could recite a single phrase in it; many of us have probably never seen it. It expresses some noble ideals, but the different nature of our practice locations demands that we create a code that reflects our relationships with all of the different people and conditions under which we practice. We have no means by which we can call delinquent members to account or to penalize them for deviation from accepted standards of conduct. There is great danger that a few derelicts in our midst will reflect poorly upon our good name and contribute further to the deprofessionalization of pharmacy. We have no way to weed them out, expose them to our scorn, and insure that they are obstructed from future practice.

Hospital pharmacists, by and large, have demonstrated a personal and collective "sense of mission" which is essential to a professional psyche. Hospital pharmacists recognize that we require (and often possess) talents and abilities which no other professional can provide. The pattern most idealized of a professional pharmacist would be one who has a close association with patients; has a comprehensive awareness of their previous medication habits; knows their allergies, sensitivities, and idiosyncrasies to drugs; extracts information about them from charts and contact with laboratory, x-ray, and other data; has access to a sophisticated source of drug-oriented information; is able to correlate that information with knowledge about the patient's physiology and disease; and recommends to physicians, nurses, and others the proper course to follow where drugs are indicated. He emphasizes and insures safety and effectiveness of drugs. The hypothetical professional pharmacist would serve as a counselor, advisor, teacher, monitor, and patient care team member who is also capable of managing traditional duties related to drug procurement and distribution. The model which comes closest to conformance with this professional ideal is the clinical pharmacist. While the need for his services exists in community practice, storefront clinics, and sophisticated HMOs, he functions almost exclusively today within the institutional setting.

Hospital pharmacists have manifested a dedication to the career concept. They have accepted a calling which has placed them in a close association with other professionals intent upon serving their patients. They recognize in their career a calling, a life devoted to good work, and they receive intense emotional and intellectual satisfaction from the rewards which are visible in renewed vigor and health of patients.

Self-centered motives cannot exist in the heart of the dedicated hospital pharmacist for he cannot profit from the accumulation of funds that might be charged for the services he provides. He escapes the slurs so often cast upon others who are accused of plundering the family fortune by unreasonable charges for drugs. Hospitals, faced with meeting ever increasing costs, are frequently singled out by the public and the government for pillaging public and personal resources, but the pharmacist engaged there in his professional work should do everything in his power to serve the interest of his patient rather than succumb to demands for more and more profits from pharmacy operations. His interest should be in the maximal use of his knowledge and in the needs of his patients rather than self-centered needs of the practitioner.

This is not to imply that the professional person refrains from seeking adequate and just compensation for his work and his knowledge. The professional and his professional association must work constantly to secure the rights and privileges that will insure his prosperity and achieve a lifestyle that is consistent with his importance and responsibility to the community.

We in hospital pharmacy have enjoyed a very special relationship with our national, state, and local associations. The ASHP, with its network of state affiliates, regional advisory panels, and local associations, has achieved general recognition as one of the most effective, responsive, and productive professional organizations in American pharmacy. It is a concentrated, cohesive group with an exceptional interest in serving its membership as well as society. It has provided a sense of identity that is unmatched by other pharmaceutical organizations and their members. It has been extremely successful in developing standards of practice to which its members aspire. Its educational programs have been uniformly hailed as the most intense, fruitful continuing education programs available. Its publications have demonstrated a commitment to the elevation of the professional knowledge of hospital pharmacy practitioners. The *American Hospital Formulary Service*, the *American Journal of Hospital Pharmacy*, and *International Pharmaceutical Abstracts* give evidence of its dedication to excellence in drug information and knowledge. That we are dedicated to the development and sharing of knowledge is evidenced by the success of the 1976 Midyear Clinical Meeting of the ASHP where the largest group of hospital pharmacists ever assembled has come together to freely disseminate the information we possess.

The ASHP has subscribed to a policy of advancing basic knowledge concerning the use of drugs in hospitals. It has assumed responsibility for developing training standards and for certifying training centers for hospital pharmacists through development of residency programs. The time has now arrived when the Society must address the basic educational component of the professional hospital pharmacist, the undergraduate curriculum. Donald Francke[11] has advanced the idea of an American School of Hospital Pharmacy. If we are to train and educate practitioners who will be required for future hospital practice in the skills, knowledge, and understanding of unique problems of rational drug use in hospitalized patients, the Society and its members must advance the development of a curriculum that emphasizes those needed qualities. No college or university currently offers a dedicated curriculum in hospital pharmacy practice. The net effect is indistinct directions for the student, confusion and bewilderment for the faculty, and a poorly prepared practitioner.

The Society and its members can wait no longer to seek the development of an institution of higher learning that will be capable of conferring both undergraduate and graduate degrees in hospital pharmacy. As the fountainhead from which new ideas, research, development, and application of the hospital pharmacist's unique talents will spring, the university should become the central forge on which all legal, ethical, moral, and educational facets of the hospital pharmacy profession are molded. Bringing together a faculty and student body dedicated to the one principle of good health for patients, especially those dependent on institutional care, would insure the essential direction and purposeful efforts that are lacking in today's pharmaceutical education.

Reversing the deprofessionalization of pharmacy can only be accomplished if each of us recognizes the fundamental role of knowledge of drugs and its dissemination to those who have need of it. I firmly believe that the pharmacist should know more about drugs than anyone. Our education certainly should prepare us to fulfill this expectation. Our entire educational experience revolves around drugs. Deplorably, few of us manifest expert knowledge in a single drug. We quickly lose the bulk of knowledge gained during our college years. Unless we are representative of the highly idealized group of clinical pharmacy practitioners, we have contact with patients only over the prescription counter. We seldom are able to see how drugs work. We cannot experiment with, evaluate, and understand the actions of drugs in sick people. We respond to the physician's efforts in these areas and are reduced to the count-and-pour status that characterizes so many of us. Our shame is that we are so satisfied with this role. We do so little to escape from it. Too many of us are satisfied to allow the process of deprofessionalization to proceed unabated.

Every day I become more convinced that every pharmacist should become a recognized expert on something. Every hospital with 10 or more pharmacists on its staff could have the world's greatest accumulation of drug experts if each of the pharmacists there was expected and required to become expert in a single category of drugs. Visualize the impact upon the status of pharmacy in the institution and the quality of its service if the directors of 50 of our largest hospital pharmacies called their staff together tomorrow and presented this speech:

You guys just can't hack it in this work. You don't know enough about drugs. There is a need for in-depth understanding of drugs by our medical and nursing staffs which they can't obtain on their own, and you sure aren't giving it to them. Generally, you measure up well to the majority of drug information requests, but the reason we are not called upon more often is that you just don't have it when it comes to expert advice. But from now on you're going to be experts and the best in the country. There are too many young kids out there looking for your jobs, and you can be damn sure that you won't have one long if you don't become the experts we expect of you. Your advancement will depend on how well you perform as the experts in your field. You will be expected to develop your own personal libraries and study like you've never studied before in your specialized field. And you will also be expected to maintain your proficiency in all other aspects of pharmaceutical service and information. We expect you to be good within six months and expert within one year.

Beginning today we are making the following assignments: You, Smith, are to become the antibiotic pharmacist. Jones, you will be the cardiovascular pharmacist; Perry's field will be in fluid and electrolyte therapy. Antineoplastic pharmacy will become your specialty, Owens. Brown will establish himself as the expert in central nervous system drugs, while Cohen will devote himself to gastrointestinal drugs. . . .

We may not be able to answer every question that arises with masterful skill, but in these fields we are going to have the most expert pharmacists in the country, and you can count on it. When our drug information center receives a question dealing with your special field of interest, you are going to be expected to respond. When there are lectures to be given or classes to be taught about your specialty, you will be the principal resource person. When our poison treatment center is faced with a problem of overdosage with one of your drugs, you will receive the call for assistance. When our ambulatory patients need expert advice in the proper management or understanding of their therapeutic programs, you will see that they obtain it.

In you we are going to witness the beginning of a new age in which the pharmacist is to assume responsibilities for patient management never before available to him. We are going to witness the rebirth of professionalism in pharmacy.

The foundation of any true profession is based on its essential social value; it will not endure if it fails to sustain public faith and confidence. Pharmacy's social value is overwhelmingly dependent on the effective use and distribution of drug knowledge. There is no evidence to suggest that economic concerns and the sale of products unrelated to drug therapy will alter the public's current low assessment of pharmacy or enhance its professionalism. The institutional practice of pharmacy offers the greatest hope the profession has for the renewal and maintenance of a viable professional base. But we must take the initiative to develop a corps of experts whose knowledge, rather than techniques, effectively serves the vital needs of man.

We have the ability. We have the knowledge, if we will only use it. We have the sense of mission and an association that provides the group identity so essential to the support of a career concept. We must achieve greater control over practitioner education and recognize the basic underlying value of a regulative code of ethics or conduct. It is essential that we establish greater bonds of commitment and respect between practitioners and patients.

If we fail to utilize effectively the knowledge we have and reject the tasks before us, pharmacy will succumb to the peril of deprofessionalization.

(For the complete list of references cited, please see page 139 of the *American Journal of Hospital Pharmacy*, Feb. 1977.)

At the time he received this award, R. David Anderson was the Director of Pharmacy Services at Waynesboro Community Hospital, Waynesboro, Virginia.

1977

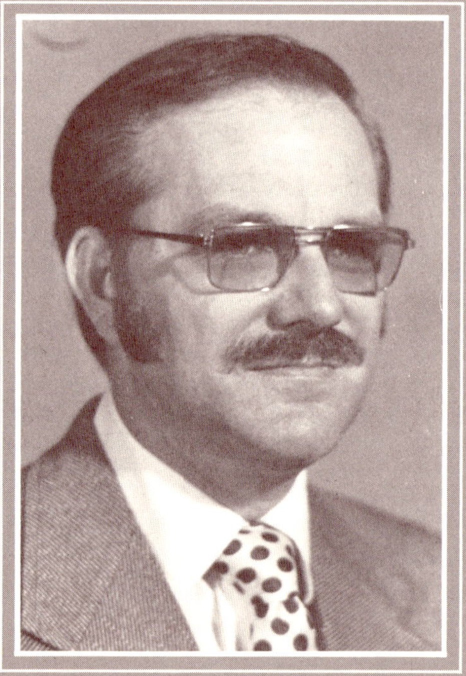

HERBERT S. CARLIN

"The future of pharmacy practice is bright if we center our activities around the patient."

PATIENT ACCOUNTABILITY —PHARMACISTS' FUTURE

Thank you for making it possible for me to receive the 1977 Harvey A. K. Whitney Lecture Award. I am indebted to my professional colleagues as well as to my mother; my wife, Ruth; my preceptor and mentor, Herbert Flack; my many professors, Drs. Brillhart, Tice, Avis, and Webster; members of the various pharmacy staffs with whom I have been associated; and my students and residents for this high honor.

I accept the award not only with a feeling of humility but with the realization that it is a symbol of achievement and progress for all of pharmacy and for its many thousands of practitioners everywhere. It is truly an honor to be shared with you this evening and forevermore.

To me, one of the most meaningful stories in the Great Book concerns the Good Samaritan. St. Luke's Gospel ends this parable with our Lord stating, "Go and do thou likewise." This statement not only provides meaning for our personal and professional lives, but it happens to be inscribed on the official seal of The New York Hospital, the institution with which I have been privileged to be associated in recent years. In reflecting on this parable, I realized that "go and do thou likewise" fits well with the theme of my message on this occasion: "patient accountability—pharmacists' future."

The satisfaction derived from service to mankind is one of the greatest rewards an individual can attain in his life. The practice of pharmacy, as a profession, should be that kind of rewarding experience. As pharmacists, our rewards are derived from our commitment to patients for whom we are responsible. The service we provide to our patients is safe and effective drug therapy.

Our expertise in drug therapy incorporates selection of drug products; recommendations about appropriate drug use; drug information; education of physicians, nurses, pharmacists, and patients; patient interviewing; patient monitoring; and the control of the system that provides for the delivery of the product to the patient.

Pharmacists must use their talents to their maximum in order to provide the comprehensive pharmaceutical services to which our patients are entitled. By doing so, the hospital pharmacist is adding the patient to the group to whom he is traditionally accountable—the hospital administration and physicians on our medical staff.

Pharmacists have always been indirectly accountable to patients when they have dispensed physicians' prescriptions with the right drug to the right patient at the right time. Over the years, we have become more involved in the total therapeutic system.

The epitome of a hospital pharmacy service 40 years ago was one that manufactured the products the physician needed for his patient. As the pharmaceutical industry developed, our attention was directed to the packaging of commercially available products which were issued to patient care areas as standard floor stock, free floor stock, or charge floor stock.

When a physician's order was sent to the pharmacy for dispensing to a hospitalized patient, it was transcribed by a nurse or a clerk and contained limited information—usually the number of dosage forms deemed necessary by the clerk. It did not include dosage information or route of administration.

We provided drug information—when asked. Rarely did we emerge from our four-walled pharmacy to determine if our services were meeting the needs of our patients. When we did appear on the patient care unit, it was to fulfill a JCAH requirement.

As we entered the sixties, things began to happen—drug information services came of age; drug interactions; then clinically significant drug interactions; parenteral incompatibilities; unit dose dispensing, centralized and decentralized; parenteral admixture programs; direct copies of physicians' orders; total parenteral nutrition; and so on. All these activities drew us closer to the rest of the health care team and, yes, to the patient.

Hospital pharmacy practice in the seventies varies from floor stock orientation to the most sophisticated of clinical care. At present, some pharmacists practice in such a manner as to constitute an underutilized health care resource. Knowing they have become stagnant and knowing they are not providing quality, comprehensive pharmacy services create a high degree of frustration within the individual practitioner. Frustration may lead to an attitude which causes loss of credibility among other health care providers. Ultimately, the loser is the patient—whose confidence and support are so essential to pharmacists' successful provision of safe and effective drug therapy.

The traditional "isolation practice," the Dutch door subterranean storeroom, has been another roadblock in our attempt to be full partners on the health care team. In recent years, however, more pharmacy services, especially in our large teaching hospitals, have been divided into smaller functional units, located strategically throughout the institution. In decentralized service, with each unit dealing with smaller patient populations, we have increased our visibility in a more personalized way to other health care practitioners, while at the same time increasing our services to patients. Suddenly they find that the pharmacist is a real person. Stripped of the veil of traditional anonymity, he now makes his personal contribution to health care.

But are we prepared to make this type of change?

Perhaps not. In some, a frustration of professional inadequacy may exist. Several options exist for us all. The way in which we exercise these options demonstrates our true commitment to the service of others. We may, of course, continue the way we always have—in isolation, even within the new environment—or we can meet the challenge by offering a personal contribution to safe and effective drug therapy.

Let's look at some of the ways we can commit ourselves to such service.

To practice "clinically"—is it merely the laying on of hands, being excellent clinical librarians, making recommendations to physicians or others that they may or may not accept? This describes much of the clinical practice within our hospitals today. For example, many clinical educators who bring their students into our hospitals have no idea or interest in the total workings of the pharmacy department. They come into the hospital, make recommendations, and leave. The physician responds to these recommendations or tries to follow up on the situation. The clinical education is long gone. The pharmacist who is accountable to the physician and to the patient for the provision of the drug product is the one with responsibility. The best interests of the patient have certainly not been met in this case. Tension develops between the physician and the pharmacy department. Future suggestions of the clinical educator may not be readily accepted, and a conflict may arise between the clinical educator and the hospital pharmacist. *The question of accountability is crucial to the provision of comprehensive pharmaceutical service and to the survival of pharmacy as a profession making a full contribution to health care.*

Comprehensive pharmaceutical services should not, and cannot, be episodic. If our pharmaceutical services are to be of value, and I believe they are—in fact, I believe they are essential to patient care—then the services should be available continuously and whenever they are needed. Consistency builds reliability, an essential component of acceptance. The ability to follow up is necessary because it leads to credibility and allows us to assess for ourselves our personal contributions to the care of the patient.

How can we attain this goal? We must consider two aspects—the environment in which we practice and ourselves as individuals.

There are many factors that influence the environment in which we practice—not the least of which are the awareness and support of the concept of comprehensive pharmaceutical services by the institution's administration and medical staff. Their initial support may not be enthusiastic or based on total commitment to the program, but they must show enough faith to allow a truly comprehensive program to develop and grow and eventually demonstrate its value.

Another contribution of the environment is the assemblage of a critical mass of pharmacists who are willing to give of themselves and form a team. This team concept must engender a mutual respect among all its members as they individually and collectively go about fulfilling their roles. Some will be administrators, some deal with distributive functions, and others with clinical activities. But all make an equal contribution to the comprehensive service. Each must be equally committed and equally accountable. Without team members who have mutual respect for one another, the objective will never be obtained.

A third aspect of the environment is an interdisciplinary team on which the pharmacist is able and willing to work as a team member. An effective interdisciplinary team is more difficult to accomplish than an effective pharmacy team. More than a decade ago, I had the opportunity to participate on an interdisciplinary team consisting of a physician, a nurse, a dentist, a physical therapist, and a pharmacist. The objective of our task force was to determine the feasibility of interdisciplinary continuing education programs. It became apparent after many weeks of dialog, centered mainly upon each individual profession's rationalization of its importance to patient care, that our project was in danger of failure. We termed these barriers to effective team work the "negativism of professionalism." Not until we focused on the needs of the patient whom we all served did we begin to work as a team and to respect each member profession's unique contributions to the overall effort of patient care.[1,2] This experience demonstrated effectively to me that patients must be the central focus of all our endeavors. *To succeed as professionals, pharmacists must be mature and realistic enough to accept a patient-centered interdisciplinary approach as the most effective and efficient method of providing patient care.*

Patient education is one good example of an instance in which an interdisciplinary approach may be most appropriate. At one time, pharmacists felt they were not giving complete services to the patient unless they personally provided the drug counseling. While we know patients are more compliant if they receive some instruction relating to their medication regimen, aren't we being provincial and unrealistic when we think only the pharmacist can provide that instruction?

A mechanism for patient education is probably already in place in the hospital. Rather than developing a parallel effort for the pharmacist's direct counseling of patients, isn't it more logical to assist the professionals already doing the job to incorporate drug education?

Our contribution in this instance would be in developing the instructional materials and supporting the other health care personnel in the educational effort. At our hospital, Dr. John Romankiewicz recently developed a patient education program through the work of two interdisciplinary committees: The New York Hospital Medical Patient Care Committee and The New York Hospital Formulary and Therapeutics Committee.

Actually, the pharmacists provided the major thrust in designing and implementing the program, but the success of the program is the result of the work of not only the pharmacists but also of the physicians, nurses, and administrators. The pharmacists provide the necessary information and train the nurses in drug education. The physicians, within their respective specialities, review the data as they relate to patients, the disease state, and the effect on the physicians' therapeutic plans. The nurses then become primary patient educators for the inpatients, while the pharmacists serve this role for ambulatory care patients.[3-5]

To make the program work, the support of administration and the cooperation of the various members of the pharmacy department and the interdisciplinary medical patient care and formulary and therapeutics committees were all required—they established the proper environment.

The second critical factor in achieving full participation in patient care, including accountability, is related to us as individuals. We must ask ourselves at least the following questions:

- Why do I want to perform this role?
- How adequate is my knowledge?
- Am I capable of being fully accountable?
- If not, how can I increase my competence?
- Am I willing to make the personal commitment of time and energy necessary to not only gain but to maintain competency?

Our motivation to perform must be based on service to the patient. There is no place for professional ego in patient care. A patient-oriented attitude, stressing service, is an essential ingredient in our prescription for personal success. And this attitude is needed by all pharmacy personnel, not just by those who have direct clinical responsibilities.

Drug and disease knowledge is, of course, essential. We must honestly assess this ingredient as we make the commitment to patient responsibility. Any area of knowledge or skill needing reinforcement should be attended to. I believe that the best method of this reinforcement is self-learning. The best impetus to self-learning is the continual challenge provided by the demands of a comprehensive daily practice. When our practice demands us to broaden our knowledge, I personally do not believe that we need laws "mandating" continuing education. The quest for knowledge and the enthusiasm I have seen this past week within the throngs of professionals—here at this largest and most comprehensive pharmacy educational program in the world—demonstrate that our pharmacy practitioners have the commitment to patient orientation and a desire for learning.

During the past 20 years or so, services that seemed to be good for patient care often were easily implemented and readily received support from administration. At present, we are constantly faced with cost justification of programs of proven patient benefit.

The entire health care system is, and will continue to be, subject to the scrutiny of the government and the public. Thus, it becomes essential for institutional practitioners to find methods to assess the quality of our contributions, not only in terms of patient care but in terms of economic cost. Without such assessment, it is unlikely there will be any expansion of comprehensive services.

Assessment of the quality of patient care is, at best, difficult. In addition, pharmacists must initiate more programs aimed at the economic justification of the numerous advances in practice that we have already nurtured and advocated. I believe this activity must be a major goal of organized pharmacy—including the American Society of Hospital Pharmacists—so that pharmacists and the profession will be able to promote and innovate practices we know to be beneficial to patients.

One serious situation which must also receive some attention is related to the rapidly decreasing availability of employment opportunities for our young pharmacists—pharmacists with excellent educational credentials and expectations for professional satisfaction.

This situation is arising because of the lack of new hospital construction, the reduction of beds within our hospitals, the reduced number of positions in schools of pharmacy, and the economic ceilings that are being placed on hospitals and which increase the competition for available funds and new programs. This brings us back to the realization that pharmacy as a profession cannot be on the periphery of patient care. To flourish in the future, the patient must be our central focus. We as pharmacists must be accountable to that patient.

Being an optimist, I know that the future of pharmacy practice is bright if we center our activities around the patient and if we make the pharmacist accountable for patient services. I see patient accountability as the primary way to satisfy pharmacists' professional needs, to increase pharmacists' utilization, and to improve pharmaceutical and therapeutic aspects of patient care while effectively reducing our frustration stemming from a lack of use of our knowledge and skills.

(For the complete list of references cited, please see page 267 of the *American Journal of Hospital Pharmacy*, Mar. 1978.)

At the time he received this award, Herbert S. Carlin was the Apothecary-in-Chief of The Society of the New York Hospital in New York City.

1978

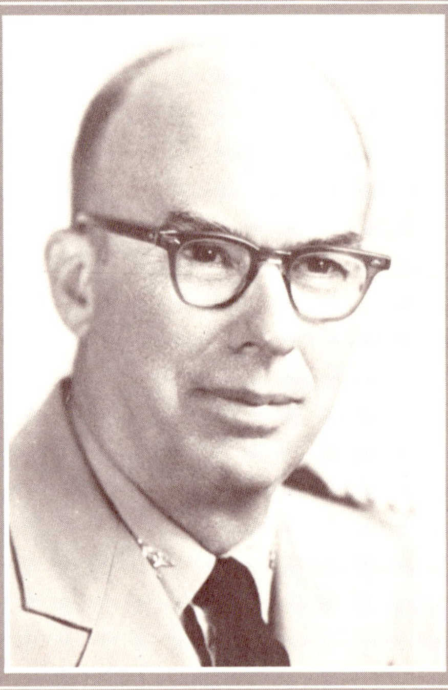

ALLEN J. BRANDS

"The patient's pharmacist is concerned with the individual patient's health and safety."

THE PATIENT'S PHARMACIST

Henry Ford once said: "The only foundation of real business is service." How true this statement is when applied to health care and pharmacy service. The word "service" is included in the term "pharmacy service" and is the very foundation upon which the practice of hospital pharmacy is based.

While a large number of drugs are stocked and dispensed in hospital pharmacies, each drug is dispensed for administration to an individual patient with a specific health problem. It must be remembered that the patient is being treated with a drug which has other actions besides those directed at the particular disease or target symptom. The patient's physical and mental well-being must be considered in treatment planning.

The assessment and treatment of patients by pharmacists go back several hundred years.[1] The general practitioner in England today is the lineal descendent of the apothecary of the 17th century. The Society of Apothecaries of England came into being in 1617, when it was constituted by the Royal Charter of James I. The Charter was drafted by Francis Bacon. At that time, the apothecaries were compounders and dispensers of medicines and assisted physicians in applying certain forms of treatment under their direction. During the first century after the Charter was granted, many members began to give advice and to supply medicines without the intervention of a physician. The College of Physicians exercised its legal powers in the endeavor to suppress this form of medical practice, but in 1703 the Society carried a test case to the House of Lords and gained a decision in its favor. Henceforth, it was recognized that the apothecaries could give advice to the sick, although they were not allowed to charge for it.

Taking advantage of the freedom the decision gave them, they studied medical textbooks to render themselves better equipped for the work before them. The result was the Apothecaries Act of 1815, which gave the Society the legal right to grant licenses to practice medicine throughout England and Wales and entrusted to it the duty of controlling that practice.

Changes in the practice of pharmacy have been taking place in hospital pharmacies in the United States, with pharmacists becoming deeply involved in the drug therapy of patients. I predict that this trend will grow because of the increasing complexity of drug therapy and the effects of drugs on patients.

The Study Commission on Pharmacy[2] emphasized that pharmacy is a knowledge system in which chemical substances and a people called patients interact. Needed and optimally effective drug therapy results only when drugs and those who consume them are fully understood. I wish to stress this reference in that the drugs and those who consume them are fully understood. When the pharmacist fully understands his patient and the prescribed drugs, we have the patient's pharmacist. The Study Commission[3] also stated that when pharmacy is viewed as a knowledge system, it must be judged as being only partially successful in delivering its full potential as a health service to the members of society.

Prior to the 1960s, hospital pharmacists had little or no patient contact, and they had little or no information concerning the problems of patients for whom they were supplying drugs. Barker[4] reported that while serving as a senior student in a hospital pharmacy class, the professor repeated an often-heard dictum "that one of the most important traditional responsibilities of the pharmacist is to prevent mistakes involving drugs." This professor's statement resulted in a study of medication errors in a hospital and a method of reducing medication errors in hospitals through the development of the unit dose drug distribution system. Over the years, unit dose drug distribution has been expanded and refined to include a systematic review of each patient's prescribed drugs for dosage and drug–drug interactions. The Joint Commission on Accreditation of Hospitals has included in its standards for pharmaceutical services a requirement that the pharmacist should review the prescriber's order, or a direct copy thereof, before the initial dose of medication is dispensed. This provides the opportunity for the pharmacist—the patient's pharmacist—to use his knowledge and skills in serving the individual patient.

Pharmacy is a profession. It is a knowledge system which the Study Commission on Pharmacy[3] reported as only partially successful in delivering its full potential as a health service to the members of society.

What is the purpose of the profession of pharmacy and the responsibilities of the individual pharmacist to a patient? The purpose and responsibilities of pharmacists are clearly stated in the Code of Ethics,[5] and I quote the preamble and first three principles:

These principles of professional conduct for pharmacists are established to guide the pharmacist in his relationship with patients, fellow practitioners, other health professionals and the public.

A pharmacist should hold the health and safety of patients to be of first consideration; he should render to each patient the full measure of his ability as an essential health practitioner.

A pharmacist should never knowingly condone the dispensing, promoting or distributing of drugs or medical devices, or assist therein, which are not of good quality, which do not meet standards required by law or which lack therapeutic value for the patient.

A pharmacist should always strive to perfect and enlarge his professional knowledge. He should utilize and make available this knowledge as may be required in accordance with his best professional judgment.

Why am I speaking of the patient's pharmacist? Wang[6] stated that with the complexity of drug therapy in current practice, it is difficult for one physician to become a leading authority of a medical center with experience and knowledge in both diagnosis and treatment. He further stated that in postgraduate medicine, the emphasis has been on diagnosis and not on treatment. Rational drug therapy means the proper use of drugs; it frequently means elimination of duplicating and conflicting drugs and the use of drugs at optimum therapeutic levels. Wang recommended the use of clinical pharmacologists for education in the treatment of patients in large teaching centers.

However, for the day-to-day patient care, clinical pharmacists have assumed much responsibility in drug therapy in many hospitals and clinics. Their clinical expertise concerns the use of drugs and choice of drugs in the treatment of disease. Now, if we take the clinical pharmacist and direct all of his efforts to the individual patient with prospective and concurrent drug use review, we have the patient's pharmacist.

What is a patient's pharmacist? What is his knowledge base? What are his duties and responsibilities?

A patient's pharmacist is familiar with the patient's medical and social history and his present health problems and ensures that the patient's drug therapy is appropriate at all times with no preventable harm to the patient from drug therapy. He speaks four languages—medical, nursing, lay, and pharmaceutical. Briefly, his knowledge base is the clinical use and actions of drugs, pharmacokinetics, optimum clinical response expected from drug therapy, monitoring and evaluating clinical response, and education counseling communication skills.

The activities of the patient's pharmacist include a prospective drug review and a concurrent drug review for inpatients and outpatients. Ideally, the pharmacist should be involved in the development of the drug treatment plan.

In order to evaluate adequately the drug therapy regimen, the patient's pharmacist must have certain information about the patient.

This includes a *drug history*. After an assessment is made of the patient's condition which is to be treated, one of the most reliable guides in selecting a drug for the individual patient is the patient's previous response to medication. A comprehensive drug history should include detailed information on daily dosage, dosage schedule, reason for using, clinical efficacy, side effects, patient acceptance, and reliability in adhering to the medication schedule. This information may prevent the prescribing and use of drugs which have been ineffective for the patient, have been unacceptable, or have caused adverse effects. It is also useful in the determination of the daily dosage and dosage schedule for those drugs in which the daily dosage and dosage schedule may vary from patient to patient. This prospective review of the drug therapy plan, using a comprehensive drug history, will eliminate problems that often develop from the drug therapy.

The *diagnosis and target symptoms* are essential in both the prospective and concurrent drug review and evaluation. The patient's pharmacist, in his prospective drug review, must be assured that the drug is indicated for the disease and target symptoms. In this review, the pharmacist should consider the relative efficacy of the prescribed drug and its cost as compared to other drugs used for the same condition. For many conditions, several drugs may be effective and available at different costs. In considering the patient's interest and health, the relative effectiveness of the drugs indicated should be of prime consideration in the decision and selection process. The patient's drug history will also have an impact on the drug selection. If the patient has had previous treatment with a particular drug for the same condition, this information, with the results of the treatment, should be considered in developing the drug treatment plan.

The dosage and dosage schedule should be tailored to the particular patient, his age and weight and other conditions that the drug therapy may affect. Too many times an average dose of a drug may be prescribed without any regard to the age or the weight of the patient.

The diagnosis and target symptoms are also necessary in the concurrent drug review by the patient's pharmacist. For inpatients, the pharmacist must collaborate with the physician and nurse in the sharing of information on the patient's progress under treatment. The pharmacist should also visit the patient to monitor and evaluate the results of the drug therapy. Has the natural course of the disease been modified as it should have been by the drug? Have the target symptoms such as fever, pain, malaise, or agitation been reduced or eliminated? Is it necessary to modify the drug therapy plan by changing the dosage or the drug because the desired results have not been obtained?

A patient interview, visual observations, physical assessment, and laboratory test results may be necessary to monitor and to evaluate the drug therapy in a concurrent drug use review. The patient's condition, the drug therapy, and anticipated results will dictate the frequency with which the pharmacist monitors and evaluates the drug aspects of his patient's care. For inpatients, this may vary from more than once a day to once a week or less often. For outpatients, the quantity of medicine dispensed would determine when the concurrent drug use review for monitoring and evaluation is done. The quantity of drugs dispensed to outpatients should be determined by when the patient's drug therapy should be reviewed and evaluated. This period, too, will vary with the patient's condition, his reliability in taking his medicine, and the drugs prescribed.

The patient's pharmacist will know whether the patient has *other diseases or conditions* that would be affected by the use of the drug and what drugs were being used concurrently. Some drugs are contraindicated, or special precautions must be taken when a patient has some chronic disease (e.g., glaucoma, impaired liver function, cardiovascular diseases). Age is of importance because of the possibility of decreased absorption, metabolism, and excretion rates. Other drugs prescribed for other conditions may interact with the new drug to decrease or increase the effectiveness of one or more of the drugs.

Adverse effects from drugs may result from known adverse reactions and allergies or adverse results from the misuse of drugs or improper dosages. The drug history is again important from the standpoint of the drugs that have caused adverse effects for the patient. The patient's history of other conditions or diseases is necessary to prevent or minimize adverse effects. If a drug must be used and it has potential for producing adverse effects, then this potential should be known by all the staff involved in the patient's care. The staff should also know the symptoms of the adverse effects.

Patient education and consultation is an integral part of the pharmacist's patient care responsibility. Education of the patient on the drugs used and drug-related aspects should begin on the day treatment is started or as soon thereafter as possible. For the inpatient, education should be a part of each visit to the patient, with a thorough review at the time of discharge of those drugs the patient will be using at home. The education should include the favorable results to be expected and the possible adverse effects. By knowing what results to expect from the drug therapy, the patient can assist the staff in determining if the desired results are obtained and when adverse effects occur.

Outpatients should receive education and counseling at each visit, even though they may have been taking the same drug over a long period of time. The *Pharmacy Practice*[7] newsletter stated that the typical level of memory retention is not high. Within two days, people forget 20% of what they have learned. Within four days, 40%; within nine days, 60%; and within 30 days, 74%. Therefore, repetition is essential.

Patient education and counseling should be done in privacy. A private consultation office has been found to be very effective in the U.S. Public Health Service hospital pharmacies. The patient and pharmacist are more at ease, and the patient has a tendency to ask questions for clarification. Pharmacists in the privacy of an office have learned of other health problems that the patient did not mention to the physician. Privacy is of utmost importance when the pharmacist is obtaining data for patient assessment to determine whether the disease is under control and the drug should be continued. Privacy is also essential in demonstrating the use of some drugs during education and counseling. The pharmacist comes to understand his patient and his problems when counseling is done in privacy, and the patient better understands, respects, and trusts his pharmacist.

The pharmacist should record in the medical record the results of his patient care activities.

First of all, the pharmacist should prepare a drug treatment plan for inclusion in the medical record for use by the nursing and medical staff. This drug treatment plan should have the drug name, dosage form, amount of each dose, time of day for each dose, anticipated length of therapy, favorable results to be expected, potential significant adverse effects and when to expect them, and laboratory tests and other physical and visible measurements with the times they should be conducted to determine the effect of the drug on the disease and to detect adverse effects. The plan should indicate action to take if adverse effects occur or treatment is not effective. This treatment plan can also be used in patient education.

When the patient's pharmacist conducts his prospective drug review, he should indicate in writing in the patient's record that the drug is indicated, the dosage and dosage schedule are appropriate, and there are no known preventable adverse drug effects, and sign his name. For the concurrent drug reviews, he should enter his findings as to the effectiveness of the therapy, the presence or absence of adverse effects, and the results of his patient education.

When the pharmacist finds a problem, it should be corrected immediately. He should take the appropriate action, which may be contacting the physician or the nurse or making the correction himself.

In conducting concurrent drug use reviews, there are three aspects to be considered: first, to assure that the disease is responding to the therapy; second, to detect any adverse drug effects; and third, to determine compliance or receipt of the drug by the patient.

The pharmacist's activities or process can be evaluated by a review of the pharmacist's notes in the medical record. Did he write a drug treatment plan? Did he review the drug therapy for appropriateness of the drug, dosage, and dosage schedule and for adverse effects? Did he provide counseling and education for the patient?

The outcome or results can be measured by a review of the patient's record to answer the following questions:

1. Was the drug indicated?
2. Were the dosage and dosage schedule appropriate?
3. Were there adverse drug effects?
4. Was the patient's disease cured or controlled in the appropriate period of time?
5. As an outpatient, did the patient comply in taking his drugs?

The American Society of Hospital Pharmacists has the right forum for the patient's pharmacist in the Special Interest Groups that it sponsors. At this 13th Annual Midyear Clinical Meeting, there are 11 Special Interest Group meetings that are concerned with patient pharmacy care. ASHP is moving forward, and pharmacists are moving forward.

The patient's pharmacist is concerned with the individual patient's health and safety. He uses his knowledge of the patient, drug actions, and drug treatment of diseases to ensure appropriate drug therapy. He collaborates with other professional staff, visits the patient for assessment and counseling, and enters his findings and assessments in the patient's medical record.

(For the complete list of references cited, please see page 315 of the *American Journal of Hospital Pharmacy*, Mar. 1979.)

At the time he received this award, Allen J. Brands was the Chief Pharmacy Officer of the Public Health Service, U.S. Department of Health, Education, and Welfare, and the Chief of the Indian Health Service Pharmacy Branch.

1979

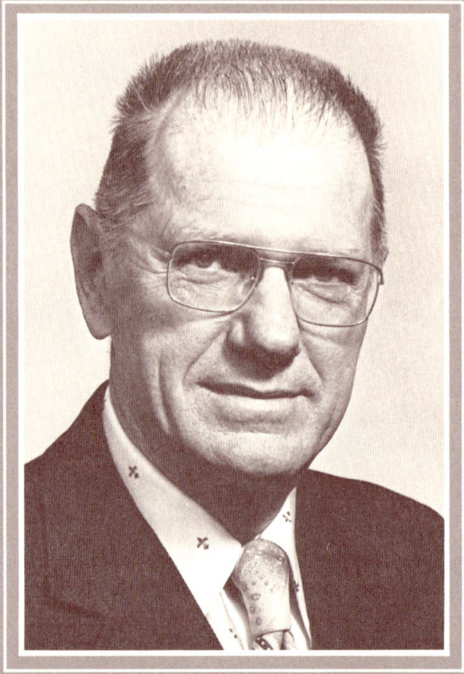

MILTON W. SKOLAUT

"I see many changes coming in our profession."

MOVING TOWARDS THE 21st CENTURY

I want to thank the Harvey A. K. Whitney Selection Committee of past recipients for the honor of selecting me to join their group. I also wish to thank the American Society of Hospital Pharmacists, the Southeastern Michigan Society of Hospital Pharmacists, and each of you for coming. Furthermore, I would not be here if it were not for the understanding, support, and encouragement of my best friend, my wife, Rheta.

Let us take a short trip back into history to review some events which may be of interest and then move forward to the year 2000, the beginning of the 21st century. Though many of you will agree with my forecasts because you happen to like what I say, while others will object because you disagree, none of us will really know the accuracy of these forecasts until the year 2000 arrives.

The first Harvey A. K. Whitney Lecture Award was given to Dr. W. Arthur Purdum, Chief Pharmacist of the Johns Hopkins Hospital in Baltimore, in 1950. I was associated with Arthur Purdum at the University of Maryland and later served as his assistant chief pharmacist at the Johns Hopkins Hospital from 1947 to 1949. Now, 29 years later, I am receiving this same award.

It is even more interesting to note that my predecessor at Duke University Medical Center also was formerly associated with the Johns Hopkins Hospital. I am speaking of I. Thomas Reamer, who worked at the Johns Hopkins Hospital for Mr. Robert S. Fuqua. In 1931, he departed Hopkins to become the chief pharmacist at the Duke University Hospital in Durham. In 1941, I arrived in Baltimore to work for Mr. Fuqua in a pharmacy internship, the forerunner of residency programs. While director at Duke, Tom Reamer received the Whitney Award in 1959. Twenty years later, I am being honored to join Tom. Hence, the Duke University Medical Center has had only two full-time directors of pharmacy, both of whom now have received the award. We are establishing quite a challenge for the next director.

I have devoted 38 years of my career to the practice of institutional pharmacy. It has been very rewarding to me, and institutional pharmacy practice is getting better, though considerably more complex. I also have served for 19 years as a member of the ASHP Executive Committee and the ASHP Board of Directors, including serving as president, vice president, and treasurer for 11 of those years. Based upon these experiences, I believe I can forecast some of our future trends, programs, and services.

Today's colleges of pharmacy are doing a better job of training students for the expanded roles now available in institutional practice. Many have developed innovative programs within the past five to seven years, and more programs are being developed or improved because of the endless, unselfish hard work of many of you. I foresee that graduate pharmacists will be able to go back to school part time or to participate in correspondence courses and complete a course with a final, short period of residence at a college of pharmacy. These programs will allow practicing pharmacists to upgrade themselves to stay competitive with new graduates, and such upgrading of practicing pharmacists can, in turn, provide stability and longevity in the professional work force.

The B.S. in Pharmacy Degree will be eliminated before the year 2000; by 1987, everyone coming out of school will have received a Pharm.D. degree. Because this degree will be the new standard, the push will be on in the early nineties to initiate another degree equivalent to the Ph.D. for a group of specialist pharmacists who will be educated to meet the needs of a total, clinically applied pharmacy practice. In the year 2000, the colleges will be graduating only 3000 new pharmacists per year, in response to both the changes in practice and the increased use of nonpharmacist assistants.

I see many changes coming in our profession—changes in responsibilities, departmental operations, and pharmacy practice. Some of these changes will be good and some will be upsetting, but one thing is certain—there will be changes.

Today, many institutional directors of pharmacy receive criticism that they hinder the new graduate intellectually and that they do not understand what is needed. In the eyes of the new graduate, some of these accusations are true, because the new graduate does not understand that the operation of a pharmacy in a hospital is extremely complicated. Budgeting and management are difficult and will become increasingly demanding with the limited funds available under constant pressures to reduce costs. We have made more progress in our practice in the 1970s than we did over the previous 30–40 years, and we are just getting started. But we must bear in mind one fact—the institution does not and will not revolve around the pharmacy, nor was it built so the pharmacist could practice.

Fortunately, in the 1990s and beyond, the young graduate will have two choices in the larger institutions—practice in a limited, specialized area or practice within the total area of pharmacy responsibility. The total service practitioners will be providing services in distribution, drug information, clinical rounding, teaching, and consultation. They also will be the ones who will clear paths for and who will assist those practicing as specialists. I believe we need to stress the practice of total pharmacy service in all institutions, but we need to assist in the further education of specialists in teaching hospitals as well. With the necessary experience and training, some of these specialists will practice within hospitals and some will move to ambulatory group practice settings.

The common criticism of medical practice is that everybody is specialized and no one looks at the whole patient. As a result, programs in which the physician is interested in the total patient are being developed (i.e., family practice). Pharmacy is moving in much the same way. Many new practitioners want to be highly specialized and actually care to know very little about the total pharmacy practice in the hospital. Yet, the hospital and the patient will be demanding total service which, in addition to excellent patient services, includes good management, reasonable costs, and liaison with the entire hospital. To meet these demands will require practitioners who can maintain good working relationships with the hospital administration and the Pharmacy and Therapeutics Committee, and who can provide careful attention to infection control, sterilization quality control, drug distribution quality control and safety, drug use review, educational programs, service and performance within prescribed standards, and productivity.

Some practitioners will want to specialize in cardiology, infectious diseases, neurology, emergency medicine, or the like, and I encourage this where conditions permit and where there is a need. Since this will be possible in only a limited number of large teaching institutions, residency and other hospital training programs will be obliged to train well-rounded pharmacists who can assume responsibility for total patient-oriented services in smaller institutions.

As patients become more familiar with health care programs and continue to demand excellence while keeping costs down, we will be expected to account for our services, our productivity, and our value to the institution and the patient. Many of us now practicing will find that our new, innovative programs will change present duties. While I do not think that pharmacists will be eliminated from institutions, other than through attrition, we will have fewer practitioners in the future than we do now. The clinical movement, or total patient service, will proceed at a quickening pace, and I see many of the specialists working with physicians in group practices. I see the pharmacist specialist as a primary drug and dose prescriber, or advisor, in the routine care of patients. As the individual pharmacist working with a group of physicians shows his credibility, he will become an indispensable member of the team.

There will continue to be individual frustration within institutions where the pharmacist practices as part of the pharmacy department. No position in any institution can be ideal in every respect. All positions have good and bad functions, because specific tasks must be performed for the patient's total care. As cost containment gathers force, hospitals will be forced to cut programs to reduce expenditures. Obviously, as most physicians will tell you, we cannot cut in the nursing department. Dietary will be fairly secure because we will not stop feeding patients. Radiology and laboratories will not be cut, because physicians feel they cannot diagnose without these services.

This leaves pharmacy, physical therapy, environmental services, operating rooms, and maintenance most vulnerable to cost-reduction efforts. Pharmacy will have to manage its operation very carefully. Pharmacists will need to know how to manage and how to budget, and they will have to justify existing services and positions as well as new programs and services.

There will be a number of large departments of pharmacy where the directorship will be split. A professional director will supervise and direct professional services only, and a nonprofessional director will handle other management functions, such as procurement, charges, inventories, and personnel management in nonprofessional matters. This nonpharmacist director will have a specialized education, such as an M.B.A. degree, and will exhibit skills in these types of responsibility.

I believe that a pharmacist, regardless of his degree or where he practices, is still a pharmacist; it can be no other way. Many pharmacy leaders have concurred and believe that we should have only one, big organization. This has not been and, without modifications, will not be the solution. We must realize that any one organization cannot be responsive to the different needs of this multifaceted profession.

Yet, we will find that we have to unite. Pharmacists must establish a successful umbrella organization comprised of a group of more specialized organizations that do not compete with one another and that can work together without requiring membership in several organizations. Whatever the names of these organizations may be, their objectives will be the welfare of *pharmacy* and the assistance of *pharmacists* in serving the public, regardless of the ways in which they provide such services.

The actual role of the institutional pharmacist has yet to be recognized by the public. By 1984, the Society will embark on an extensive program of educating patients about the pharmacist's contributions to their health care in the institutional setting.

Let us review the Society's membership and future trends. The current membership is over 18,000. Of this number, approximately half are active members and the rest are first-, second-, third-, and fourth-year pledges, students, and others. With the ASHP programs and services now being provided, I predict that the total membership will level out at 21,000. However, if the Society is successful in broadening its role through extending institutional practice into home health care, I then predict that by 1987 our total membership will be 25,000 and by the year 2000 it will be 40,000. There will be an amazing shift of membership categories by this time. A large number of the members will be technicians and technologists, representing individuals with two levels of training and legal recognition.

The technologists will be legally recognized as associate pharmacists. A number of schools will be offering programs for two-year technologists or associate pharmacists by 1986. By 1995, there will be at least 42 states licensing these individuals. Technicians, however, will continue to be trained in institution-based or noncollege programs and will have certification recognition by many state boards of pharmacy.

The ASHP must continually review its responsiveness to the practitioner's needs. As the ASHP gets bigger, members may perceive that the Society has become more remote. Even with our efforts through deliberations of the Councils, SIGs, and the House of Delegates, we must continually reexamine our organizational structure to determine if it truly is responsive to the interests of the majority of practitioners.

The Society has to become even more active in the legislative field, but the state societies will have the greatest opportunity and need for legislative involvement. The ASHP can only continue to stress and assist in sensitizing members to the importance of local and state involvement. The members themselves must actively encourage state chapters to increase awareness and participation in legislative and agency regulatory matters.

As a reminder of the Society's growth over the last 25 years, let me cite several treasurer's reports. In 1955, when I was vice president, Treasurer Sister Mary Rebecca reported an income of $11,250 and expenses of $13,515 with a savings account of $1,020. In 1963, when I was president, Treasurer Sister Mary Berenice reported the income as $303,432 and expenses of $317,325. In 1968, my first year as treasurer, I reported an income of $883,985 and expenses of $874,023, while the 1979 income and expenses will exceed $4,080,000. The treasurer's report in the year 2000 will report an income and expenses of over $20 million or, possibly, as high as $25 million. With the many new membership-directed programs, ASHP dues will be $215 per year by the year 2000.

Hospitals will embark on communication programs directed to the public that are based upon sound marketing principles. Hospitals will be forced to listen to patients, their families and friends, and consumer groups and then to respond by providing imaginative, appropriate, and useful health programs. Many hospitals will establish regional and local advisory groups, as well as being required to respond to citizen awareness groups.

I believe that the 7000 hospitals existing in 1979 will decrease to 5600 by 1990 and to 5100 by 2000. Hospitals will not be necessary in every small town, but those hospitals that do remain will expand and prosper by referrals from the ambulatory health centers that will be operating in the small towns.

Consumers will continue to demand improved regulatory protection as drugs and services provided by the pharmacist are more closely scrutinized. The pharmacist will become more responsible for drug product selection, less concerned about trade names, and more knowledgeable about bioavailability and quality consistency, and will improve patient compliance by proper counseling, recommend appropriate drug therapy, and control the delivery of that product to the patient.

The successful institutional pharmacy practitioner of the future will benefit from:

1. Improved education, including individualized residency programs,
2. Commitment to a total pharmacy service, including specialized services,
3. Commitment to membership support of the ASHP in return for broader organizational support and services to the members, and
4. Changes in expectations of practice from physicians, colleagues, and the public that will open entirely new roles and opportunities for our pharmacists.

At the time he received this award, Milton W. Skolaut was the Director of Pharmacy at Duke Hospital, Durham, North Carolina, and Adjunct Professor at the School of Pharmacy, University of North Carolina, Chapel Hill.

1980

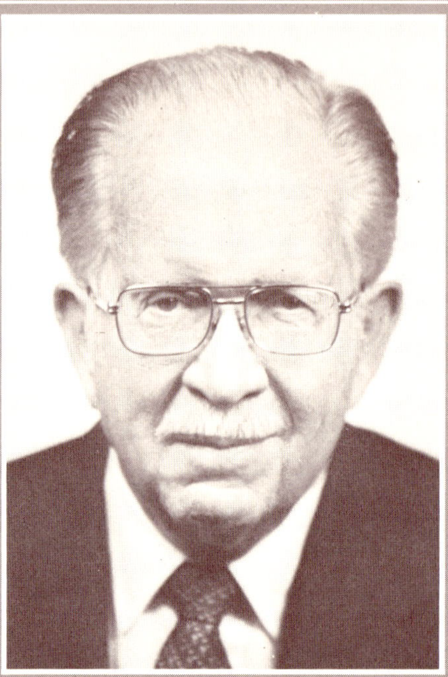

DONALD C. BRODIE

"A theory dealing with the practice of pharmacy. . .could be useful in directing the course of our future."

NEED FOR A THEORETICAL BASE FOR PHARMACY PRACTICE

We are gathered this evening to pay tribute to the memory of Harvey A. K. Whitney. Some of us here knew Harvey Whitney when he was chief pharmacist at the University of Michigan Hospital and can match the name with the man; some of us know only the name. In either case, we come together each year with a resolve to perpetuate his memory by creating an environment of admiration, respect, and reverence for a hospital pharmacist of many talents.

Harvey Whitney was a man who could motivate and stimulate people; during the course of his career, he developed a cadre of disciples who carried his philosophies and goals for hospital pharmacy practice wherever they went. Some of these are with us this evening. Harvey Whitney had a keen sense that permitted him to detect deficiencies in the pharmacy curriculum of his day in light of the needs of students who would practice in hospitals. Harvey Whitney was the founder of the American Society of Hospital Pharmacists; he was its first president. Harvey Whitney was a man who made things happen; he inspired people; he shaped reality, both conceptually and physically. His career was a living example of the admonition:

Don't go where the path leads, rather go where there is no path and leave a trail.

We revere and honor his memory this night.

I have entitled my address "Need for a Theoretical Base for Pharmacy Practice." Actually, I had hoped to include some comments on pharmaceutical education with particular reference to the needs of hospital pharmacy and a few thoughts for the future, but the constraints of time made that totally impractical. I concluded that for this occasion the idea of a theoretical base was the most appropriate of the three ideas, and I am leaving the other two to some future time.

We have passed over the threshold into the 1980s. The only certainty of today is the uncertainty of tomorrow. Our nation probably has never entered a decade with more formidable issues to be solved than those that lie ahead in the 1980s. One of the issues of particular concern is the entire spectrum of problems involving health: changing roles of health professionals, the cost of health care and cost containment, health manpower and the use of support personnel, the role of government in health care delivery, the impact of computers and high technology, and the numerous problems in bioethics resulting from recombinant DNA research.

For the profession of pharmacy as a whole, the central issue will continue to be the acceptance of the fact and reality of change and the determination to take an active role in shaping that change. The alternatives seem obvious: pharmacy either accepts what the future brings or works to shape the future in accordance with what pharmacists want that future to be. One of the difficult problems will be the identification of changes before and as they occur and the development of strategies to deal with them. One strategy that is available to us is the development of a theoretical base for pharmacy practice. To my knowledge, pharmacists have never been challenged by the idea that there might be a theory (or a family of theories) dealing with the practice of pharmacy and that such theory or theories could be useful in directing the course of our future.

I am defining "theoretical base" to mean an intellectual framework designed to serve the purposes and needs of future planning for pharmacy. The framework or structure is based on empirical information that is consistent with data available to support it either in the literature or elsewhere. You will sense from this definition that we are dealing with a structure composed of concepts and other sets of abstract ideas that, when brought together, form an ideal state. In fact, Dickoff and James,[1] in their definition of "theory," emphasize the abstract nature of theory:

> *. . . a conceptual system or framework invented to some purpose; and as the purpose varies so too must vary the structure and complexity of the system.*

What a worthy objective for the profession were it to begin building a theoretical base for pharmacy practice during the decade of the eighties. Such an effort will not lead to a neatly bound compendium entitled "A Theory of Pharmacy Practice." Rather, it will be in the form of a series of ideas, statements, hypotheses, and other forms of abstraction. When statements about pharmacists and pharmacy can be interrelated and describe a causal process (relationship), they can be studied, documented, and tested. If empirical data can be derived from causal processes and combined with existing data, they can be presented to members of the pharmacy profession for study, modification, and adoption. Where existing data are not adequate, research will be necessary to provide the documentation. What we are striving for is to develop a conceptual base in the form of ideas, constructs, and statements which describes, clarifies, and strengthens the societal position of pharmacy and its practitioners. It is part of the scientific body of knowledge about pharmacy developed by pharmacists in keeping with the purposes of pharmacy. In his introductory statement to his *Primer in Theory Construction*, Professor Paul Reynolds[2] states:

A scientific body of knowledge consists of those concepts and statements that scientists consider useful for achieving the purposes of science.

As our statements and concepts lead to tangible evidence that documents the purpose and needs of pharmacy, they begin to shape the framework which ultimately will encompass the theoretical base of pharmacy practice.

The construction of models of professional behavior is a useful step in the development of a theoretical base for pharmacy practice. Models, representations of reality or some hypothetical state of reality, are designed to provide clarity, understanding, and guidance. Models have been useful in studying social systems, such as systems of evaluation or patterns of human behavior. They can be constructed to represent new or modified roles for health professionals as a means of examining their proposed utility and general acceptance. A model for pharmacists, for example, would emphasize those contributions unique to pharmacists because of their education and training, such as monitoring drug therapy, applying pharmacokinetic principles to the design and adjustment of dose regimens, providing drug information to physicians and patients, and maintaining individual patient records of drug usage. It would include activities being developed by selected pharmacists in the care of certain classes of patients (oncology) in hospitals and ambulant patients in the out-of-hospital setting and the reciprocal relationships between physicians and pharmacists designed to improve the level of patient care. The model would include those activities that are at variance with traditional pharmacist functions, such as the prescribing of drugs as currently being done legally on an experimental basis in California.[3]

In each instance, the uniqueness of the pharmacist's contribution to society would be emphasized as well as the desire and confidence pharmacists have in serving societal needs. Obviously, such a model would represent an alternative to pharmacists' traditional behavior and, if it were constructed, could be studied to determine its acceptability by present-day pharmacists, the public, and other health professionals. The degree of acceptability would provide justification and guidance to the profession for developing the modified role specified in the model. Similarly, it would guide the schools of pharmacy in adjusting the pharmacy curriculum in keeping with the new role.

If pharmacists were to begin construction of a theoretical base, they would find a useful guideline in the generally accepted pattern of professional behavior usually referred to as the paradigm for the professions. The literary form in which the paradigm is presented will vary from scholar to scholar, but there is general agreement in terms of behavioral characteristics. I have chosen a model adapted from one presented by Argyris and Schon in their text, *Theory in Practice: Increasing Professional Effectiveness:*[4]

1. *An ideology—based on the original faith professed by a profession.*
2. *An ethic—that is binding on the practitioners of a profession.*
3. *A body of knowledge—unique to a given profession.*
4. *A set of skills—which, when combined, form the technique of a profession.*
5. *A guild—of those entitled to practice a profession—the brotherhood.*
6. *Authority—granted by society as a form of professional respect and licensure or certification.*
7. *An institutional setting—where a profession is practiced in a standardized environment such as a hospital, courtroom, pharmacy, and church.*
8. *A theory—based on the societal benefits derived from the faith professed—the ideology.*

Historically, the prototypical professional was the priest who practiced as a multiprofessional in an undifferentiated way, serving as minister, judge, healer, and teacher. In time, the professions of theology, law, medicine, and education were differentiated from the priesthood as secular institutions. The process of differentiation has been replicated many times in history with the growth of knowledge and skill where today we recognize some 200 professions, more than 50 of which are in the health field. Pharmacy was differentiated from medicine in the late Middle Ages and stands today as one of the autonomous health professions with a very specific mission in society.[5] That mission, however, has suffered from the lack of definition over the past 50 years as the responsibility for making medicines has passed to the pharmaceutical industry. Some questions have been raised by social scientists and others regarding the professional status of pharmacy because of the passive attitudes and behavior of many pharmacists, the environment in which much pharmacy is practiced, and the apparent belief that the boundaries of the pharmacist's social responsibility are circumscribed by the act of pharmaceutical dispensing. These matters should be of concern to us as we begin to think of a theoretical base for pharmacy practice.

Because the professions have their roots in religion, Palmer[6] was prompted to say:

A professional, as I understand it, is supposed to profess, to testify, to bear witness to some sort of faith or confidence or point of view. Traditionally, at least, it was only because he did so that he merited being called "professional."

Thus, medicine professed health, law professed justice, education professed truth, and the ministry professed salvation. And pharmacy —what did pharmacy profess? We have difficulty with this question in today's world. We do not have a clear picture of nor do we communicate with conviction that which we profess. As a result, the transformation of what we profess into a professional ideology seems distorted or in some way is incomplete. A question that has nagged me for years deals with the idea that at one time pharmacists did make a strong testimony of commitment to society that ultimately was transformed into an ideology for the profession. In the mid sixties, I was searching for an answer by identifying a mainstream function for medicine, law, theology, and other professions; I could not identify one for pharmacy. In the report of the Commission on Pharmaceutical Services to Ambulant Patients by Hospitals and Related Facilities,[7] I wrote:

Does pharmacy practice have, in a historic sense, a mainstream component as have other professions? Has it had one only to lose it to time, science, technology, and social change? Has it had one only to lose it to professional neglect, such as over-indulgence in nonprofessional activities, or, perhaps, an attempt to serve the public on a part-time basis? Has it had one that in time has become so ill-defined in its outline that both practitioner and layman alike have difficulty in identifying the distinguishing marks?

I am forced to acknowledge that the faith pharmacists professed in my time has not led to a strong professional ideology that generates confidence in the values that are inherent in the services pharmacists provide. That ideology must be strengthened and restored for the 21st century envisioned by Alvin Toffler[8] and other futurists. No doubt, some of the historic ideology has eroded with the industrialization of pharmacy, which stripped the practitioner of many creative functions unique to him.

Without a clear ideological component in the professional paradigm, the task of constructing a theoretical base for pharmacy practice is made difficult. The ideology, fully developed, envisions a better world because of the availability of drugs and drug-related services delivered by pharmacists who are educated and trained to fulfill these societal needs.[9] Because of the availability of these services, society is the beneficiary; without them, the welfare of society is in jeopardy. As we think about our professional ideology and plan construction of a theoretical base for professional practice, there is yet another component that lacks clear definition in the minds of most people, including pharmacists. That component is an identified and articulated professional purpose. During my search for identity of a mainstream function for pharmacy, I proposed that drug-use control was that function:

. . . the sum total of knowledge, understanding, judgments, procedures, skills, controls, and ethics that assures optimal safety in the distribution and use of medication.

This concept gave us light at the end of what seemed, at the time, to be a badly obscured tunnel. Richard Penna[10] commented recently that this concept provided a ray of hope to "younger pharmacists" and "identified what pharmacists should be doing in serving the health needs of the American public." Is the concept of drug-use control our professional purpose? What is the object for which pharmacy exists? Is that object essential for the welfare of society or is it a convenience? I believe there is general agreement among pharmacists that their role in society is the delivery of the drug component of health care, but just what the limits of that role are is a question for which there is as yet no universal agreement. The answer, in my opinion, will direct the future course of pharmacy in our time. If that role expands as a result of progressive and responsible behavior, the slope of the curve of professionalism will be positive; if pharmacists choose to retain their traditional behavior, the slope almost surely will regress.

Pharmacists' behavior has changed perceptibly since World War II, undergoing the greatest change in the 1960s with the emergence of an expanded clinical role. If one lists the services pharmacists are providing today, he would find that they could be arranged in one of three categories:

1. Services mandated by law, rule, or regulation.
2. Discretionary services provided by a majority of pharmacists.
3. Discretionary services provided by a small minority of pharmacists.

He would find that there would not be a consensus among pharmacists that they should provide all the listed discretionary services. Even if the list were submitted to hospital pharmacists on the one hand and community practitioners on the other, still there would not be agreement among those in either group. But if the profession seeks guidance in the development of an expanded clinical role for its practitioners, it must rely particularly on its acceptability by pharmacists in addition to that by the public and other health professionals. This leads to a researchable question: What is the degree of consensus among pharmacists, consumers, and other health care providers on the acceptability of an expanded role for pharmacists, including the clinical services assumed in the current model?

The following[a] or some such list of pharmacists' services can be used to determine the degree of consensus. Whatever list is used, it should contain those clinical services already provided by pharmacists (to assess the minimal level of consensus) and a brief description of each service (to aid respondents). These services, incorporated into a scientifically designed and tested questionnaire, can be submitted to an agreed upon population of pharmacists, consumers, and physicians in order to answer two questions: Should the service be provided by any health professional? Should pharmacists provide the service?

1. Compounds and dispenses prescriptions.
2. Assumes custodial care and responsibility for the distribution of controlled substances.
3. Explains the directions for use of prescription medicines at the time of delivery of prescriptions to ambulant patients.
4. Delivers package inserts (PPIs) to patients at the time of delivery of estrogens and progestational agents.
5. Establishes and monitors a system to insure proper storage for perishable pharmacy items such as insulin and other biological products.
6. Selects the manufacturing source of drug products to be purchased under generic names.
7. Maintains prescription profile records for ambulant patients.
8. Refers to prescription profile records prior to dispensing refill prescriptions.
9. Obtains a drug history on selected inpatients and ambulant patients.
10. Conducts drug-use studies at periodic intervals using computer printouts and other sources of data.
11. Develops guidelines for the use of antibiotics.
12. Applies pharmacokinetic principles in determining or modifying the dose of selected drugs.
13. Provides patient counseling on an individual basis or through some form of mass media.
14. Provides formal and informal consultations with physicians regarding patient drug therapy problems.
15. Applies selected physical assessment techniques in evaluating patient responses to drug therapy.
16. Provides supplies and appropriate counseling services in the use of ostomy appliances and other surgical and sickroom supplies.
17. Provides emergency services such as poison information, cardiovascular pulmonary resuscitation, and counseling regarding the appropriate use of drugs in emergent situations.
18. Reviews periodically the use of drugs in nursing homes in accordance with professional and legal standards.
19. Participates in home health care programs with public health nurses.

20. Interprets drug levels for selected drugs in order to obtain optimal benefit in drug therapy.

Assuming that a scientifically valid study is conducted and the results showed a consensus ranging from 55 to 70% in support of pharmacists assuming an expanded role, what significance might these results have? They surely would lend support, confidence, and direction to the profession in its efforts to improve the utility of its practitioners. On the other hand, if one or both of the nonpharmacist groups believed that pharmacists should not provide the services, it would lead to an understanding of reality and simultaneously provide guidance in developing long-range strategy to shape that reality. But, in addition, such a study would contribute to the development of a theory for pharmacy practice. I have used this example because it illustrates how the profession of pharmacy can relate "theory development" to planning for the future. It places future planning in a broader frame of reference than we are accustomed to using.

The worth of pharmacy to society is judged by the actions and services of its practitioners. These actions justify or deny its recognition and acceptance as a profession. Pharmacists provide action; they are doers; they, as other professionals, define their scope of social concern through a more or less standardized pattern of professional behavior. They create, construct, and maintain reality. But the true professional does more than create, construct, and maintain the status quo. He shapes and changes reality and has before him those purposes that have been "invented" or "created" by and for his profession. Dickoff and James[1] summarize professional purpose as follows:

> *. . . a professional cannot just watch, cannot just do, and cannot just hope or dream . . . A theory for a profession or practice discipline must provide for more than mere understanding or "describing" or even predicting reality and must provide a conceptualization specially intended to guide the shaping of reality to that profession's professional purpose.*

You in my audience tonight—pharmacists, scientists, and researchers—have the ability and the capacity to shape and change that reality; I challenge you to commit yourselves to such a goal because you have the vision and discipline to do so. But a theoretical base for pharmacy practice cannot be perceived according to traditional views of the world as we know it today. Our professional purpose and ideology must be perceived and articulated in view of that world we believe lies ahead. No one knows precisely the dimensions of that world, but futurists are beginning to give us a glimpse of some of its characteristics. Alvin Toffler[8] says:

> *Today, four clusters of related industries are poised for major growth and are likely*

to become the backbone industries of the Third Wave era, bringing with the, once more, major shifts in economic power and in social and political alignments.

Those industries—electronics and computers, space exploration, ocean exploration, and genetic engineering—all will have an impact on the future practice of pharmacy.

Futurist Robert Theobald[11] said in 1978:

We should recognize that we must move away from our industrial/mobile society toward a communication/community society. This shift will require modification in our social patterns which will be at least as great as those which occurred between the agricultural era and industrial era but they will take place far more rapidly. One of the most worrying aspects of the present period is the failure to understand the speed and scope of the microelectronic revolution which will change so much of our lives in the next decade.

Mr. Theobald's last sentence reminds us that the "future is now."[12] I am going into that future with hope and optimism notwithstanding the negative signs that surround us. I believe that you as hospital pharmacists and the Society which directs your professional destinies can share in my confidence. The experience, the successes, and the failures of the past justify our approach to the future, with the anticipation that the problems we find there will be solvable and that we can solve them. And that being so justifies our hope and confidence for continued growth.

(For the complete list of references cited, please see pages 53–54 of the *American Journal of Hospital Pharmacy*, Jan. 1981.)

At the time he received this award, Donald C. Brodie was Professor Emeritus of the University of California and Adjunct Professor of Medicine and Pharmacy at the University of Southern California, Los Angeles.

1981

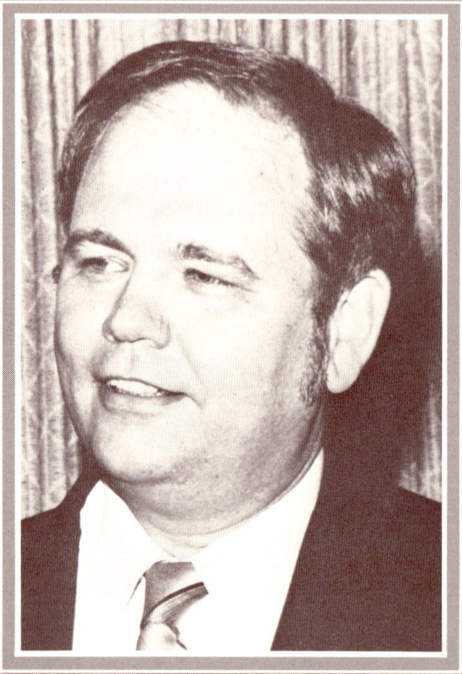

KENNETH N. BARKER

"There will be no time for pseudopharmacy."

PSEUDO-PHARMACY PRACTICE AND THE FUTURE

I am very grateful for this award. This will always be one of the most significant events of my life.

I've spent most of my career in research, on topics having to do with the evaluation of systems and organizations. I assume my receiving the award had something to do with that, and so I will speak to you as a researcher observing hospital pharmacy, its practice, and its organization.

My topic will be the future and a change we must make to get ready for it.

The future is coming. It's rushing at us with some startling changes.

You have surely heard by now that America is growing up. Already there are more retired people in the United States than the total population of Canada. By the year 2025, there will be 85 million Americans over age 55.

The net effect is that the average patient will have more illnesses, and more money to spend on them. He will also be better educated, demand better care, and raise more hell when he doesn't get it. What else can you expect from someone who has his mortgage paid off, his kids through college, and no boss to please? What does he do for aggravation?

We are in the midst of a communications revolution. While our newspapers have been losing circulation, in Japan and in Great Britain, and soon in Atlanta, TV users can push a button to request the display of a dozen different data services, such as stock market quotations, ball scores, and theater reservations.

The decline of the post office is in sight, as secretaries begin typing letters that are transmitted by phone line to a cathode-ray tube (CRT) or printer in the addressee's office. And the French are eliminating the phone book and replacing it with a CRT in each home.

The communications revolution will enable many people to work at home. Already, half of the 2000 Western Electric employees in their Northern Illinois plant work at home. This will not only save enormous amounts of time and gasoline involved in commuting but also help bring families back together, to *work* together.

Home microcomputers will be as common as indoor plumbing. While you are at work, your computer will take your grocery list and call the foodstore computers all over town to shop for the best prices.

Shortly, we will be manufacturing drugs in space, which offers gravity-free electrophoresis and a super supply of vacuum.

In his book *The Third Wave*, Alvin Toffler[1] describes the rise of the "prosumer," a term meaning the consumer who produces that which he consumes. Every "do-it-yourselfer" is a prosumer. This includes the people already checking their own blood pressure in coin-operated machines, mothers who learn how to take throat cultures themselves, and the housewife who buys a "smart" electric sewing machine. Instead of a pattern, she buys a cassette with a program on it that will sew the dress for her.

The most disturbing change of all is the accelerating pace of change itself.

Consider speed. It was not until 1784 that man finally traveled as fast as 10 miles an hour on a steam locomotive. Less than 200 years later, men in space capsules circle the earth at 18,000 miles per hour.

For the vacuum cleaner, electric range, and refrigerator, it took 34 years between the time they were invented and became widely used. But for later inventions, such as the electric frying pan and television, the span was only eight years. Technology feeds upon itself. Each new development makes more developments possible.

The number of scientific journals and articles is doubling about every 15 years. In part, that is probably because 90% of all the scientists who ever lived are alive today—publishing like crazy—all trying to get tenure.

The scariest part of it all is that I'm not really talking about the future. Everything I've mentioned is already here, in one stage or another.

Are we ready to face the future? How well have we hospital pharmacists responded in the past? How good have we been at adopting the innovations needed to cope with new demands upon us?

To evalute our past performance, I propose we use the "Theory of the Diffusion of Innovations." This theory has to do with the process of the spread of a new idea from the time of its origination to its ultimate widespread adoption or demise. This process might take about 10 years, for example, as it moves through the five stages of:

1. Awareness.
2. Interest.

3. Evaluation.
4. Trial.
5. Adoption.

For a case study, there are several different innovations in hospital pharmacy practice that we could examine. I propose to use unit dose dispensing.

The unit dose dispensing concept was first proposed at the end of the 1950s. To set the stage, here is a brief idea of the world of hospital pharmacy in those times.

Only 47% of hospitals had at least one pharmacist on a full-time basis in 1952.

The news section of the ASHP *Bulletin* reported that Paul Parker was appointed chief at the University of Chicago Clinics. It also said a graduating intern, named Clifton J. Latiolais, would receive his Master of Science degree in June. (I think he made it.)

A column in the journal called "Therapeutic Trends" discussed the drug Aureomycin. You could also read George Archambault's article "Complete Hospital System for Control of Narcotics, Hypnotics, and Other Drugs."

But, most of the articles in the fifties had to do with bulk manufacturing. Someone later called that period the "bulk manufacturing decade." A typical journal article dealt with the topic "The Use of Propylene Glycol as a Substitute for Glycerin." Alan Beck presented pictures of a simple automatic bottler.

During the fifties, people were concerned about the nursing shortage—that's the previous one, not the latest one. Near the end of the fifties, it was discovered that 25% of nursing time was spent handling medications.

In 1960, the dimensions of the medication error problem became known, and the demand for innovations in drug distribution fell upon us. The response was the unit dose dispensing concept. It moved quickly through the early stages towards adoption, fueled by money from large Public Health Service grants and strong support from ASHP.

By the mid-sixties, it seemed as if every pharmacy had a pilot study of a unit dose system.[2–5]

Conducting a pilot study became such a fad that our research group was asked more than once to come to a hospital and "put on" a pilot study, though there were no real plans to go further if it worked. We could have played more cities than "The Sound of Music" if we had wanted to.

Unfortunately, after these pilot study "road shows" closed, everybody went home, so to speak. In 1975, Wallace Werble, the editor of *The Pink Sheet*, spoke at a meeting of hospital pharmacists and asked, "Whatever happened to unit dose?"

The theory of the diffusion of innovations tells us that the rate of adoption of an innovation is usually affected by the five factors shown below:

1. Advantage to adopter.
2. Compatibility with cultural norms.
3. Complexity.
4. Divisibility (can be tried piecemeal).
5. Communicability.

The president of ASHP in 1975 was Fred Eckel. Fred said he thought the problem was the first factor.[6] He laid the blame on pharmacists who dragged their feet after they discovered that unit dose dispensing was hard work. He suggested that many hospital pharmacists were giving only lip service to implementing new pharmacy programs.

My own experience supports Fred's observations about lip service, which I call "pseudopharmacy."

Have you ever gone to visit the pharmacy of one of the authors of a journal article to see for yourself the new system he wrote about?

I visited a famous proponent of the formulary system to find that his hospital didn't have one.

I visited a pioneer drug information center to discover that they now answer only two requests per week.

I visited a famous IV admixture service to discover they prepare admixtures only upon request, between 8 a.m. and 5 p.m. and only on weekdays.

How about a "total unit dose system" that does not include controlled drugs or IVs?

But there might be good excuses in these cases. Besides, everybody knows, to paraphrase the old song, "It ain't necessarily so, it ain't necessarily so, the things that you're liable to read in the *Journal*, they ain't necessarily so!"

Big deal!

Does it really make any difference?

In 1975, a 12-year-old boy in our town was hit by a car. He spent five hours in surgery and eight days in a coma. After that, he was hospitalized for several weeks.

One day the boy's mother found a little card on the floor of his hospital room. It was a medicine card calling for kanamycin injection. She gave the card to the doctor, who mumbled "I never ordered that." But then he said: "Don't worry, it probably did him some good." But the boy was already having difficulties with his hearing, discovered when it was noticed he could no longer hear the sound of the floor cleaning machine in the hall outside his room.

The boy was my youngest son, Doug. He was a victim of a series of medication errors which occurred because the nurse put the wrong patient's name on a medicine card. The hospital was considered the best in town, but their "unit dose system" didn't include patient profiles and injections were dispensed in multiple-dose vials.

As I stood in Doug's hospital room, I was stunned. My next thought was this: 14 years later, nothing has changed. This is what I saw in 1961 while observing nurses for medication errors for my master's thesis.

All of those papers published, the conferences held, the publicity—nevertheless, a patient in one of our better hospitals, claiming to have "unit dose," could still receive a drug like kanamycin injection by mistake for *four days*. And what if we hadn't found the card?

Pseudopharmacy—it does make a difference when it gets to you personally.

In 1977, we got a chance to take a good close look at a "state-of-the-art unit dose system" in a collaborative study with Joe Harris at Sinai Hospital in Detroit.

As part of a three-year study, we had a pharmacist accompany selected nurses as they prepared their medications and then witness the actual administration to the patient. The observer's notes, telling what was actually done, were compared with the physician's orders on the patient's chart to identify medication errors. The results revealed an error rate of 9%, not the 3% or less that was achieved with the systems tested 10–15 years ago.

Why? Here is some of what we found.

Recall that the original concept for a unit dose system included this key feature: *dose dispensed at the time each dose is due.*

A major source of errors under their system was where the correct unit dose was delivered to the nurse, but she nevertheless misused it in some way. Look at the right of Table 1, the number at the top. Note that 40 errors were of this type. Could this have something to do with the frequency of cart exchanges per day?

How important is it to deliver unit doses only at the times they are due? When the frequency of deliveries is reduced to twice a day, or even once a day, how does this affect the error rate?

Listen to this. During a five-day period, one patient suffered six omission errors and one wrong-dose error.

Table 1. Nursing Errors by Source and Error Type

	Number of Errors by Type						
Source	Omission	Dosage	Extra	Unordered	Route	Other	Total
Medication Nurse							
Administration (correct dose delivered to nurse)	18	14	2	3	1	2	40
MAR alterations by nurse	6	0	0	0	0	0	6
Borrowed (unordered) dose	0	0	1	0	0	0	1
Floor Clerk							
Pulled records too soon before discharge	1	0	0	0	0	0	1
Order put on wrong MAR	7	0	0	6	0	0	13
Order omitted from MAR	2	0	0	0	0	0	2
Total	34	14	3	9	1	2	63

The nurse accidentally dropped an Isordil tablet on the floor when passing the noon medications. To replace it, she reached in the drawer and took the dose already there for the next time, sent along with the first dose. She did not order a replacement. The evening shift nurse, not finding her dose in the cart at the time it was due, thought that it was discontinued and omitted it.

The omission of a dose of Atromid-S was similar. Instead of taking it, the patient left it on his breakfast tray and the nurse saw it go into the garbage. To replace it, she took the next dose from the cart, sent in advance as per usual practice, and gave him that one. As a result, the evening nurse found the drawer empty. She told the observer this had happened the night before but she did not get around to doing anything about it. The dose was never given.

In another case, the order said "Lasix 80 mg in the a.m. and 40 mg in the p.m." At 6 p.m. the nurse looked for the 40-mg dose, and it was not on the cart. Right then, however, she discovered a bag containing the 80-mg dose for the next morning, sent up in advance. So she gave that 80-mg dose to the patient.

There was much more, but the lesson we learned is this. When the cart exchanges are infrequent, you can no longer rely on the cart to automatically present the nurse, on schedule, the next dose due and, perhaps more important, only the dose that is due. The result is more errors.

And so, at Sinai Hospital we looked at some of the modern compromises that have been introduced into the original unit dose systems tested in the sixties, and they don't look very good. At Sinai, major changes have already been approved.

But that prompts me to ask: Where are all the studies that proved that deliveries once a day are just as good?

Let's look at the 1981 *ASHP Statement on Unit Dose Drug Distribution*,[7] published just last August. Three elements basic to all unit dose systems are listed:

1. Single-unit packages.
2. Ready-to-administer form.
3. Not more than 24-hour supply[a] of doses delivered.

Setting aside the first two elements, where did element number three come from?

Did it get there, for example, because many chief pharmacists want it to be true so that they can claim to have unit dose systems without paying the price, as Fred Eckel had the courage to suggest in 1976?

That little superscript "a" on point number three refers to a footnote which read as follows:

In long-term care facilities, a larger supply of medication (e.g., 48 or 72 hours) may be acceptable.

When was that shown to be true?

We did a study last summer observing for medication errors in 58 nursing homes across the country. We found no statistically significant differences between the error rates for those nursing homes claiming to have unit dose and those who said they didn't have it.

Do these findings mean that unit dose dispensing systems do not reduce medication errors in nursing homes? Or could it simply mean that their systems have been "watered down" so badly they don't work?

It seems to me that, as it stands, the new *ASHP Statement on Unit Dose Drug Distribution* is pseudopharmacy, however well intentioned it may be.

I am not charging that this is deliberate. I believe that mostly it is not. Ambitious chief pharmacists want to have the best and the latest, and that's good. When they can't afford it, that's sad. But when they slip into pseudopharmacy, that's bad.

You probably think by now that this is a lecture on ethics, but that's not my main point. The future we face won't allow us the luxury of the time and resources that pseudopharmacy consumes. Regardless of whether it's right or wrong, we can't afford it anymore.

The future is rushing upon us, and we may not like what we see. And we won't be able to cope, taking "time out" for pseudopharmacy.

What will it look like?

In the future, many of our hospital outpatient pharmacies may look like chain drugstores. In fact, they may be units of major drug chains.

Unbelievable? Undesirable? Consider these facts.

Today with the nation's political shift towards conservatism, government is abandoning its dominant role in health care. It wants to shift leadership to the private sector and let the marketplace determine medical prices and services.

The new Secretary of Health and Human Services, Richard Schweiker, has said, "Competition is our highest priority in the health field."

Hospitals have listened. At the recent convention of the American Hospital Association, several sessions dealt with such topics as "how to change a nonprofit hospital into a for-profit hospital," "the hospital department of marketing," and "hospital market research."

The new model for hospital administrators will be that of the 40 for-profit corporations that are in the business of owning and managing hospitals. Examples are the Hospital Corporation of America, Humana, and Lifemark. They now own roughly 15% of the nation's community hospitals and half of the psychiatric institutions. By the end of the decade, they are expected to own or manage 33% of the nation's hospitals.

Proprietary hospital chains have begun taking over management of public facilities also. For example, Hospital Corporation of America

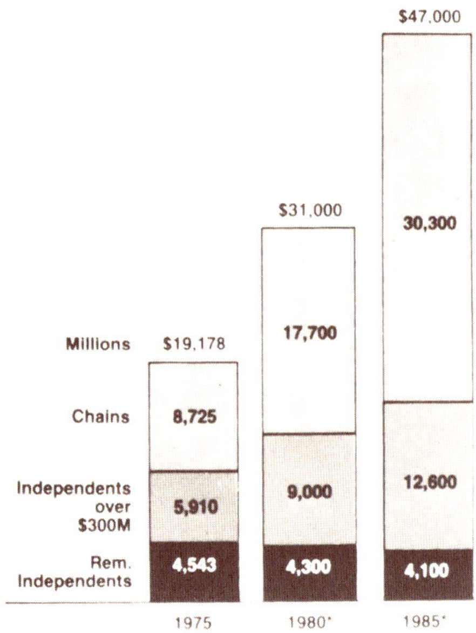

Figure 1. *Projected dollar sales of drugstores by type (*estimated). (Source: Nielsen Review.)*

acquired franchises to operate 10 public hospitals this last year alone. Cook County Hospital in Chicago is now being managed by Hyatt Medical Management Services.

Include the government hospitals, such as the Veterans Administration. This last year, the Office of Management and Budget issued Directive A76, ordering all agencies of the federal government to identify those services that can be contracted out. And they were instructed to do it wherever a bidder can do it at less cost than the government agency.

After the bids come back, will we see VA outpatient pharmacies run by Eckerd, or Peoples, or Rite-Aid in the same way that Morrisons and Marriott now provide food service in many of our hospitals?

Are the drug chains interested in this business? Why not? If the name of the game is dispensing prescriptions at a competitive price in an open market, would you expect them not to participate? In a game they know how to play so well? As you can see in Figure 1, they are already on their way to dominating all drugstore sales in this country and are rapidly increasing their share.

What can we expect to find in an outpatient pharmacy run by a chain or one that has to compete with a chain? The answer is: (a) a philosophy based on maximizing profit, and (b) careful attention to consumer demand.

In trying to predict what chains will do, this should be clear: the consumer will be in control. They will try to give the consumer whatever he wants and can pay for, regardless of what others may think that he needs. And the chains have read the studies showing a growing demand, by patients, for more information about their drugs and for direct personal contact with the pharmacist.

Counseling booths of various designs have been seen in hospital pharmacies and some community pharmacies for more than 10 years. Figure 2 shows an idea of the counseling area of the outpatient pharmacy of the future. This new design features an attractice environment designed for a primarily female clientele. It includes provision for the storage and distribution of patient package insert information plus the following other features:

1. An area for private conversation that does not make the patient feel cornered or trapped.
2. Both pharmacist and patient can adjust their physical proximity to each other in the design of this seating and desk.
3. Wheelchair access.
4. Built-in audiovisuals.
5. The pharmacist can still view the rest of the store while he counsels.

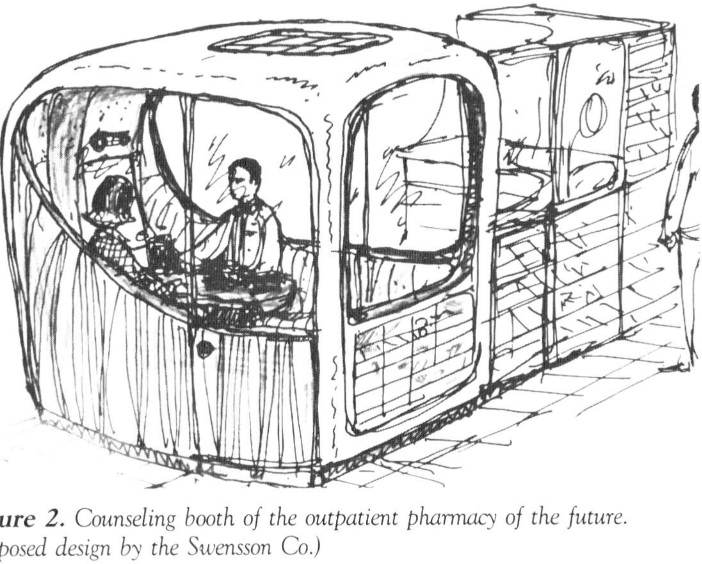

Figure 2. *Counseling booth of the outpatient pharmacy of the future. (Proposed design by the Swensson Co.)*

But do you notice the biggest difference? The design was inspired by the ornate sedan chairs used by the rich in Victorian England. That makes it interesting, perhaps even fun. This is the marketing of pharmacy services to the consumer, which we are going to have to learn to do.

Regarding nonprescription medications, recent studies have made it clear that the advice of the pharmacist can be the single most important factor affecting their sales. Customers often walk right past the supermarket and on into the pharmacy to purchase the very same product. In this design of the future, the pharmacist is only steps away from the nonprescription drug sales area.

The chains are aware that today people are turning to perform for themselves service heretofore performed only by physicians. For example, patients began doing their own laboratory tests in 1970 when the do-it-yourself pregnancy-test kit hit the market. Now, across the land, ordinary people are learning to handle stethoscopes, conduct breast self-examinations, and even pap smears.

An abundance of self-help information has become available, including books which enable a patient to diagnose his own ailments.

Another area of the future outpatient pharmacy I foresee is a self-medication station (Figure 3). This self-service center is located in front of the nonprescription drug display. It provides references to be used by customers for self-diagnosis and self-medication. Customers

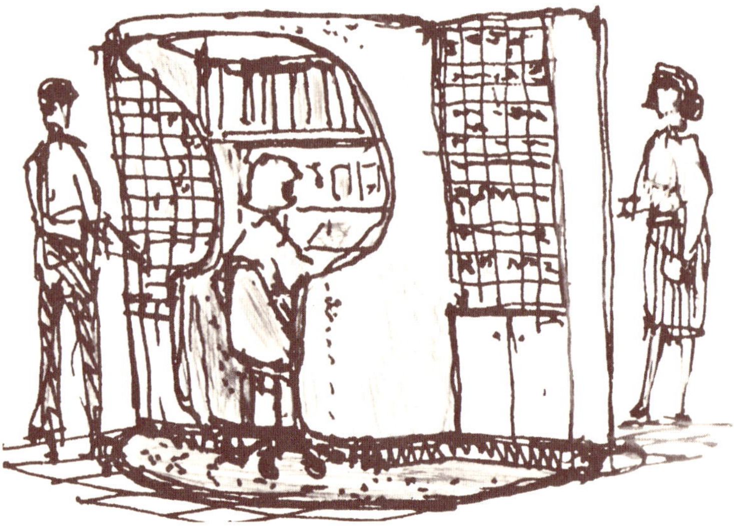

Figure 3. *Self-medication station of the outpatient pharmacy of the future. (Proposed design by the Swensson Co.)*

will also find a store catalog to help them find the drugs and devices they decide they need.

The benefit to the patient is a reduction in the number of trips to the doctor. To the pharmacist, it offers the opportunity for a patient–pharmacist relationship which is out from under the physician's authority over prescription drugs and self-supporting.

In the future, it will be the consumer who will largely influence our destiny, displacing the physician and the administrator to an important extent.

My next vision of the future I call "the disassembled pharmacy" or "the decentralization of almost everything."

Toffler describes how the philosophy of decentralization is spreading everywhere, explaining the tax revolt and the demand for "neighborhood power," the new trend in schools of architecture on designing communities to be self-sufficient, and the rush of large corporations to break their departments down into smaller, more autonomous profit centers.

The floor plan of the central pharmacy of a modern 600-bed teaching hospital is shown on the left of Figure 4. On the right is that same central pharmacy area in the future, as I see it. The shaded areas will no longer be needed. The only functions that will remain centralized will include the packaging of unit doses, the manufacturing of hyperalimentation solutions, quality control, and the receiving and storage functions.

Drug distribution is already being decentralized in the mobile pharmacy teams that are currently gaining popularity.

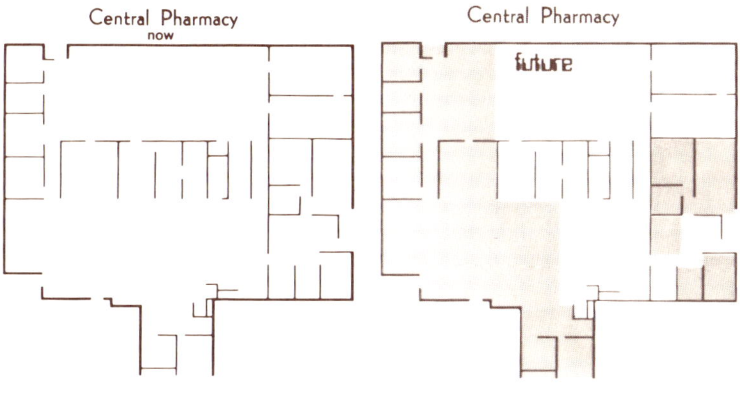

Figure 4. *Floor plan of the central pharmacy of a modern 600-bed teaching hospital now (left) and in the future (right); the shaded area will no longer be needed.*

In the future, the director of the pharmacy, secretaries, and clerks will all go home—"not together"—and spend much of their time at computer consoles and teleconferencing equipment in their homes. They will come to work occasionally for meetings and coordinating sessions and to attend the office party. Otherwise, the advent of low-cost communications and teleprocessing equipment will eliminate the need for elaborate office suites. Only one or two all-purpose rooms will be needed.

Toffler refers to the trend towards work at home as the advent of the "electronic cottage."

Certainly it's not difficult to envision the drug information center being operated by a pharmacist and his or her spouse out of their home and serving several different pharmacies on a contract basis. That is, or course, unless they are eliminated entirely by the new system just announced by the American Medical Association, which will let any physician access the database for *AMA Drug Evaluations* in Chicago. Their contract with General Telephone calls for this to be up and running in 1983.

The clinical pharmacist practitioner of tomorrow will have plenty of interaction with the patient and the medical team. That is, his computer will interact with theirs. The clinical pharmacist, completely freed from the central pharmacy, has a "glorious" future ahead, performing the function of clinical maintenance man.

His role will focus on servicing his own computers, which will interact with the medical team computers in prescribing and monitoring drug therapy. He will service the bedside computers as they teach the patients, interactively, how to take their medications. He will service the patient's home computer by transmitting, by phone line, the program it will need to remind him when to take his drugs. It will also monitor his compliance.

The clinical pharmacist will need to go to a patient's bedside of course—to service the patient's implanted drug devices. He could end up like the Maytag repairman, with little left to do. Of course, the patient will probably always prefer a human being at the interface with all these machines.

My last vision of the future I label simply "the pill machine."

I predict that, in the near future, all routine prescriptions will be filled by machine. I think it will happen this way.

Back in the 1950s, a multidose dispensing machine called the Brewer machine was introduced. At that time, hospital pharmacy reacted violently to this threat of automation, and the Brewer machine was soon put in its place by the state boards of pharmacy.

Since that time, the automation of dispensing has returned, on silent "cat feet" if you will, while we have been playing pseudo-pharmacy, and we are now about to be consumed by this big kitty before we realize it's hungry.

Consider the outpatient pharmacy department at a VA hospital in California. The pharmacists are out front receiving the prescriptions. They then pass them through a slot to be filled by technicians in the backroom. When filled, the pharmacists hand them out and counsel the patients.

The dose counting machine is in wide use throughout military pharmacies, and its use is spreading throughout other large outpatient pharmacies. The next generation model is completely controlled by a computer. We are evaluating one of these units in our laboratories right now.

My point is this. We already have computer-operated storage and counting equipment and computer-printed labels. The patient profiles are in the computer. The only people left in the filling process are the technicians, and they don't have state boards to defend them the way that pharmacy boards defended pharmacists against automation in the late fifties. It should only be a matter of time before the dispensing of routine medication is completely automated, leaving maintenance of the machines as the only task requiring human intervention.

The potential impact of this on patient care is receiving little attention, if any. If we study it and find that it's good for patient care—that's good pharmacy. If we just let it happen because nobody cares, that's more pseudopharmacy.

A comment on predicting the future before I go on. The only thing for sure is that pharmacy is not "at the crossroads." That analogy is out of date. Straight-line projections don't work because the future is becoming so disorderly. Once a trend is apparent, people now quickly react to it, never exactly the way you expect. And that alters the outcome.

Medicare and Medicaid did a lot for pharmacy—what will happen to pharmacy when they are diminished next year? How badly will the growing surplus of physicians threaten clinical pharmacy? It is on the way towards eliminating the physician's assistant.

It has never been more difficult to predict the future, or more important to try.

To get ready for the future, we will need flexibility and speed. We must prepare ourselves to deal with these new developments quickly with positive proposals that will stand the closest scrutiny. If they do not withstand it, we must discard them just as quickly and move on to find alternatives that will. There will be no time for pseudopharmacy.

How can we avoid it? How can we eliminate this endemic disease of creeping self-deception? I would prescribe regular doses of good objective feedback in the form of a continuing, critical review and analysis of our policies and programs. But who should do it?

The official statements and guidelines of the Society are effective mechanisms for producing the motivation to speed the adoption of our innovations. But who should we ask to review them, to tell us whether they are still valid and effective, or ever were? Who will play the devil's advocate?

ASHP has always been blessed with the kind of leadership we needed—first to survive, and then to grow. Now we are engaged in the next phase of any successful organization. It's called "coping with success." And we need to give our leaders a new tool to help them with this task.

My proposal is that the Society create, fund, and operate a small, new, and very different organizational component for which I have coined the named Policy Analysis Laboratory.

The Policy Analysis Laboratory (PAL) should be a function of, and report to, the ASHP House of Delegates. It should not be a function of the ASHP staff or Board for the following reasons. The obvious one is that it must be completely free to analyze and criticize current policies and programs. Not so obviously, the ASHP leadership must be equally free to disagree with the PAL, without obligation for its conduct, and to continue with those policies and programs felt to be important.

Nobody is perfect, and this new body will not be either. We are looking only for a second opinion here, not a new "medical team."

Though initially the ASHP leaders and staff may view this idea as "just something else to harass them," I think they will find it particularly helpful when dealing with "unpopular realities that need to be faced." If leadership can be defined as "the art of persuading people to forget what they want and seek what they need," then we can see why it is pretty rare. The Policy Analysis Laboratory can help our leaders by providing independent confirmation of those things we do not want to hear, but *need* to hear, from a perspective wider than pharmacy.

The PAL staff can consist of one person—the director—with authority to create ad hoc advisory panels, plus a secretarial and travel allowance. It should be a revolving position, attracting the best and the brightest for perhaps a two-year period. He or she will need access to the resources of a university and could be located in Washington, though not at ASHP headquarters. Of course, access to all ASHP documents, correspondence, and meetings is essential. Perhaps a foundation would fund this office, for the initial years at least.

A model of the organizational component I have in mind would be a cross between that offered by the Government Accounting Office (GAO) and the Brookings Institution. The GAO was established to give Congress an independent investigative body for the analysis of programs carried out by the administration. The GAO has one of the best reputations in Washington. Best of all, it really works. The Brookings Institution was established to offer to the government an independent policy review and analysis body, drawing upon the universities and expertise outside the government. The Brookings Institution is a success also.

I see no reason why ASHP can't emulate these models and many good reasons why it should.

What should be the first assignment of PAL once created? That would be for the House to say. In the face of the pressure to hold quality constant at the lowest level of cost, plus the loss of all of those university clinical positions previously supported by the capitation funds that are now being eliminated, my preference would be a review of the justification of the various clinical pharmacy services.

That is my one proposal and recommendation. We need a Policy Analysis Laboratory to fight pseudopharmacy.

ASHP has a remarkable history of professionalism for an organization of its size. In terms of leadership, we have lived in the land of giants. And from its stature, ASHP derives its most valuable resource —its appeal to the best in us all.

Now it is time for ASHP to take the lead again and do what no other pharmacy organization has yet dared to do—create an independent body to evaluate its own programs. Some old-fashioned virtues are involved: Honesty with ourselves, and courage to face the truth. Such virtues are stylish again I hear.

The cynics in Washington say you can fool some of the people some of the time, and that's enough. But it is not when we are fooling ourselves. As the old song says, the fundamental things apply as time goes by—but time is moving faster.

In closing, I thank you for this honor, and I want to recognize the following people, particularly Bill Heller, to whom I owe so much; Louise, Brad, Linda, and Douglas; my parents; William M. Heller; Warren E. McConnell; Ben F. Cooper; Don and Gloria Francke; Robert H. Henry; Janet D. Maiuro; Paul F. Parker; Joseph F. Stringer; and my colleagues and staff at Auburn University and the USP.

(For the complete list of references cited, please see page 265 of the *American Journal of Hospital Pharmacy*, Feb. 1982.)

At the time he received this award, Kenneth N. Barker was Professor and Head of the Department of Pharmacy Care Systems at Auburn University School of Pharmacy, Auburn, Alabama, and Director of the Drug-Related Analysis Research and Evaluation program.

1982

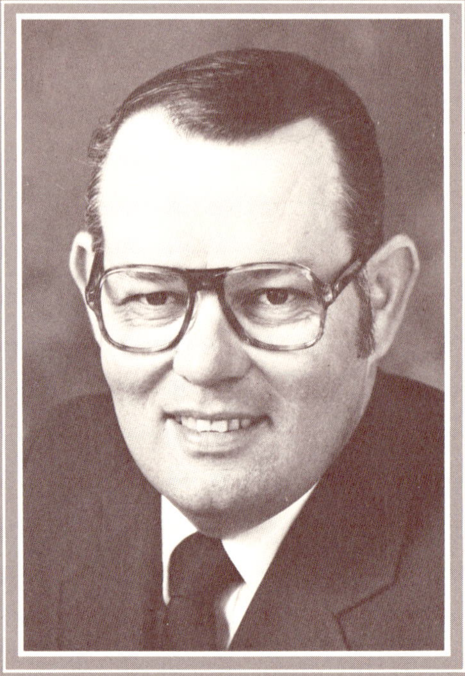

WILLIAM E. SMITH

"The 1980s is a decade of rapid change in the financing of hospital care."

CLINICAL PHARMACY IN THE 1980s

Will clinical pharmacy services in hospitals survive the 1980s? My answer to that question is "yes." I would like to share with you some aspects of my yes answer and identify what hospital pharmacy practitioners and pharmacy educators need to do differently in the 1980s to ensure that clinical pharmacy services will survive and thrive.

Beginning in the mid-1960s, patient drug history interviews, pharmacist participation in patient care rounds, adverse drug reaction reporting, patient drug therapy monitoring, answering drug information requests, and patient discharge drug counseling interviews provide specific examples of pharmacists' clinical activities. Will these services continue to be provided and supported financially in the remaining years of this decade? Current rapid changes within hospital care, catalyzed by the continually increasing costs of that care, make it mandatory that hospital pharmacists assess the past and the present to plan for the future of clinical pharmacy services.

What has been learned since the beginning of the clinical pharmacy movement in its modern context? The hopes and aspirations of the pioneers of pharmacists' clinical services focused on a desire to contribute to quality patient care by using their drug knowledge, to be respected professional colleagues of physicians and nurses, to be respected health care professionals, and to achieve a high level of personal satisfaction with their chosen profession.

The professional literature of the mid-1960s documented many patient drug-related problems in hospitals. The problems included medication errors,[1–2] adverse drug reactions,[3–5] prolonged hospitalization as a result of adverse drug reactions,[3–5] drug–drug interactions,[6] drug–laboratory test interactions,[7] IV admixture incompatibilities,[8] and drug-induced diseases.[9] The pioneers of clinical pharmacy reasoned that, given an opportunity, pharmacists located in patient care areas could reduce and prevent many of these drug-related problems.

Fortunately, there were some physicians, nurses, and hospital administrators who were interested in improving drug-related services and expanding the role of pharmacists, and they allocated resources to pharmacists to let them demonstrate what they could do. From the beginning, pharmacists were confronted with the challenges to justify their performance, determine costs, and prove the benefits. Skeptics and critics were plentiful and included physicians, hospital administrators, and hospital pharmacists.

What has been accomplished? What can be stated with confidence in 1982? More pharmacists are providing clinical services than ever before in university hospitals and large and small community hospitals. Even so, clinical services are not provided to patients and physicians in even a majority, let alone all, of U.S. hospitals.[10] More pharmacy students are provided clinical clerkship learning experiences than ever before. Even so, too many students question the future use of their clinical education. Postgraduate educational programs on clinical subjects are plentiful, and the number of postgraduate clinical residency programs increases each year. Pharmacist participation in clinical drug research is increasing. International interest in clinical pharmacy continues at a high level. Clinical services, education, and research by pharmacists are at the highest level ever.

What are the principles, the givens, the truths of the past 15 years that will be the basis for expansion in the 1980s? Each of these will be discussed in turn.

Pharmacists can provide effective clinical services if given the time, opportunity, and drug information support. Performance requires knowledge of drugs and their effects on people. It also requires the skill to apply knowledge and the ability to communicate and to work well with others. A desire to perform and a commitment to serve the drug-related needs of patients, physicians, and nurses whenever required are essential. Drug information support gives the clinical staff more time to provide services and also helps expand the scope of clinical practice.

Physicians will support and use the pharmacist's clinical services.[11-14] Drug knowledge and skill are the basis for a good working relationship with physicians. Knowledge must be specific and accurate; the information must be available and reliable. Physicians must believe that the pharmacist's knowledge and skill will assist them and benefit their patients. Pharmacists and physicians must respect each other's roles and responsibilities.

Nurses will support and use the pharmacist's clinical services.[11,12] Knowledge and skill also are the basis for a good working relationship with nurses. They, too, must believe that the pharmacist's services will assist them and benefit their patients. As is the case with physicians, these professionals must respect each other's roles and responsibilities.

Clinical services provided by pharmacists are accepted as appropriate for reimbursement by private and government third-party payers. Precedence has been set in many different parts of the country for pharmacists to be paid for clinical services by third-party payers, and various methods have been developed for the payment of clinical services.[15,16]

Patients do benefit from the pharmacist's clinical services. Reduction of drug toxicity, drug incompatibilities, inappropriate use, interactions, and adverse reactions occur daily in clinical programs.[12] Specific examples of pharmacist-regulated therapy that have been documented and evaluated include lower rate of bleeding complications with heparin therapy, lower incidence of nephrotoxicity from the use of aminoglycosides, reduction in serum drug concentrations of no useful clinical value, and reduction in IV aminophylline toxicity.[a]

Well-planned and managed clinical pharmacy services are cost effective. Studies that have included the costs for both clinical pharmacy services and drug distribution have resulted in lower patient per day costs.[11] Reduction in drug-related problems results in lower patient costs.

Other things we have learned include the following:

- Pharmacists' activities for a comprehensive clinical service are greater than can be provided by a pharmacist in a regular workday. Supplying the combination of all clinical opportunities described in the literature exceeds an 8-, 10-, or 12-hour workday. Priorities must be established so that the most essential clinical activities are provided.
- Financial resources are limited. No pharmacy department will receive all the financial support desired for personnel. Again, service priorities must be established.
- Many hospitals cannot support decentralized pharmaceutical services; space for satellite pharmacies in the patient care areas may not be available. More often, the number of patients per nursing unit may be too small to support a decentralized service. For those hospitals, a centralized drug system with pharmacists in the patient care area only for selected clinical services will result.
- Use of pharmacy technicians to perform many of the drug distribution tasks is essential to help free pharmacists for clinical services. Financial resources will not support one group of pharmacists for clinical services plus another group for drug distribution services.
- A centralized drug information service and a pharmacokinetics service are necessary to support and extend pharmacists' clinical services; these areas require specialists and specific reference resources.
- Computer technology is of great assistance for drug distribution services. Maximum benefit of this technology has not yet been demonstrated and achieved for pharmacists' clinical services.
- The demands on pharmacy management are greater for a clinical pharmacy program than for a traditional one. Requests for

resources are greater and more complex. Pharmacist and physician interactions are frequent, and conflict can occur. Pharmacists in clinical practice need and request greater support to achieve their needs and expectations. The management decisionmaking process of the hospital or hospital system needs to be thoroughly understood; methods must be developed by the pharmacy director to substantiate requests for needed resources.

In summary, we have demonstrated that a clinical pharmacy program will improve the quality of patient care in hospitals by reducing patient drug-related problems. We have demonstrated that clinical pharmacy services can be provided on a cost-effective basis. We have demonstrated that physicians and nurses will support the clinical pharmacy program and use the pharmacist for drug information. We have learned that the implementation of a successful clinical program needs well-educated and committed pharmacists and competent managers. Together, staff and managers can successfully implement cost-effective services to the benefit of patients, physicians, nurses, and pharmacists. It has been a challenging and exciting period for the profession of pharmacy.

The development of clinical pharmacy coincided with a massive influx of dollars into hospital care. Government expenditures through Medicare and Medicaid plus private health insurance have resulted in unparalleled growth of inpatient services in U.S. hospitals. Many hospital management decisions for resource allocations before 1980 included revenue generation as an important part of decisions to implement new services, and revenue generation was used as an essential part of requests for approval to implement clinical pharmacy services. Revenue generation is no longer the dominant factor of the hospital decisionmaking process in 1982. Expense management, the operational cost for doing business, is the dominant factor. Business, labor, and government have made it clear that they will no longer support the continually high annual increases in hospital charges and costs regardless of the perceived benefits.

The implementation and expansion of clinical pharmacy services in the 1980s will be challenged by six external forces bearing down on the hospital. These include: (1) federal and state government regulations and amount of payment for providing care to Medicare and Medicaid patients, (2) price competition for government and privately insured patients, (3) extension of cost limits to ancillary departments, (4) a physician surplus, (5) medical liability and risk-management requirements, and (6) accreditation and licensing requirements. Hospital pharmacy managers must develop a complete understanding of these external forces and their probable impact on hospital financial activities. Hospital pharmacy departments have already experienced reduction in staff and service programs, denial of requests to implement or expand clinical services, and freezing of institute, education, and other budget items. These negative experiences—and I suspect more are yet to come—will test pharmacists' belief in and commitment to providing clinical services for patients.

Four components of this new financial management era that will affect hospital pharmacy services most directly, in my opinion, are cost control, new technology, physician surplus, and new drugs.

In many states, hospital budgets are being controlled by governmental rate-setting commissions. Other states are experimenting with price competition and contract bidding for patients with the goal of reducing hospitalization costs. It is clear that the increase in hospital budgets from year to year will be less than what has occurred in the past decade. At the same time, the desires, wants, and needs of the medical staff and each hospital department for financial support for personnel, capital equipment, supplies, and services will far exceed available resources. The hospital pharmacy department will be forced to "compete" more effectively for limited resources with the medical staff and departments of pathology, radiology, nursing, information systems, and others.

The pressure to control and reduce costs has accelerated the need for changes in hospital organizational structures and relationships. Corporate reorganization, multihospital relationships, and group purchasing programs are examples of such changes. Patient enrollments in HMOs are increasing, and the number of patients with private health insurance will decrease. How these changes will affect hospital pharmacy in total is not yet clear. It is certain that physicians and patients who have a financial stake in limiting use of health care services will lead efforts to reduce use of drugs, as well as other diagnostic and therapeutic services.

Cost controls will have a particular impact on those hospital departments that have a substantial supply cost component in reimbursement formulas; pharmacy is such a department because of the cost of drug products. Dollar limits will be imposed on ancillary departments. Pharmacy department funds are allocated for net revenue, cost of drug products, and services provided by personnel. The greater the increase in the cost of drugs, the less money will be available for personnel, unless the hospital decides to reduce net revenue. Thus, as drug product costs go up, clinical services personnel drop. The cost of drugs in U.S. hospitals is increasing each year. Successful strategies by hospital pharmacy managers to limit the increase in the cost of drugs are essential for the continued development of clinical services, despite promotional efforts and tactics by pharmaceutical companies. Decisions about drugs to be used in the hospital must be based on the best scientific information available. Efforts to block or undermine objective drug formulary decisions of a hospital and medical staff must be resisted vigorously.

Pharmacy managers must identify and explain the differences between financial resources required for drug product costs and those for clinical services. We must help hospital management, third-party payers, and government agencies understand the difference between these two components as dollar limits are applied to the pharmacy department. Without pharmacists' clinical services, total patient costs will be greater.[11]

Organ transplant surgery, CAT scanners, automated laboratory systems, and hospital information systems are examples of expensive technology developed during the past several years. New forms of technology—expensive technology—will continue to be developed and financially supported. Some examples include nuclear magnetic resonance to eliminate the traditional roentgenogram, additional automation of the laboratory, hyperthermia controlled by computers for selected oncologic conditions, and CAT scanners for interventional procedures in neurosurgery.

These technologies should result in better patient care; they will require substantial capital allocations. How hospital management decides to support particular technologies, or how much technology can achieve the same objective, will influence resource allocation decisions for all hospital departments. You may be certain the pharmacy department will be affected.

The pharmaceutical industry has predicted a "new era" in drug therapy with many important advances in new drugs and drug delivery systems. There were more than 25 new drug entities approved in both 1981 and 1982. Over 160 drugs were in the FDA approval process as 1982 drew to a close.

Initial experiences with recent new drugs include the following three factors: (1) costs are three to five times more than existing similar products; (2) pharmaceutical manufacturers used aggressive and extensive promotional practices; and (3) physicians, nurses, and pharmacists have difficulty in keeping up with the new information. To illustrate these factors, Pharmacy and Therapeutics Committees are strained to decide which new drugs should be added to the formulary, drug product costs per patient day are increasing at rates exceeding 20%, and prescribers are confused about which new drug to use because of the amount and type of new information.

Patient needs for safe and effective drug therapy have not changed. The drug-related problems identified in the mid-1960s exist today in too many U.S. hospitals. For example, in recent years articles have identified problems of inaccurate dosage calculations in pediatrics by physicians and nurses,[17] a high rate of medication errors,[18] theophylline-induced seizures in accidentally overdosed neonates,[19] and nosocomial bacteremias.[20,21] The new drugs add complexity to drug use in hospitals. Traditional drug systems and interprofessional relationships must be modified to meet patient needs. In my opinion, new drugs will accelerate the implementation of clinical pharmacy services; safer and more effective patient drug therapy will result.

Many more physicians will be in practice by 1990 than at present. Authors on the subject of physician surplus predict and describe how the relationships—including financial—among physicians, as well as between physicians and hospitals, will change. Economics of health care, income, and consultation fees will dominate the discussions and decisions associated with these relationships. The physician surplus will contribute to hospital and medical price competition and to the deregulation of the health care industry.

Physicians exert a strong influence on hospital operations and resource allocation decisions. More physicians are expressing concerns about costs for each line item charged in the hospital, including drugs and pharmaceutical services. Questions are being asked about pharmacy department costs and patient charges and how these charges can be reduced. Pharmacy's answers must candidly include the point that changing physician demands can help reduce pharmacy operational costs. The reduction of inappropriate prescribing, prescribing of high-cost drugs that are not more effective than less expensive drugs, and widespread use of orders for p.r.n. drugs by physicians would lower pharmacy operational costs.

A physician surplus could have an impact on clinical pharmacy services. Drug therapy monitoring and patient assessment by pharmacists could revert back to the physician. As more physicians become available and there is less work for them to do in direct patient care, conflicts for drug therapy consultations and associated fees could develop. More physicians could resist the development of the pharmacist's clinical role.

In summary, the financing of hospital care is in the initial stages of a revolution. Patients, government, business, and labor have made their message clear: reduce the spiraling costs of hospital care. Patients' needs for quality clinical services must not get lost in this financial revolution. The needs of patients, physicians, and nurses for clinical drug information and safe medication systems will be greater in the 1980s than ever before, but we have to document this. Experience and personal opinion will not protect the progress we have made.

The expansion of clinical pharmacy services to all hospital patients who need them in this era of price competition, coupled with new drugs and technology, presents unique challenges and opportunities to pharmacists and pharmacy educators. How well hospital pharmacy practitioners and educators recognize the opportunities and develop specific methods and strategies to prepare, perform, and defend cost-effective clinical services will determine how many patients in U.S. hospitals will receive the benefits in this decade. To help ensure success, I offer the following comments for your consideration and appropriate action.

Hospital pharmacy societies exist to promote the interests of their members. I suggest a more important reason for their existence is the development and expansion of clinical pharmacy services for patients in hospitals. I challenge each and every organized hospital pharmacy society to develop a strategic plan committed to the implementation of clinical services for patients in all hospitals within its specific geographical area. This strategic plan would include (1) identification of patients who need clinical services; (2) the best method to provide and document the services; (3) resolution of the technician-use question; (4) recognition of the political, legal, and economic hurdles to overcome; (5) identification of educational programs needed for both staff and managers; and (6) active solicitation of physician, nurse, and hospital management involvement and support to achieve the objectives.

I do not believe the standard method of society operations of councils, houses of delegates, and boards of directors can be successful in meeting this challenge. The subject is too big and complex to tolerate the slowness of usual society program development. What I am recommending is for each society to develop a special study group or task force of pharmacy managers and clinical staff who will meet several times a year for the two to four years required to develop a comprehensive strategic plan. If hospital pharmacy societies at all levels accept this challenge, state societies could use the findings of each local society and the ASHP could use the findings of each state to develop an overall national strategic plan.

As each society makes such a commitment, many aspects of society operations will be clarified. Programs for continuing education, residencies, and pharmacy student teaching will be clarified. The needs of the membership will be better met by the society. I hear over and over again that hospital pharmacy societies do not meet the needs of the members. What is more important than helping the members cope with their daily practice and prepare for the future?

Without competent and effective management, clinical services will not be successfully developed, implemented, and maintained. To ensure that adequate resources are allocated for clinical services is a pharmacy management task. It is unfortunate that the Board of Specialties of the American Pharmaceutical Association and self-proclaimed clinical expert groups exclude hospital pharmacy management from its ranks. Hospital pharmacy management is a specialty within pharmacy; it has a unique body of knowledge and skill requirements to contribute.

Schools of pharmacy are not preparing graduates for management positions. At the minimum, schools need to identify students with the aptitude and potential for leadership and provide them with principles of management in their educational program.

The profession's rush to clinical practice has also decreased the number of residencies with management emphasis. The American Society of Hospital Pharmacists needs to accelerate the development of standards for an advanced residency in management.

Seven specific areas of clinical pharmacy management need study and review; these areas are the following:

1. The hospital management's decisionmaking process, including how decisions are made and by whom and what data and justification are required for a program proposal.
2. The working relationship between the director of pharmacy and immediate supervisor, including the requirements for a good working relationship.
3. The proper location of the pharmacy department in the hospital's organizational structure, specifically determining if pharmacy is a clinical or material department and to what level of management the pharmacy director reports.
4. Management methods to produce both financial and clinical results, including a good work-measurement system.
5. Methods to increase productivity of the staff, including how computer technology and other techniques can be used most effectively for clinical services and drug distribution systems.
6. Developing essential skills to function effectively in interdisciplinary situations.

Hospital pharmacy societies must play an important role in developing and fostering greater management expertise within hospital pharmacy. In my judgment, this demands a high priority of attention by society leadership.

The first step for successful implementation of a clinical pharmacy program is a definition of the services to be provided. This definition must be made by the pharmacy staff. If the pharmacy staff does not know what it wants to do and why, how can hospital management, medical, and nursing staffs be expected to support the proposed changes? The definition will include each clinical activity to be provided by pharmacists, as well as the expected benefits for patients, physicians, and nurses. With these definitions and a personal commitment to succeed, pharmacy managers and staff can be successful.

"How to study your own hospital" and "what patients need clinical services" are two questions that need better answers before clinical services will expand in hospitals. It is important to realize that hospital specificity determines what and how services are provided. People in key management positions (administration, nursing, pharmacy, and medical staff leadership) and hospital goals, objectives, and facilities are all important factors to be considered in the design of cost-effective services for a hospital. As a result, pharmacy management must develop methods for studying any hospital that will produce the best program design for that hospital. Data to be collected and analyzed will include (1) patient types and number of patients per service, (2) number of hospital service areas, (3) systems for the delivery of drugs and number of doses administered per patient day by dosage form and by time of day, (4) medical staff visit patterns to the hospital, and (5) pharmacy department workload and facilities. These data will translate into decisions of centralized versus decentralized systems, scope of unit dose drug packaging programs, personnel requirements, and impact on nursing time and that of other hospital personnel. This is an excellent topic for seminars, resident projects, and graduate student research.

Inherent in the question of which patients need clinical services is the suggestion that not all patients need pharmacists' clinical services. Those who do need clinical services need to be identified; knowing the number and type of patients will determine a reasonable staffing requirement and, therefore, costs for services. This is a selective approach that fits well with the era of cost limits, and it is an approach that I believe hospital management will support. A study of a hospital patient population should focus on selected drugs: drugs in which dosage is affected by quick changes in patient status, drugs that require serum concentrations, drugs that interact with other drugs, and drugs that could have a toxic effect on blood, kidneys, or liver.

Comprehensive and cost-effective clinical pharmacy services require extensive use of pharmacy technicians. Quality patient care and the vested self-interest of our profession can no longer tolerate failure to resolve the use and training of technicians. Hospital pharmacists cannot let the archaic attitudes and thinking of many community and hospital pharmacists, state boards of pharmacy, pharmacy organizations, and employee pharmacist organizations block the proper and necessary use of pharmacy technicians in hospitals. Every industrialized country in the world uses pharmacy technicians in providing pharmacy services. Technicians are used extensively in the manufacture of drugs and intravenous solutions. Yet, as soon as the drug product passes through the door of a pharmacy, only a pharmacist can look at, handle, count, and package the drug products. Restrictive ratios of one technician and one pharmacist for inpatient services must be resisted. Flexibility is needed to determine pharmacy department staffing in the 1980s and to ensure the growth and development of our profession in clinical practice.

Most clinical pharmacy programs have not yet evolved to the extent that the combination of clinical services and distribution is greater than can be provided by a single pharmacist. If more pharmacists cannot be hired to expand clinical pharmacy services, then distribution tasks must be delegated to pharmacy technicians. Pharmacists must realize that wherever the level of technician performance is drawn, the pharmacist's capacity is also defined. The less technicians are allowed to do, the less pharmacists will be able to do.

Pharmacy education is entitled to accept some of the credit for the successful implementation of clinical services. Without a pharmacy education that gave sufficient confidence to the pioneers of clinical services, the accomplishments of the past 15 years would not have been realized.

The challenges before pharmacy education are even greater if clinical pharmacy services are going to be fully effective. These challenges include three elements: knowledge-in-depth, research, and service.

Clinical pharmacists require the broad knowledge and skills of a generalist in the use of drugs. Specific knowledge, or knowledge-in-depth, is also required. Clinical teaching must include assignments that require the student to learn at least one subject in great depth. The student must experience the time required, the amount of literature to be reviewed, how to make judgments on the subject matter, and the self-confidence that results from knowledge-in-depth. The skills developed from this experience will be used throughout the graduate's career as drug information changes.

Greater participation by schools of pharmacy in research to help implement changes in professional practice is needed. It would be helpful if schools of pharmacy would take more of a lead role in the needed research. It must be recognized that research limited to university hospitals is not sufficient. Research in large, medium, and small community hospitals is also required.

Each school of pharmacy that uses hospitals as sites for student teaching should assist in the development of comprehensive clinical services. Students need to learn in environments where the clinical faculty members perform the services the students are being educated to provide after graduation. Credibility is lost when the services at the teaching sites are less than complete.

Teaching, research, and service are the responsibilities of a school of pharmacy. Faculty members need to recognize the importance of clinical services to their own personal growth and support. Without continual growth and success in the profession, how long will pharmacy education and, therefore, faculties continue to be supported? When faculty members finally realize the importance of the success of clinical pharmacy, many conflicts within pharmacy education can be resolved, and educational programs will advance.

Pharmacy is a service profession, and the pharmacist's mission is to serve the drug-related needs of patients, physicians, and nurses. Drug therapy in the modern hospital is a primary modality of patient care. Most hospital patients receive drugs, and the number of drug orders and doses prepared and administered is staggering. The pharmacy leadership in each hospital should ask the following questions: What are the drug-related problems in my hospital? What are the alternatives for solving these problems? What are the roles for the pharmacists in my hospital? I am confident that clinical pharmacy services is the answer to these questions.

The 1980s is a decade of rapid change in the financing of hospital care. It is a decade of opportunity for pharmacists. Clinical pharmacy services can reduce costs, increase hospital efficiency, and improve the level of patient care in a cost-effective manner.

A clinical pharmacy practice brings its own rewards to the pharmacist. To be an expert in the clinical use of drugs presents a lifelong challenge of learning and self-study. It brings professional respect from physicians and nurses and places the pharmacist in the mainstream of caring and healing. A career in clinical pharmacy is an open-ended opportunity for those who seek its rewards.

(For the complete list of references cited, please see page 229 of the *American Journal of Hospital Pharmacy*, Feb. 1983.)

At the time he received this award, William E. Smith was the Director of Pharmacy and Central Services and Assistant Administrator at the Memorial Hospital Medical Center of Long Beach, Long Beach, California; Clinical Professor at the School of Pharmacy, University of Southern California; and Assistant Dean and Associate Clinical Professor at the University of California School of Pharmacy.

1983

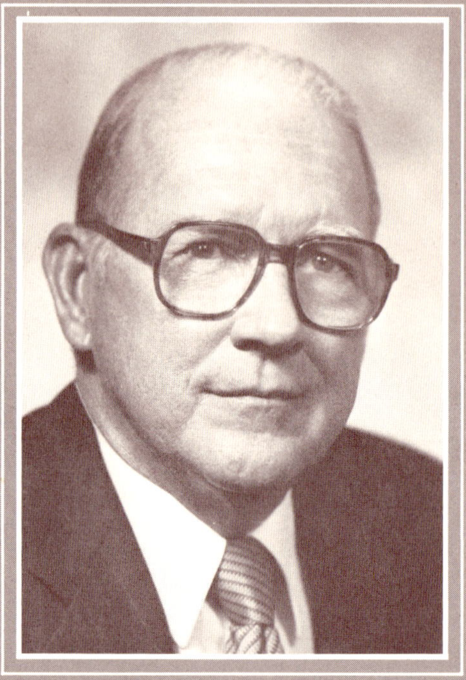

WARREN E. McCONNELL

"Start thinking now about what our roles should be 5–20 years from now."

A 20–20 VISION: ALTERNATIVE FUTURES FOR HOSPITAL PHARMACY

Since the future is the realm of infinite possibilities, we can never know all the things that might come to pass within its domain; all we can do is to make a few forays into that awesomely vast and incomparably fascinating territory.

Edward Cornish, *1999—The World of Tomorrow*

Several months ago, I happened upon a review of a book entitled *The Post-Physician Era: Medicine in the Twenty-First Century*, by Jerrold S. Maxmen.[1] The title itself was enough to capture my attention, but reading the review really sparked my interest. The author of the book is a physician. This fact seemed particularly important. Here was a physician speculating that medical doctors will become virtually extinct in another 50 years! This started me thinking: If there will no longer be any doctors around in another 40 or 50 years, what about pharmacists? With no doctors, what will we be doing in 2025? So, when I learned last February that I was to give this address, the first topic that came to mind was hospital pharmacy's future.

Since this is ASHP's 40th anniversary year, I thought it would be interesting to look 40 years into the future, when ASHP would be twice its present age, and speculate what the status of hospital pharmacy would be then. It was not just coincidence that 40 years from now is just about the time that Maxmen predicts the obsolescence of all physicians.

A word about the title of this address. Some simple arithmetic will quickly tell you that 40 years takes us to the year 2023. You will forgive, I hope, the liberty I took in choosing to title my talk "A

20–20 Vision," but to call it "A 20–23 Vision" just didn't seem to get the point across.

Perhaps you are wondering why we should bother to examine what might happen 40 years from now when we cannot even predict with any known degree of accuracy what will happen 10 years from now, or five years, or even one year. Is not studying the future just a waste of time? Maxmen[2] observed that:

> *Exploring the future can be interesting because we and our children are going to spend the rest of our lives in it. . . . By focusing upon specific future developments, one can begin to evaluate their relative desirability. . . . [By] anticipating the potential consequences of a projected development, one is afforded the opportunity to assess its desirability thoroughly* before *the event occurs. Consequently, individuals or society can be better equipped to adopt constructive policies and to avert potential difficulties. Because we are too often unprepared to cope with the consequences of scientific innovations we hastily make decisions that we learn to regret. Studying the future can help to minimize this problem.*

Of all the allied health professions, I believe pharmacy has less control over its destiny than perhaps any of the others. This is even more true for hospital pharmacy than for other branches of the profession. Hospital pharmacists provide their services at the pleasure of—and sometimes at the displeasure of—consumers, physicians, nurses, hospital administrators, pharmaceutical manufacturers, and occasionally other health professionals. Thus, if we are to examine realistically the future of hospital pharmacy, we cannot do so in isolation. We must look at it in the context of the entire health care system and the world around us. And we cannot simply extrapolate our past and present knowledge and experiences to arrive at a forecast for the future. We must wade into unknown waters.

The most difficult aspect of futures research is the impossibility of accounting for all the variables affecting the issue under study, not to mention predicting what changes may occur in the important ones we can identify and how they will interact. The only way around this difficulty is to establish certain premises beforehand. In exploring alternative futures for hospital pharmacy, I have made the following assumptions:

- There will be no world catastrophe, such as nuclear war or an ecological disaster.
- The population of the developed countries will continue to have adequate food and housing.
- The world economy will stabilize at no worse than its present level.
- There will be no major cultural upheavals in the developed countries.
- Natural resources will be sufficient to sustain technological growth.

Although these conditions may not hold, I shall not speculate on the results of their failure to do so.

To set the stage for projecting hospital pharmacy's future, I shall first take a look at some of the major trends that affect society today and will most likely affect the health care system. I shall then examine trends in the health care system in this country that will have an impact on hospital pharmacy practice. And, finally, I shall describe two scenarios for future health care systems and speculate how hospital pharmacy will fare in them.

Few developments have had as great an impact on the lives of people in our generation as television and computers. Automation or electronic communications play a role in almost every activity in which we are involved, whether at work, at home, or at play. And we hear from all sides that we are only on the threshold of what we can expect in the future.

Clement Bezold,[3] Director of the Institute for Alternative Futures, which is located in Washington, says we are in a communications revolution and dates it from about 1950 when home television receivers first became relatively affordable. John Naisbitt,[4] author of the recent book *Megatrends*, explains that we have moved from an industrial society to an information society. A recent article by Dwight Tousignaut[5] describing automated literature-retrieval techniques brings this point home most vividly.

In the next 20–40 years, we can expect to see technological developments in the applications of computers and microelectronics that will dwarf by comparison developments up to this time. In the health care field, obtaining a medical history will not require the intervention of a physician.[6] Instead, the patient will use an interactive computer terminal programmed to elicit the desired information. The patient will enter information into the computer by keyboard, by use of a light pen, or through a touch-sensitive screen. Alternatively, the patient may provide the same information from home using a Touch-Tone telephone as an interactive "terminal" instead of a keyboard. He will indicate his answers to questions generated orally from a central computer by keying responses using the phone buttons and a predetermined code. It will be possible for the computer to modify its clinical interview in response to various nonverbal signals, such as pulse, blood pressure, or response latency.[7]

Eventually, interaction between the patient and computer may be entirely by voice (speech recognition) without the need for a keyboard or phone set. The patient's medical history, as a part of the medical record, will be permanently stored in a central computer file accessible to authorized persons from anywhere in the country—or the world, if need be. Maxmen[8] calls this computer file a national medical data bank (NMDB). A person's record will be created at birth and updated each time he interfaces with the health system. It will also be reviewed systematically and periodically to purge inaccurate, irrelevant, or outdated information.[9]

We can also expect that most diagnostic procedures, such as complete blood counts, urinalyses, various functional tests, roentgenograms, ECGs, and EEGs, will be ordered, performed, and interpreted by computers without the physician even entering the picture.[10] Wireless sensing devices will be used for remote transmission of ECGs, EEGs, vital signs, and so on. Videophones will be used to transmit visual images of roentgenograms, ECGs, and the like between health facilities or health personnel.[11] Interactive television will permit "face-to-face" communication between a patient and a remotely located health professional, or between health professionals themselves for consultation purposes. Eventually, by using interactive television or videophone or by pushing the appropriate buttons on his Touch-Tone telephone, a patient's medical requirements will be met in many circumstances without his ever leaving his home.[12]

It has already been demonstrated that computers can outperform physicians in diagnosing a wide range of illnesses. In the 21st century, all diagnoses will be performed by computer.[13] Treatment decisions, likewise, will be made by the computer, and, following drug therapy, patient-monitoring functions will be computer controlled.[14] The final disease-oriented function of the physician—rendering a prognosis—is simply a matter of probabilities and readily adaptable to computer programming.[15]

We may expect that automated methods will also be applied in so-called preventive-health activities (wellness programs). This has already been demonstrated in several automated multiphasic screening programs around the country. Computers will also prescribe prophylactic treatments in wellness programs and will be used in conjunction with interactive television as the primary medium in health education for the public.

Since the health care industry exists because of illness, our attention naturally focuses on technological developments in medical diagnosis and treatment. Even though these scientific advancements do save lives, the impact on the overall health status of the population of the United States is negligible. For example, the U.S. Surgeon General's Office estimated that for the year 1976 more than two-thirds of the U.S. mortality was attributed to unhealthful lifestyle and environmental factors. Less than a third was because of human biological factors and inadequacies in health care.[16]

There has been a decided shift in the last decade or two in the average American's lifestyle and values away from institutional help to self-help.[17,18] Changing attitudes towards health are reflected in the increased numbers of people who, for example, regularly exercise, changed dietary habits, reduced use of tobacco, and shifted from drinking hard liquor to wine. In addition, more and more businesses and corporations, including hospitals, are implementing employee fitness and wellness programs. Several companies and a few hospitals are providing health-hazard appraisal services for their employees.[19] In a health-hazard appraisal, individuals answer a battery of 300–400 questions about their living habits and health history. The answers are compared with computerized statistical tables that assess the health risks and benefits associated with the person's particular lifestyle and history. The objective of the appraisal is to use statistical methods and epidemiological data to motivate an individual to change his lifestyle to achieve a gain in life expectancy.

The self-help trend in the health field is further exemplified by the dramatic growth in sales to the public of such items as do-it-yourself pregnancy test kits, sphygmomanometers, stethoscopes, otoscopes, specialized convalescent devices, and so forth. An increasing number of women are opting for natural childbirth, home deliveries, and deliveries by nurse midwives instead of by obstetricians. More families are choosing hospices over hospitals so family members with terminal illnesses may live out their final days in a home-like atmosphere. In general, individuals are assuming more responsibility for their own health, reducing the number of visits to the doctor, cutting short their hospital stays, or choosing alternatives to use of the hospital.[20]

The holistic-health movement, which focuses on health maintenance rather than illness care, represents a growing popular challenge to established health policies and practices. The holistic-health movement stresses the necessity of restructuring the social environment to achieve and maintain health effectively.[21] Spokesmen for the movement argue for establishment of a "healthy public policy" to replace our "public health policy."[22,23]

The trend in changing personal attitudes and lifestyles is already having an effect on the health care industry. Clement Bezold,[24] in his book *The Future of Pharmaceuticals*, cites the trend as a factor to be considered by pharmaceutical manufacturers in their long-range research and development planning. Jeff Goldsmith,[25] President of Health Futures, Inc., points out the possible future effect of this trend on the consumption of health services, particularly the potential decrease in hospital usage.

If the self-help trend continues, and if individuals continue to assume greater responsibility for their own well-being, we can expect a decrease in the use of drugs in general. At the same time, there will be increased demand by the public for health education to make it more self-reliant in health matters. Hospital pharmacists, therefore, will find their roles gradually shifting to assume this public education responsibility. As the home computer and interactive television become more common, however, health education will be provided through these media and the educational role of the pharmacist may then diminish.

In 1900 the leading causes of death in the United States were influenza and pneumonia, tuberculosis, gastroenteritis, and heart disease.[26] Today they are heart disease, cancer, stroke, and accidents.[27] The change reflects several factors, including the discovery of antibiotics and advances in nutrition and environmental conditions. As life expectancy has advanced because of these and other developments, the incidence of the disorders of the elderly, such as cancer, stroke, and heart disease, has increased.

Over the next 40 years, the number of so-called acute organic diseases will diminish substantially.[28] Although infectious diseases will not be eradicated entirely, they will have been largely controlled through new antibiotic therapy, diminished transmission resulting from lower disease incidence, and discovery of new prophylactic immunization measures. The problem of resistant organisms will probably have been solved.

Cardiovascular and cerebrovascular problems will probably still plague us unless hereditary factors, psychosocial stresses, and dietary traits can be better controlled; however, many cardiac dysfunctions will be effectively treated with new therapeutic agents. Allergies will increase because of the proliferation of new biologic substances, synthetics, and additives encountered in foods, water, pharmaceuticals, clothing, and other materials. Environmental pollutants—biochemical, radioactive, and sound—may pose some of the most troublesome health problems in the future unless more effective means can be found for their control.

By the turn of the century, vehicular and industrial accidents as leading health problems should be yielding to control. Accounting for this will be automated vehicular and traffic control systems and computer-controlled (cybernated) manufacturing systems replacing humans in the production lines.

Psychogenic illness will constitute one of the greatest, if not *the* greatest, health problems as we move into the 21st century. The "future shock" syndrome—Toffler's[29] "disease of change"—will be the primary causative factor. Stresses arising from the individual's attempts to cope with rapidly changing needs, values, and goals will be responsible.[30] Most difficulties will be traceable to group maladaptations and rejections as our society becomes less individualistic and more group oriented. Changing family structures and male–female relationships will be important factors. Too many choices and lack of choices will be sources of stress and frustration. Automation and cybernation in the workplace will result in large increases in leisure time for a vast majority of the population, and this will be particularly stressful to many.

Bezold[31] lists the increasing proportion of elderly as one of five major trends and issues that will shape the future of health care. According to official projections, the number of Americans 65 and older, now about 25 million, will rise to more than 55 million by

2035. Unless the birth rate increases substantially, elderly persons will compose nearly 20% of the total population, compared with 11% today.[32] The "old old" (age 75 and over)—the group with the most illness and disability—will outnumber today's 65 and over by the year 2040. The growth in the elderly population probably will mean increasing demand for hospital services since elderly individuals consume almost four times as much hospital care per capita as the national average. This demand will be determined, in part, by trade-offs with aftercare alternatives to hospitalization forced by strained federal budgets and the changing health status of this segment of the population.[33]

As medical advances prolong life, chronic illness will become a greater problem. Undoubtedly, some elderly Americans will require nursing home care, but some will be cared for at home with the aid of electronic monitoring devices and telecommunication hookups with central health facilities. Hospitals are likely to broaden their service offerings to elderly persons by providing for day hospitalization (day care) for geriatric patients and by providing home health care services. Smaller hospitals may open "swing beds," which can be converted from acute care to long-term care as needed.

Much ongoing research today focuses on the action of individual cells in an effort to discover more about the basic functioning of the human body. Because immunotherapy promises to be useful for such a wide range of diseases, much current research is targeted on the human immune system. Current studies include continuing investigations of the interferons, the immune system's role in tissue rejection in organ transplantation, immunologic prevention of tooth decay, the relationship between the immune system and the aging process, and the development of vaccines for prophylaxis against parasitic diseases.[34]

Research on neurotransmitters—molecules that mediate brain activity—may turn out to be major breakthroughs. About two dozen neuropeptides have already been discovered, and there are perhaps hundreds more.

In the area of birth control, it is claimed there is so much research going on that by the year 2000 there will be a large selection of safe pharmacologic techniques from which to choose.[35]

We are only beginning to scratch the surface in our research on genetics. Protein synthesis is the goal of most current genetic engineering efforts, but future possibilities for development of new therapies and preventive measures for disease are almost limitless.[36]

Discovery and refinement of the technique for producing monoclonal antibodies promise to bring about revolutionary changes in the understanding and treatment of diseases. They are already being used with success in research on cancer, heart disease, multiple sclerosis, viral diseases, and disorders of the human immunological defense system. They may also be used as drug conveyers in organ-targeted therapy, as drug-carrying vehicles to neutralize overdoses of drugs or to desensitize patients with allergy, or as a monitoring system to trace drug effects. Highly specific antibodies may also be used for preparing improved vaccines for use against specific types of cancer, such as malignant melanoma.[37]

We can expect to see development of new and unique drug-delivery systems. Controlled-release technology is likely to be made much more sophisticated and reliable. Alternatives to drugs, such as electrical stimulation, are being studied. Nuclear magnetic resonance (NMR) as a diagnostic alternative to conventional roentgenograms and the computerized axial tomographic (CAT) scanner will soon be in common use.[38]

As the patterns of illness are modified by the medical, social, and technological developments we have described, the patterns of treatment will also change. The trend towards greater self-reliance of the individual in health matters, the shift of the health care system from illness care to health maintenance (wellness), the improved health and physical condition of the public in general, the reduced incidence of disease, the availability of more effective drugs for a broader spectrum of illness, and the technological developments that will permit patients to be treated at home will mean that many fewer people will be hospitalized and that ambulatory care will greatly increase.

The runaway escalation of health care costs in the last few years has put hospitals under tremendous pressure to reduce their expenses. William Smith,[39] in his Whitney address last December, described the situation facing hospitals and some of the implications for hospital pharmacy. Goldsmith,[40] in his book *Can Hospitals Survive?*, states:

> *The health care industry in the United States is undergoing profound structural changes which will alter the role the hospital and the physician play in rendering medical care. As this structure broadens and diversifies, alternatives to acute care hospitalization will become increasingly attractive economically. The more rapidly hospital costs escalate, the more rapidly these trade-offs will be forced by health insurers. . . [T]he rising price of hospital care will encourage growth of ambulatory services, alternative delivery systems, and aftercare for the nation's elderly. As costs increase, competitive pressures within the hospital industry will intensify to the point where many hospitals, perhaps hundreds, may be forced to close, and as many as several thousand others may be absorbed by large hospital management firms. . . .*

The impact of this trend on hospital pharmacy—and hospital pharmacists—may be substantial indeed, especially in hospitals forced to close and those taken over by management firms.

Now that I have reviewed the major trends shaping the future health care system, we should have a better image of the context within which the system will metamorphose. I shall now examine future hospital pharmacy practice in the context of this changing health care system.

In subscribing to the concept of clinical pharmacy, hospital pharmacy has cast its lot with the health care team; therefore, the future of hospital pharmacy practice may be determined in large measure by whatever happens with the health care team, particularly with respect to the clinical aspects of our practice.

The current concept of the health care team identifies the physician as, if not captain of the team, then certainly its dean. So the future of the physician and his role on the health care team should give some inkling of what the future has in store for the hospital pharmacist.

Two incisive expositions on medicine and the health care system in the 21st century are Maxmen's *The Post-Physician Era,* which I cited earlier, and a book entitled *The Future of the Health Sciences: Anticipating Tomorrow,*[41] by Stanley Lesse, a physician who is editor-in-chief of the *American Journal of Psychotherapy* and currently on the faculty of neurology of the College of Physicians and Surgeons at Columbia University. The two books were published in 1976 and 1981, respectively.

These books are not science fiction; they are serious dissertations with substantial documentation from the literature to back them up. In the preface to his book, Lesse states that he has "... attempted to develop a future health science model that will be a reflection of the interrelated social, demographic, and technologic forces that will mold it." Maxmen stated as his objective in writing *The Post-Physician Era*: "By proposing the eventual replacement of a physician-centered model by a medic-computer model, I hope to present an innovative, viable and desirable alternative solution to the American health care crisis." The future health systems proposed by Maxmen and Lesse are strikingly similar. Both are based on highly sophisticated automated and cybernated[a] (computerized) systems that will perform more efficiently most of the functions of the contemporary physician. Both proposals emphasize health maintenance rather than illness care. Both authors predict the demise of the physician within the next 40 or 50 years.

The two physician authors suggest that private medical practice will disappear during the first decade of the 21st century. By the turn of the century, the vast majority of physicians we train today, they say, will become what Maxmen calls "medics" and what Lesse calls "health technical experts." These medics will work as assistants to sophisticated automated devices that will take over many, if not most, of the tasks now carried on by today's highly specialized physicians. There will be generalist medics and specialist medics. The latter would require further training to learn about such things as psychotherapy, delivering babies, setting fractures, and so forth. Some medics will be diagnosticians; some will be trained as therapists. The medic–computer team will replace the general practitioner and the clinical specialist of today. In combination with the automated systems, the medics will interpret and apply procedures that are suggested and planned by higher level health professionals.

Lesse and Maxmen see the need for one or two higher levels of health manpower that will have overall conceptual and operational responsibility for the health system. They will be generalists, not specialists. They will supervise the programming of the automated diagnostic–treatment system and the health record–memory banks and have responsibility for their attending medics. They will be humanistically oriented cyberneticists. They will be programmers, consultants, teachers, and researchers, but of a different order from what we now associate with these terms. They will *not* be comparable to today's physicians and their education will be vastly different from present-day medical education.

Charging that today's mammoth medical centers are one of the greatest deterrents to the future progress of American medicine, Lesse and Maxmen propose that the formal physical structure of future health practice be greatly simplified. Since the primary focus of the future health system will be prophylaxis and health maintenance, design of facilities will put heavy emphasis on automated diagnostic and health-maintenance technology.

The types of facilities and numbers of each will be planned to take into account the emphasis on health maintenance and self-care, lower incidence of acute illness and injuries, new therapeutic developments, increased elderly population, and other factors I have already described. With no need to accommodate the requirements of doctors, the facilities can be planned and operated at much lower cost and greater efficiency.

Maxmen's concept of how the transition from a health-team model to a medic–computer model will occur is particularly interesting. He believes the public's experience with nurse-practitioners, nurse-clinicians, and physician's assistants (and we could add clinical pharmacists) will influence the likelihood of future patients accepting the "medic." He thinks that, as physicians continue to withdraw from active patient care under a health-team model, the public will become less dependent on physicians' services; furthermore, as paraprofessionals increasingly use computers in providing clinical services, patients will become accustomed to receiving treatment from machine-assisted allied health personnel. He believes also that physicians will actually facilitate their own obsolescence because they are not suited by temperament to perform tasks that can be delivered more readily and more effectively by a medic or by a computer. Because physicians are not going to *want* to do something that a medic–computer symbiosis can do better, they may actually facilitate the development of a medic–computer model.

What can we say now about hospital pharmacy practice 40 years in the future?

Let us assume for the moment that Lesse and Maxmen are correct and that by the year 2025 automation has progressed to the level of sophistication they forecast and that physicians have become extinct, replaced by the health personnel they describe.

What will happen to the clinical functions performed by today's institutional pharmacist? Of the 10 activities listed in the *ASHP Statement on Clinical Functions in Institutional Pharmacy Practice*,[42] I suggest that all but one will have been automated or turned over to medics. Such functions as taking medication histories, drug-therapy monitoring, patient education, and drug prescribing have already been described in our discussion of future trends. It requires no stretch of the imagination to envision similar automation and delegation of other functions, such as pharmacokinetics consultations, medication administration control, detection and reporting of adverse drug reactions, conducting drug-use reviews, and so on. The only function for which a higher level person might be required is initiation and participation in research, which would remain a responsibility of the clinical pharmacist or a similarly qualified person.

Since there will be no physicians, what will happen to the health care team with which clinical pharmacists identify today? It appears that the only one of today's health professionals in the hospital who will still be needed 40 years from now is the technical (bedside) nurse —the licensed practical nurse. The professional nurse will disappear along with the physician. So, too, will the physician's assistant. Maxmen suggests that during the transition period from the health-team model to the medic–computer model, nurses who wish to perform clinical services could become medics. Physician's assistants, on the other hand, might be in a natural position to help in the conversion, after which there would be no place for them. So, the health care team, as we know it today, has disappeared along with the physician, the professional nurse, and the physician's assistant.

What will happen to the nonclinical functions of the hospital pharmacist? In my opinion, these will disappear long before the clinical functions. Most of the technical functions related to compounding and dispensing have already been automated or turned over to technicians. The administrative functions, such as record keeping, purchasing, and inventory control, can be performed by nonpharmacists and computers, as well as by pharmacists. Management activities likewise do not require pharmacists' unique knowledge and expertise.

Drug information service activities, which some may call clinical functions but which in my opinion are largely technical, will probably be completely automated before the end of this decade. With the departure of the physician and with automation of medical diagnosis and treatment, the clinical function of the drug information pharmacist—interpretation of the literature—will be in slight demand. The only consumers of this service will be medical researchers and "health academicians" involved in programming the automated systems, and they will either do their own literature interpretations or obtain the needed information online from national or international "literature interpretation centers."

Earl Joseph,[43] editor of *Future Trends*, which is published by the Minnesota Futurists, identifies five basic periods of the future:

1. Now and the immediate future: up to one year from now.
2. The near-term future: one to five years from now.
3. The middle-range future: five to 20 years from now.
4. The long-range future: 20–50 years from now.
5. The far future: 50 years or more hence.

Joseph makes two points he believes are important in long-range planning: (1) the world that we shall experience in five to 20 years is being shaped by decisions made now, and (2) almost anything can be done in 20 years. To illustrate the latter point, Joseph reminds us that, once the decisions were made, only four years were needed to build the first atomic bomb and only eight years to put man on the moon.

We need to start thinking now about what our roles should be five to 20 years from now, not by extrapolating from the past and present but by looking 20–50 years into the future and then working back from there. Our objective should be to think of what we as health professionals can contribute to the needs of the future health system as we think it will be.

The kind of thinking and planning we must do will not be easy. And it may be quite stressful. We will have to consider the possibility that, if we wish to have a meaningful role in the future system, we may not even be called pharmacists or clinical pharmacists. Educational requirements for our future role may be entirely different from today's pharmaceutical education. There may not be any pharmacy colleges.

The planning needed cannot be done in isolation by pharmacy alone. It must be a joint effort involving all the health disciplines and those outside the health disciplines as well. It will call for uncommon statesmanship—of a kind not often witnessed. It will be a lengthy process; in fact, it must be a continuing process. Plans must be perpetually updated as new knowledge or evidence comes to light.

If, as Earl Joseph claims, there is little we can do now to change the course of things during the next five years, we can shape our future beyond that time if, beginning now, we commit our creative energies to participating in planning for change. American hospital pharmacy has never lacked forward-thinking leaders. The man in whose honor this award was established, Harvey A. K. Whitney, was one of these. Dr. Arthur Purdum was another. And Dr. Don Francke. I am confident that we hospital pharmacists can meet the challenges that lie before us.

(For the complete list of references cited, please see page 1322 of the *American Journal of Hospital Pharmacy*, Aug. 1983.)

At the time he received this award, Warren E. McConnell was Special Assistant in the Executive Office of the American Society of Hospital Pharmacists, Bethesda, Maryland.

1984

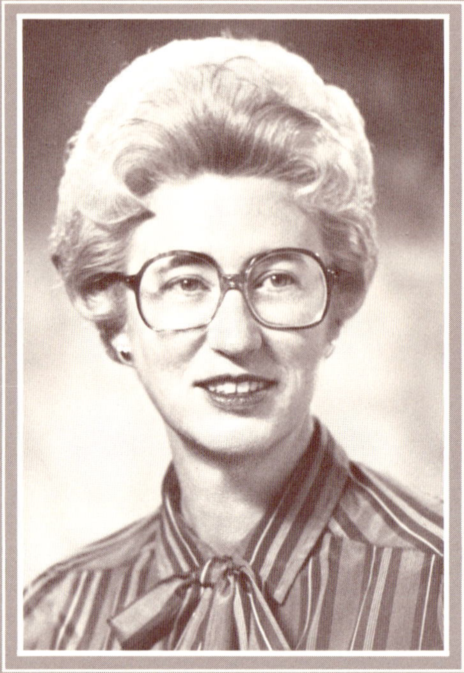

MARY JO REILLY

"We have rededicated ourselves to a professionalism which finds its fulfillment in serving."

OLD DREAMS, YOUNG HOPES

Having celebrated my 20th anniversary as a member of the ASHP staff last March, I began several months ago a journey of retrospection that has helped me to formulate the thoughts I will share with you this evening. If I struggle to find the words and the proper voice to express those thoughts, it is not a dilemma of language but of emotion and persona. There are many in this audience and on this dais to whom I am grateful for having always tried to make the mountains seem low; the crooked, straight; and the rough places, smooth. Between us there is a depth of understanding that words need not reach, perhaps cannot. For me and for my family, thank you all for sharing this evening with us.

You honor this evening, in a break with the Harvey A. K. Whitney Lecture Award tradition, not an innovator but an implementor, a facilitator, an enabler. And in so honoring me, you honor all ASHP staff—past, present, and future. All our staff bear their white ribbons with pride and with few aspirations to anything but utility.

I have had on my desk for many years a quotation by William Blake, "He who would do good must do it in minute particulars... For art and science cannot exist but in minutely organized particulars."[1] I and many others of our staff have tried to serve our profession in minute, organized particulars.

I have been privileged to work side by side with six past recipients of this Whitney Award. I know personally and have worked in a variety of capacities with more than 20 others. These associations and those I have had with so many ASHP officers, Board members, leaders, and members have afforded me a unique perspective on the continuum that is ASHP and American hospital pharmacy.

The Society is 42 years old this August—middle aged. Middle age is a complicated thing. It means growing up; it means being at the heart of the matter; it means it is time to reexamine the past and replot the future. It can be a time for reorientation or for a last grand fling at the fading fantasies of youth.

There is a certain insistency in middle age. Time becomes quite different. The sense of "this is it" bullies us into a state of semiorganization. It is not enough to "plan" to stop smoking, get in shape, or get straight with the underwriters. We must do it now. We become more aware of the challenge of simple maintenance. The back must be bent with discipline or cease to bend at all. We begin to appreciate the long view. We begin to understand the meaning of phrases such as "it takes time" and "set in your ways" and "you have your whole life ahead of you." I suppose the difference between middle age and the next, less agreeable, stage is the fact that in middle age we can still believe that next year will be better.

In the fifth decade of its age, ASHP is undergoing its expected midlife crisis. Crisis connoting not a catastrophe, but a turning point, a crucial period of increased vulnerability and heightened potential. Those who pioneered our professional Society and our practice of hospital pharmacy fashioned a Society and a practice dedicated to certain values, and those values have always been the center of life at ASHP. One role of a mature ASHP is to maintain that abiding sense of the past—to be the custodian of the dreams. ASHP must hold the old values while we collect the new, young hopes. Dreams and hopes, old and new, must be matched to the possibilities for progress as we present a confident face to the future.

The challenge is to sort out the qualities we want to retain from our childhood models, to bind them with the qualities and capabilities that distinguish us now as a mature profession, and to fit all of this back together in broader form.

The original 1942 ASHP Statement of Purpose, which served us so well in our youth, was revamped into a new constitution and bylaws in our 21st year, 1963. For more than 20 years, the 1963 documents offered us, through our young adulthood, a certain stability and a set of commonly accepted professional and cultural values. But life is a continuum, not an accumulation, and "well enough" will rarely let itself be let alone.

For those of us who have grown up with the Society, our perception of ASHP does not change much as time passes. After all, we are always with ourselves, peering into the mirror most mornings and evenings, and changes come slowly, with subtlety. If we run across a photograph of ourselves—or a membership or budget report—of 10, 20, or 30 years ago, we are reminded of how much we have changed; but once the picture is out of sight, it is quickly out of mind.

A mature ASHP has earned the right to new sensations, emotions, and opinions. We do not have to bend with every political or cultural wind. We do not have to believe that the world was invented in the 1960s. We can allow others the fierceness of their opinions and the right to be inconsistent—just as we allow ourselves to be inconsistent. That tolerance is a function of maturity. We have more reference points now than were available to us 20 years ago. We have a better sense of what is temporal and what is enduring than we had 20 years ago.

In our 40th year, we began a revision of ASHP's governing documents. Throughout this project, we have embraced our original purposes and values and at the same time reexpressed our mission as a Society in relation to contemporary needs. We have rededicated ourselves to a professionalism which finds its fulfillment in serving. We are committed to fostering rational drug use and pharmacy practice innovation in pursuit of quality patient care. Such a goal cannot be achieved by people who are afraid to pay the cost, feel the exertion, stretch, change, move, and accept the pain that may be involved. We must help each other respond to the demands and responsibilities of our success. We rely on the vigor of each member's contribution.

Perhaps it is my own middle age—my 20th anniversary with ASHP, planning for the 25th reunion weekend of my pharmacy school class —that has set me on this course of looking both backward and forward. I recently realized, too, that all my favorite young movie stars—Jane Fonda, Robert Redford, Dustin Hoffman, Mary Tyler Moore—are 46 years old. "Oh well," said I, "1937 was a very good year."

In hospital pharmacy, in 1937, Spease offered at Western Reserve University the first academic program combined with a residency. The first hospital pharmacy residency program, conducted by Harvey A. K. Whitney, was already 10 years old. Whitney, in 1937, had his residents attend clinical staff conferences, grand rounds, and autopsies—an unusual occurrence in a hospital in 1937 and a dream, perhaps, for the future of pharmacy by a man whose vision became his legacy.

The very first Whitney Lecture I ever attended was in 1960. Tom Foster was the recipient of the award, and the title of his lecture was "The Expanding Role of the Hospital Pharmacist as a Member of the Health Care Team."[2] Mr. Foster envisioned participation in clinical research; leadership in disaster planning; involvement in the development of intelligent, practical, and economic prepaid health care plans; and leadership in confronting the socioeconomic challenges presented by geriatric and catastrophic disease problems. He saw in the future hospital pharmacists playing a vital part in formulating public and professional opinions and attitudes on health issues. His 24-year-old dream is reiterated in the hopes of today's practitioners.

For many of us, it is only the present that matters, the imposition of the dreams of others and the struggle to realize our own. But if we examine things more closely, I think we shall find that tradition and irony have their own system of circulation, their own sense of fulfillment and surprise. What we describe as change is really continuity. The answers of one generation become the questions of the next. Let me describe what I mean by using as an example an area of practice close to my own heart—drug information services.

As the ASHP was founded in 1942, one of its stated objectives was "to disseminate knowledge by providing for interchange of information among hospital pharmacists and members of allied specialties and professions." Information service of some description, then, was identified very early in our Society's history as a basic value of our profession.

As early as 1945, the editor of the *Bulletin of the American Society of Hospital Pharmacists*, Don Francke, editorialized, "The pharmacist should be a consultant to the physician."[3] Until the early 1950s, though, emphasis in hospital pharmacy was on integration of pharmacy with administration and on providing services to nurses. In the 1950s, our literature began to reflect ways the pharmacist might function in programs of drug evaluation, thus providing more service to the medical staff. In the mid-1950s, the audit of pharmaceutical services in hospitals (*Mirror to Hospital Pharmacy*) first showed that drug information services were provided or that pharmacists would like to provide these services in a very high percentage of hospitals. The audit recommended:[4]

> *that hospital pharmacists more fully recognize the importance of their role as consultants on matters pertaining to drugs, that they commit themselves to the task of improving their ability to assume this role, and that they make efforts to assemble and organize the bibliographic resources to enable them to perform this function. . . .*

By 1959, two important documents were under development, and between 1959 and 1964 these were adopted by ASHP in conjunction with other organizations including the American Hospital Association, American Medical Association, and American Pharmaceutical Association. The *Statement on the Pharmacy and Therapeutics Committee* and the *Statement of Guiding Principles on the Operation of the Hospital Formulary System* formally acknowledged agreement among the medical and pharmacy professions and hospitals that achievement of rational drug therapy requires an organized program, that drug information services are essential to the conduct of this organized program, and that the pharmacist has prime responsibility for these information services.

Our professional literature around the time these official policy statements were being developed suggested some specific types of drug information services—some dreams and hopes of the late 1950s and early 1960s—making ward rounds with physicians; evaluating manufacturers' literature; assisting in double-blind, placebo-controlled studies; and consulting in pharmacologic problems and therapeutic problems such as therapeutic uses, therapeutic equivalents, and comparisons.

The study by Barker and McConnell at the University of Florida in 1961,[5,6] confirmed by studies of Heller and Barker at Arkansas[7-12] and Tester, Black, and colleagues at Iowa,[13-15] showed that the incidence of medication errors in hospitals was much higher than anyone had realized. These studies also suggested the value of having pharmacists working more closely with physicians and nurses and knowing more about how and why drugs were being prescribed and how they were handled on nursing units. These studies led to the advent of unit dose drug distribution systems, which freed the pharmacist to associate with physicians and nurses—to leave the pharmacy and follow the drug, to investigate what went on in nursing units and patient care areas. Hand-in-hand with unit dose systems were development of pharmacy-based IV additive programs, receipt of physicians' original orders by the pharmacy, and development of patient profiles.

A group of practitioners examining and improving the distributive aspects of institutional practice intersected with the group interested in drug information services, each making a unique and necessary contribution to modern pharmacy practice. Practitioners who shared basic values were pulling together in the same direction.

Pharmacists were now out of the pharmacy because of improvements in distribution systems. Realizing the improvements in patient care that would result if drugs were used more intelligently, and armed with the official sanction of involvement in therapeutics, the pharmacist as drug information expert came into his own. The clinical need for drug information was identified and characterized, and practical techniques and services were developed to provide support of rational therapeutics. The early drug information pharmacists helped us gain access to the total drug use process and therapeutic decision-making.

One of the primary characteristics of the health practitioner's need for drug information is the random manner in which it occurs. Usually, physicians, nurses, and pharmacists need information in relation to a specific problem in a specific patient. This need for information is best accommodated by data, not by documents. Ideally, drug information should be available in time to be used in making decisions about treatment of the patient.[16]

Any response to the drug information needs I've just described must involve several components. Considerable effort must be exerted in developing an information store. Some method must be developed to retrieve bits of data about drugs in a short period of time and, similarly, specific patient data must be available to the decision maker. A specialist is needed to organize and centralize existing drug information and to assist in selection, coordination, and dissemination of information.

By the mid-1960s, there was a cadre of pharmacists who considered themselves drug information specialists. In 1964, the ASHP held a Special Conference on Drug Information Services in conjunction with

ASHP's Committee on Drug Information Services. This Conference and subsequent committee meetings signified the early recognition of a clinical role for the hospital pharmacist and the changing character of drug information needs that accompanied the pharmacist's increased involvement in direct patient care.

This contribution by drug information pharmacists set the course for a generation of practitioners and offered us hope for a new kind of pharmacy practice. It suggested new ASHP products and services, new guidelines, statements, and standards of practice.

It has been said there are three ways to get something done: do it yourself, hire someone, or forbid your kids to do it. Our profession's "kids" in the late 1960s and early 1970s would not be denied. With determination, our kids aspired to use their drug knowledge to contribute to quality patient care and to become respected members of the health care team. And they did. It has been a decade since the fever of pharmacy's youth culture burnt for itself and for our profession a unique and permanent place in American health care. While there is no antidote for that special enthusiasm of youth, many doors had to be opened by those in the practice establishment, who recalled their own dreams for our profession. Your professional Society developed standards of practice that incorporated principles that were once dreams, then hopes, and, finally, reality. At that important crossroad, we all saw a path to a new beginning—an opportunity to make ourselves more.

Through ASHP you have recently revised the 20-year-old statements on the formulary system and the Pharmacy and Therapeutics Committee to make them more contemporary. We no longer have a separate statement on the hospital pharmacist and drug information services—that concept has been incorporated into all of our standards of practice. Indeed, the Report of the Study Commission on Pharmacy in 1975 concluded that pharmacy should be conceived basically as a knowledge system and suggested that the greatest potential for our profession is in developing, organizing, and distributing knowledge and information about drugs.[17]

It is quite an amalgam of old dreams and young hopes that together sum up the complicated experience of middle age. As a Society and as a profession, we are finding that middle age has some advantages, or at least some consolations. There is a perspective that age alone affords. While vigor may wane somewhat, so do the foolish purposes in which it was sometimes employed. The presumed slights that were once so affronting in adolescence and young adulthood are suffered more tolerantly in the middle years. Conclusions are not reached in haste. The generation that so hotly contested the issues of the sixties and seventies is now given to long looks and sober consideration.

Middle age is a period of transition. It can be a period of reevaluation, a period of new hopes, or a time of early despair. It represents an opportunity for reflection on our dreams and hopes, for gauging our further course in life.

One of the major challenges of our middle age is the computer and related technology and the transition it is causing in all our lives. Continuing with my drug information service example, computers and related technology have changed substantially the way we now approach information-handling needs. Fresh tracks must be laid, novel approaches taken to enable us to work the available technology we know is at our disposal. Beginning with large-scale computational and business applications, the use of computers has spread to information retrieval and database management. At ASHP, we have developed a host of drug information resources and conducted instructional programs to help advance a practice in transition. We have recently announced the availability of our new generation of drug information resource—Drug Information Fulltext—an online database service geared to management of an impressive store of drug information and to rapid retrieval of data of a random nature. The experts tell us that in the future we will see a proliferation of knowledge-based systems such as Drug Information Fulltext, the "expert systems" that are intelligent computer programs using knowledge and inference procedures to solve problems difficult enough to require substantial human expertise.

Pharmacy will be one of the professions regularly using computers. We are confident that a computer is just another tool to help us do our jobs. Such diverse professionals as lawyers, engineers, librarians, and medical practitioners all use the computer with equal facility, not because computer science is part of their academic training but because their basic communications skills are well developed. In an information-oriented age, we must be able to communicate ideas, problems, descriptions, and solutions. We must be able to speak and to write concisely, to express ourselves clearly. As an editor, it seems I've been making that same plea for years and years. If we are to remain respected health professionals, we must be able to communicate effectively. It is a basic challenge of our times to improve our education system in many areas, but none so important as linguistic and logical skills.

One final comment.

We hear so much today about containing health care costs. Every day we hear, "Health care stands out as the single most inflationary factor in the American economy today," and "$321 billion annual cost of health care delivery—10% of the gross national product—is too much." How are we to decide how much is too much to spend on health care?

The successes of the medical system are being dealt with in the political system. Everyone agrees our resources are not unlimited. The problem of increasing costs will only worsen as research labs, pharmaceutical companies, and makers of diagnostic equipment continue to turn out new methods and new products. These innovations can help save lives that are now doomed, but they will make tomorrow's health care costs even higher than today's.

Today's care is complex, sophisticated, and effective. Our system of health care offers achievements, capabilities, and hope once deemed unobtainable. As John Alexander McMahon of the American Hospital Association has pointed out, we have set a high and visible standard and created an expectation of quality from which we cannot now retreat.[18]

What we must strive to achieve is the same and better quality for less money. Our ability to do that will depend on all professions, and indeed all individuals throughout the system, altering their behavior and targeting, refining a bit more sharply, their role in the system. We must trim the excess without cutting into the essence. We must above all maintain a caring environment in the face of technological assault. Any endeavor of the healing professions is valued because of its ability to affirm the dignity of the human person and life and to build a human community by its respect for the sanctity of human relationships. There must be a heightened sensitivity among all health professionals to the dignity of patients and their families.

As a mature profession, we have an obligation to arrive at and take responsibility for those difficult, uncomfortable decisions that must be made as we take a hard look at the complex of problems associated with cost versus quality.

ASHP's new governing documents state that ASHP was formed "to foster rational drug use in society such as through advocating appropriate public policies toward that end."[19] As one of the sobering responsibilities of middle age, ASHP has an obligation to take this more active role in the public policy debate. You, as individual members of a mature profession, must do the same.

Patient protection in all drug-related areas will be a continuing need. "High tech" drugs providing specialized therapy tailored to individual patient needs will be highly beneficial but very expensive. Pharmacists will need to take a proactive role in drug use policy development, analysis, and enforcement. Important issues are going to be determined by someone: why not by those of us who are best qualified to present a balanced and patient-centered perspective? Middle age is the time of maximum influence—of necessary thinking by knowledgeable people. Now it is time that we claim the authority we have earned.

We must see to it that our public policy decisions are based on wisdom and morality, not expediency. We must provide that deeper and more comprehensive perspective that goes beyond pure science and technology.

Whatever our decisions, they must be made in a caring atmosphere. That is the health professional's contribution to the decision process.

And what if we continue to be successful in saving and prolonging more lives at an acceptable financial cost? Finding the solution to a problem changes the nature of the problem. The next challenge will be in evaluating handicapped or impaired persons—those with transplants or with implantable pumps, those with serious illnesses who are undergoing successful long-term treatment—and restoring them as functioning members of society. What are the medical requirements for handling these workers, and what physical adjustments to the workplace are necessary? We need more creative approaches to employment of the handicapped and a review of public policy issues and the responsibilities of employers and employees.

It's a dilemma. No matter how much we do, we will never do enough. And what we don't do is always more important than what we do.

One of the real hazards of middle age is having to view the world through bifocals. Near and far vision are quite clear, but the midrange is blurred, the image jumps. There is that distance between close up and far away that bifocals don't correct for at all: speedometers, prices on supermarket shelves, papers across a desk.

Exactly how we approach the tough issues of the next decade may be a little blurred right now, a jumpy image. One thing is certain: our leaders must call forth the creativity from us all. They must listen with an understanding ear, speak with simplicity and directness, and give value to the presence and contributions of all. As a Society, we must reaffirm the goodness that we have been, we are, and are becoming.

Above all, we must refuse to be victimized by apathy and discouragement. We must avoid a climate of undue seriousness and apprehension, even though we live in an anxious age. There must be room for joy and celebration and laughter and good fun as we go about the serious tasks we have undertaken.

For life is about getting better. Ideally, we have learned from our past. We keep moving forward, seeking out new ways of doing things, new things to do. We have learned that willpower and intellect alone do not overcome all obstacles. We have some experience now with many techniques for facing challenges and change; we have modified many of the assumptions and illusions of youth. We are willing to make a few mistakes and to learn from them. We cannot deny what experience has taught us. The best we can do in life is to discover what we are good at and then build on our strengths. We come to approve of ourselves quite independently of other people's standards and agenda. We have given each other the courage to experiment with our lives and have arrived at a point of dignity worth defending —we have achieved a measure of integrity. Mind and heart can at last be united in judgment, and it is this improvement in the exercise of judgment that is one of the most reassuring aspects of middle age.

Many have contributed to our profession and to our professional Society to bring us to a secure and stable middle age. Hubert Humphrey once said, "before the reality lies the dream," and how obvious that is as we view our own rich heritage as a profession. There are still needs unanswered, unresolved, unextinguished. It is for the future to fulfill those hopes.

(For the complete list of references cited, please see page 1535 of the *American Journal of Hospital Pharmacy*, Aug. 1984.)

At the time she received this award, Mary Jo Reilly was Senior Vice President of the American Society of Hospital Pharmacists, Bethesda, Maryland.

1985

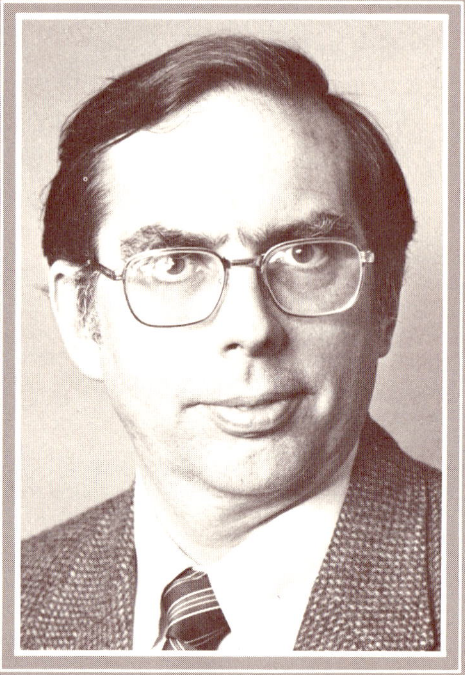

FRED M. ECKEL

"Research should be directed at understanding the unknowns in the practice arena."

RESEARCH: CORNERSTONE OF PHARMACY PRACTICE

Ladies and gentlemen of the dias, officers and members of ASHP, and friends.

To be recognized by one's peers is always a professional high point in a career.

To be cited with such kind words by people you respect makes the recognition more satisfying.

To be honored for professional accomplishments that were done out of enjoyment and benefited me more than anyone else makes such an award undeserved but truly appreciated.

My deepest thanks to the Harvey A. K. Whitney Selection Committee for bestowing this honor on me.

I would like to divide my address into three parts tonight: reflection, response, and shared recognition. Everyone expects the Whitney awardee to make a scholarly address, and I will try to comply. However, having successfully traversed my midlife crisis with most of my hair entitles me to some introspection and reflection. Finally, this honor is not singularly deserved; I must share this recognition with others.

Although I never knew Mr. Whitney, I entered hospital pharmacy when his memory was very much alive. My initial professional interactions were with individuals who lived through those early years of organizing hospital pharmacy. These hospital pharmacy leaders were committed to what they were doing and willingly shared their goals, beliefs, and experience with us neophytes. This early professionalization experience helped make hospital pharmacy into a lifelong commitment for me. Starting in hospital pharmacy in the early 1960s allowed me to mature with it, contribute a small part to its growth, and benefit immensely from the association. Pharmacy is a great profession. It has provided me with opportunities to serve others, one characteristic of a true profession.

Early hospital pharmacy leaders were willing to put the needs of others before their own. This resulted in the establishment of hospital pharmacy as an accepted component of pharmacy education, practice, and research. Our hospital pharmacy forefathers had a commitment to the cause of establishing hospital pharmacy. I am concerned that some of us have lost this commitment. For some, "What can the profession do for me?" has replaced our forefathers' concern of "How can I advance our profession through service?" It is common to see pharmacists moving from job to job, apparently in pursuit of some elusive goals. Not realizing their dreams, they become disenchanted. Although a move is sometimes necessary to advance a career, I am convinced that real contribution to the advancement of hospital pharmacy requires the establishment of a strong foundation. This requires a commitment of effort over a substantial period of time to see results.

In an age where materialism is a way of life, when individuals believe commitments can be broken when the going is rough and everyone wants immediate rewards for their efforts, hospital pharmacy needs to rekindle and maintain those attributes of Harvey A. K. Whitney and others who brought hospital pharmacy into a leadership role in pharmacy education, research, and service. If hospital pharmacy practitioners can learn once more how to put the needs of others before their own needs, then we shall continue our position of pharmacy leadership.

One of the most memorable Whitney addresses to me was that of Albert Lauve in 1964. He spoke from his heart and conveyed a sense of professional commitment which I wanted to emulate in my career. He expressed my thoughts when he said:[1]

> *Young pharmacists, take heed. My years offer me the protection of experience, but they also offer me the fruits of observation and retrospect. Society recognizes the contributions our profession has made and continues to make. It wants more of the same. Do not be overly concerned or tempted to cast aside the enduring rewards of professional satisfaction for the temporary and fleeting pleasure of material rewards.*

I too challenge our young pharmacists to the development of their careers through a lifetime of service to others.

Some younger pharmacists continue to be concerned about our profession. They see so much that needs to be done and may become discouraged. "How can you feel so positive about our profession?" they ask. Age and experience have some advantages. They allow one to look retrospectively and see how far pharmacy has come. All of pharmacy, but particularly hospital pharmacy, has made substantial progress. In 1960, my initial interest in hospital pharmacy occurred because most hospital pharmacists did not have to work nights and weekends. How our responsibilities and activities have grown! My professional pride is strengthened by our progress. My professional commitment is challenged by the opportunities still waiting to be met.

Those of us who recognize how far our profession still has to go to strengthen our service to society wonder how we can get there faster and go farther than seem possible now. Rather than concerning ourselves with the whole problem, we need to focus on the part that we control. The old "divide and conquer" adage works as well in this arena as in any other. If all of us only concerned ourselves with enhancing pharmacy's role in our own sphere of influence, much professional progress would be made. We shall reach our professional destination faster if we focus our energies on improving our own situation. However, progress in our individual practice must be made within an overall philosophy of practice that is common to us all. Our individual efforts will not lead to overall professional enhancement unless we are guided by the same professional service philosophy.

How to advance our profession further is of equal concern to pharmacy practice. My personal belief is that it will require a renewed appreciation for the role of research—the quest for new knowledge and the development and evaluation of new services. Because our professional goals can be extended further only as new knowledge is generated to support new advancements, research must become the cornerstone of pharmacy practice.

I wish to offer a sequence of thoughts that focus attention on the value of research as an essential component of pharmacy practice:

1. Research accomplishments assure prestige and influence and result in more resources to a profession whose education is university based.
2. Pharmacy as a profession is clearly differentiated, and this differentiation fosters a needed division of labor.
3. Pharmacy as a profession lacks adequate resources to accomplish all of its goals unless each segment cooperates and integrates its efforts.
4. The purpose of a university is to engage in scholarly efforts to advance knowledge.
5. Pharmacy practice faculty must develop the appropriate research skills and be engaged actively in this advancement of knowledge to support advances in pharmacy practice.
6. Pharmacy practitioners must respect and support this research effort and assist the educational process by assuming a growing role in classroom and experiential teaching.
7. The acceptance and implementation of this relationship will bring an enhanced professional image for pharmacy, professional growth for the individual practitioner, and health advances for society.

Now let me develop these seven ideas further.

In 1980, William S. Apple observed that many of pharmacy's brightest minds were entering the clinical pharmacy area rather than the pharmaceutical sciences. He lamented this trend because in his sphere of influence, Washington, DC, and the halls of Congress, pharmacy's credibility derives from the pharmaceutical sciences that underpin the profession.[2]

I believe, also, that a scientific foundation is essential for the pharmacy profession. Rather than lament the growth in clinical pharmacy, we need to expand the scientific foundation of clinical practice to assure continued acceptance of our professional role.

Each of us can recall breakthrough advances in science that captured the minds of the public and helped establish or maintain the eminence of some professions. These dramatic technological developments really lend credibility to a profession. These scientific contributions win professional acceptance and, more importantly, societal respect and support. This results in governmental, philanthropic, or individual willingness to finance such activities. Pharmacy needs such support now, and it will become more important in the future. The profession of medicine is an example of practitioners benefiting from the contributions of medical research. My first thought then is that research accomplishments assure prestige and influence for a profession.

The concept of pharmacy as a differentiated profession was clearly developed in *Pharmacists for the Future: The Report of the Study Commission on Pharmacy*.[3] Although recognizing a common purpose for pharmacy, the report stated that:

> *A pharmacist must be defined as an individual who is engaged in one of the steps of a system called pharmacy.*
> *. . . A pharmacist is characterized by the common denominator of drug knowledge and the differentiated additional knowledge and skill required by his particular role.*

Our own professional organization, the American Society of Hospital Pharmacists, recognized the differentiation occurring in hospital pharmacy with the creation of Special Interest Groups (SIGs). Today, there are 11 different SIGs: Administrative Pharmacy Practice, Adult Clinical Pharmacy Practice, Ambulatory Care Pharmacy Practice, Clinical Pharmacokinetics Practice, Drug and Poison Information Practice, Geriatric Pharmacy Practice, Intravenous Therapy Practice, Nuclear Pharmacy Practice, Oncology Pharmacy Practice, Pediatric Pharmacy Practice, and Psychopharmacy Practice.

Since all pharmacists do not emphasize the same professional activities, the need for a common, unifying purpose that all pharmacists understand and follow is critical. Pharmacists must follow a similar philosophy of practice as they pursue their specific interest area if our profession is to be strong.

The thought that I want to develop about our professional differentiation is that each pharmacist cannot be expected to do all professional functions well. We need to accept our colleagues and to respect their professional contributions. We need to support them in their efforts to advance the profession because the differentiation in pharmacy fosters a needed division of labor.

The need to recognize this division of labor is made more critical because our profession lacks adequate resources to do everything we would like to do. In an ideal situation, each segment of pharmacy could be all things to all people. Unfortunately, this ideal situation does not exist. Prospective reimbursement systems have brought new pressures to reduce costs in hospitals. Many pharmacy departments are trying to hold on to existing programs instead of proposing new ones. The loss of federal capitation programs for pharmacy education and the possibility of further diminished federal dollars to support health education have severely constrained many pharmacy school budgets. The future does not appear bright for an influx of new resources. My third thought then is that pharmacy as a profession lacks adequate resources to accomplish all of its goals unless each segment cooperates and integrates its efforts.

Some people will find my next thought controversial. I suggest that the purpose of a university is to engage in scholarly efforts to advance knowledge. Dr. Jules Lapidus, a former professor of pharmaceutical chemistry and graduate school dean, stated that research in its broadest sense is the only reason for a university.[4] Our own University recently completed a special study in connection with its reaccreditation by the Southern Association of Colleges and Schools. The forward to the Report states that:[5]

The University is a center for learning. Most colleges and universities would make the same claim. But a research university differs in this respect: beyond the learning transmitted to students, there is the learning that transcends the current wisdom marking the various disciplines. This University is dedicated not only to the transmission of knowledge, but also to its extension.

The word "knowledge," however, is not self-defining. Nor are the words "scholarship" and "research." Sometimes they are used interchangeably. Sometimes they seem to imply different processes and outcomes. This Steering Committee, therefore, uses the general term "scholarly work" to designate the means by which a university becomes a great center of learning. That work ranges from the disciplined collection of data, through research that adjudicates contending theories, to the critical and creative activities that expand understanding so often provided by the humanities and the performing arts. Scholarly work will vary between disciplines and even among scholars within a given discipline. That variation is a source of strength insofar as differing perspectives engender new lines of inquiry, new prospects of understanding.

We have defined a research university as a center of knowledge-creation as well as knowledge-transmission, and this dualism of function may mislead. We do not mean that the transmission and creation of knowledge need be carried out by different persons, in different places, and with different resources. A great center of learning is distinguished by a pervasive spirit of inquiry that permeates classrooms as well as libraries and laboratories, and that animates students as well as faculty. In such a center of learning, teachers do not perform scholarly work despite their obligations to students: they do that work, in part, because of its contribution to their teaching. Conversely, teaching advances scholarship by raising questions that necessitate further research.

Two recommendations of the University of North Carolina at Chapel Hill's Self-Study Committee further support my thought of the research role of a university:[6]

The research mission must be recognized and articulated as a central and valuable pursuit of the University, and the means to succeed in that mission should be provided.

The first and most important criterion for tenure, promotion, and salary advancement in the faculty ranks must be demonstrated scholarship of high quality.

Society has recognized and identified that there is something special about a university. It expects something different from a university than it expects from other institutions within society. What society expects from a university is this concept of scholarship. Webster defines a university as an "institution of higher learning, providing for teaching and research."[7] So from a historical perspective, society looks at a university as something unique and expects it to engage in research.

John Weaver made this point as he addressed the faculty of Ohio State University in 1964:[8]

We cannot fail to keep our faith with a credo that in a university, truth and understanding is, in the first instance, pursued for its own sake and its own sake alone. Here in academic halls must be the shielded place where the world protects the smokeless fires of creativity so that they may burn and cast their steady light. If we are to protect these fires, we must of necessity protect our scholars of the faculty, of whatever scholarship persuasion, from the frantic array of intramural and extramural activities that increasingly divert them from basic academic pursuits. We must create and hold inviolate, opportunities for contemplation, reflection, growing depth of understanding. These to-be-treasured opportunities for the mind are too easily, too often sacrificed on the altar of momentary expediency.

The Argus Commission of the American Association of Colleges of Pharmacy concurred that scholarship and research are necessary for pharmacy education:[9]

It is the primary position of the Argus Commission that Faculties at Colleges of Pharmacy share the responsibility for conducting scholarly activities along with their colleagues in other disciplines for the advancement of knowledge, and for the benefit of mankind.

Universities do have a special responsibility in the area of scholarship. Schools of pharmacy, as university-based institutions, have that same responsibility.

In introducing this thought, I suggested that some people will not agree. My own initial academic career started with a different perspective. I was going to show the University faculty how pharmacy education should be conducted. As a practitioner-educator, I was going to change the system by emphasizing the delivery of service as a basis for my teaching role. This was more important than a research base, I thought. How I have changed! I still believe in the importance of the practitioner-educator in the education of a professional, but I now realize the critical importance of the clinical scientist who is engaged in a scholarly effort to broaden the knowledge base underpinning our practice base.

This leads to my next thought. Pharmacy practice faculty must develop the appropriate research skills and be engaged actively in this advancement of knowledge through research endeavors. These research endeavors must be directed at addressing practice-related issues.

There are at least three reasons for engaging in research according to *Pharmacists for the Future.*[10] First, it is the means by which faculty members continue their own self-directed learning, assure their long-term competence, and demonstrate to students that life is a continual learning process and that a degree is not the termination of the educational process.

Second, it is a means by which new knowledge is generated. There is some feeling in our society that we may have too much technological advancement. Other people think that new technology must be proven to be cost-effective before it is introduced. I think we are entering an era when we are going to focus more on research and the strengthening of our technological developments.

Finally, the purpose of research is to solve problems. Those of us in practice recognize that an increasing number of practice problems demand resolution.

P. O. Williams, speaking on medical education, agreed with these purposes for research:[11]

Research assures that students realize that knowledge is not static. That knowledge is a growing process. Two, it's a means to improve teachers by making them less dogmatic. Three, it insures that the knowledge progresses on a sound basis proven by scientific experiment. And four, it leads to discoveries that will improve the health of man.

When pharmacy practice or clinical programs were initiated in the School of Pharmacy in the mid-sixties, their purpose was to bring the practitioner-educator into academia, to meet an unmet need in the education of pharmacy students. We said that all other health professions trained their students at the bedside. Physicians took their students to the bedside. Veterinarians took students to the cageside. Nurses trained at the bedside. Pharmacy, on the other hand, terminated its professional activity in a simulated laboratory in a college of pharmacy. The experiential learning required to prepare pharmacy students for practice was the responsibility of boards of pharmacy, not schools of pharmacy.

We needed a change and that need resulted in the introduction of a practice component into the curriculum. We appointed faculty members who saw themselves as practitioners, who understood the practice environment, and who could communicate that practice environment to the students. Clinical pharmacy was described as the area within the pharmacy curriculum that dealt with patient care with emphasis on drug therapy. The acquisition of new knowledge was felt to be secondary to the delivery of patient care. It is interesting that as we created departments of pharmacy practice or clinical pharmacy, we were not especially concerned about new knowledge. We wanted the clinical faculty to be concerned about teaching students what we already knew so that they could become more effective practitioners. We only wanted these faculty members to help students develop appropriate attitudes and specific skills utilized by the pharmacist.

Since the 1960s, there has been a dramatic change in the practice of pharmacy and its educational system. What we did then is no longer an appropriate goal and direction for pharmacy practice departments.

We need to be assured that our pharmacy faculty members are teaching what is current now, not what was current when they were trained. In 1963, as I moved into a faculty position, I was very critical of my colleagues who were using outdated examples. I do not want pharmacy practice faculty using examples of outdated drug interactions or adverse reactions. What is the best way to assure that our faculties stay at the forefront of new knowledge? Is it through providing service, or is it through providing and being engaged in research, or through at least a balance of both activities? Although we could probably receive a lot of argument on this point, my position is that the arena of research will assure the professional competence of faculty and a scientific foundation for our practice.

Although my thesis is that research is the critical activity, I feel that this research should be directed at understanding the unknowns in the practice arena. This means that pharmacy practice faculties must maintain a practice component in their educational effort. In this way, their research plan can be directed towards practical applications.

How can this be accomplished in an era of diminished resources? Pharmacy practitioners must respect and support this research effort by faculty and develop their own scholarly approach to their practice. Pharmacy practitioners can assist the educational process by assuming a role in classroom and experiential teaching.

Pharmacy practitioners need to respect pharmacy practice scientists, and pharmacy practice scientists must respect practitioners. One of my great concerns as I talk with practitioners is the attitude, "Oh, those academicians are in their own world, doing their own things, unconcerned with the profession, lost to society." Educators have a similar attitude. "Those practitioners are out there, only interested in today, not looking into the future."

Well, the truth is that both groups are concerned with the profession and are committed to resolving our problems. We need somebody who can interface between practitioners with their interests and demands and the basic scientists with their interests and demands. It is my suggestion that pharmacy practice faculties who maintain a practice base and are involved in a research effort can fill this role.

But more importantly, in hospital pharmacy we are moving into a new era. The talk about cost containment makes us aware of our limited resources, leading to the need to define better the pharmacy practice–research interface.

I suggest that departments of pharmacy practice place greater importance on the generation of new knowledge by emphasizing their faculty members' research responsibility. In an era of limited resources, this change in emphasis does not compromise the education of pharmacy students if our pharmacy practitioners serve as practitioner-educators in their practice site and the classroom.

Why should pharmacy practitioners accept an increasing responsibility to assist schools of pharmacy in the education of pharmacy students? The students' presence in the practice arena provides stimulation to the practitioner. Their inquiring minds challenge the status quo and encourage practice improvements. The self-image of practitioners can be enhanced by their teaching role. They may even receive formal recognition through a faculty appointment.

But these are not my real reasons for making this suggestion. My real reason is that as college faculty members move towards research responsibilities, we will need the practitioner to complete our students' education. The practitioner brings skills, insights, and abilities to the student, whether through an occasional lecture or in the continuation of the academic externship programs in which many are already involved. Coincident with that is the need for pharmacy practice educators to make a commitment to scholarship in a way that generates the new knowledge and provides the new insights that can solve practice problems.

I have given you reasons why I think a university-based educational program ought to be engaged in research since society expects it. The profession needs knowledge to solve its problems. Who will do that? The people who ought to be doing that are the people who make a commitment to be academicians. They do that by choice. As they make that choice, they ought to be nurtured to pursue this responsibility.

My last thought is that this new relationship will lead to an enhanced professional image for pharmacy, professional growth for the individual practitioner, and health advances for society.

We need to accept the differentiation that exists between people who assume faculty positions and those who accept practice positions. We need to learn to support and encourage each other in the face of our differences in order to achieve the common good. If we can do so, the profession itself, of which we are proud and to which we are committed, will find a way to move into the 1990s in a manner that will truly meet society's needs and expectations. More importantly, this research commitment will give recognition and societal acceptance to the profession.

Now let me share this recognition being accorded me with the others who share it with me. In honoring me this evening, you honor so many who invested themselves in my development. Any recognition I earned occurred because I surrounded myself with bright hardworking people. You honor all these colleagues in recognizing me.

From my parents, I received the ability to believe in the worth of human endeavor, a faith that is unshakeable, and the realization that a commitment to a cause is worthwhile. I share this recognition with them posthumously.

My pharmacy heritage is rich. My first Whitney Award banquet was in Chicago in 1961. Herb Flack, the award recipient, even bought my ticket. Herb's hospital pharmacy enthusiasm provided the spark to start my career. Clif Latiolais took me as an enthusiastic but inexperienced young man and kindled that spark into a flame. From them, I gained an appreciation for hospital pharmacy's past and a dream about its future. How fortunate for me that I met these leaders during my impressionable years. To them, I express my thanks; with them, I share this honor.

Finally, let me publicly recognize my family and its support. At times, my wife Peggy thought I was married to pharmacy instead of to her. I share this award with her and thank her for keeping the home in order during my frequent absences. My two teenagers, Sarah and Stephen, have added a continuing joy to my life. Sometimes they did not understand my absences, but their love was always felt. I share this award with them also.

To each of you, my thanks for sharing this evening with me.

(For the complete list of references cited, please see page 1723 of the *American Journal of Hospital Pharmacy*, Aug. 1985.)

At the time he received this award, Fred M. Eckel was Professor of Hospital Pharmacy and Chairman of the Division of Pharmacy Practice at the School of Pharmacy, University of North Carolina; Associate Director of Pharmacy Services, North Carolina Memorial Hospital, Chapel Hill; Research Associate, Health Services Research Center, University of North Carolina; and a Director of the American Foundation for Pharmaceutical Education.

1986

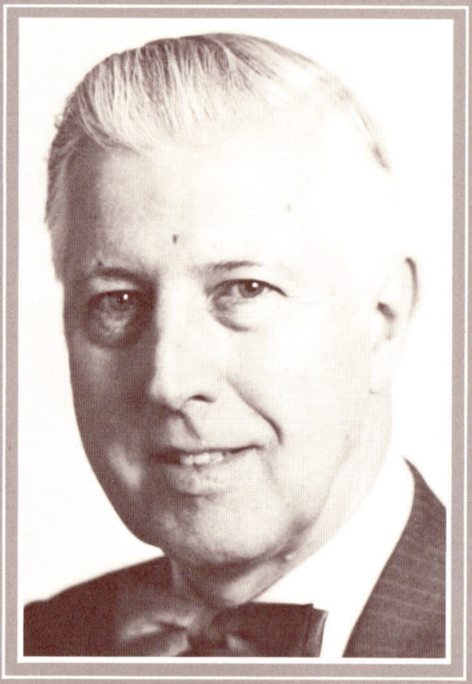

JOHN W. WEBB

"What specific actions do you have for your own personal growth?"

THE ART OF GROWING PROFESSIONALLY

Whitney Award recipients have the privilege of talking on a topic of their choice. With your indulgence, I would like to spend the next few minutes talking about you.

You are all aware of the polls showing that pharmacists are highly respected by the public. If that were a recording, you could listen to it for hours and even play it for your friends. However, on the flip side it seems that no matter which journal you pick up, it will have at least one article urging you to be better. By repeated exposure to such reproofs, it is easy for us to develop a collective guilt. This may explain why one psychiatrist observed that pharmacy leads the professions in self-denigration. By our own standards, we are never satisfied with our performance.

While everyone seems happy to tell you to be better, few tell you how. One basic rule of performance reviews is to recommend specific actions rather than speaking in vague general terms. We are all sophisticated enough to know this, but in your personal performance review what specific actions do you have for your own personal growth? This is an appropriate occasion to use past Whitney Award recipients as our quality assurance standard. It has been my good fortune to have met each one, so I can tell you some of the actions they took and you can see how yours compare.

First, they were willing to accept help from others. The most obvious is family support. Those of you who were at last year's banquet may remember that Fred Eckel expressed this thought in his closing remarks. I am not as disciplined as Fred. I cannot wait until the end. I would like to pause right here to thank my wife and family for the support that they have given me through the years. In my innocent youth, I thought that all families gave support; but I have sadly watched more than one person with great talent waste years in hibernation before the spouse and family came to realize the need for professional growth.

Next, most of them had a mentor. A mentor will advise and guide you, show you some shortcuts, and help you to interpret the information which repeatedly inundates you. A mentor will teach you how to think properly, help you to shed much of your provincial thinking, and give support to your moral character. H. A. K. Whitney was a mentor to Don Francke who, in turn, was a mentor to such well-known personalities as Bowles, Latiolais, and Phillips. Don Brodie and Herb Flack are other examples of outstanding mentors.

Those of you who find a good mentor are most fortunate. I had two: Ellsworth T. Neumann, M.D., an outstanding hospital administrator, and Dr. John T. Murphy, one of the country's leading hospital pharmacists. He was also Lou Jeffrey's preceptor.

Dr. Murphy was repeatedly an active candidate for the Whitney Award, but he always withdrew his name from nomination if the honor required giving a talk. As I stand in front of this august body, it is easy to understand his thinking. His reluctance to speak before large groups kept him from receiving due recognition. I would like to accept this award in his memory.

It has been stated that one grows by association with something bigger. Whitney Award winners have a history of associating with professional organizations. They must have heard the same remark that you and I have heard: "What can they do for me?" In addition to the obvious educational programs, societies offer committee members and officers the opportunity to gain experience in group dynamics, public speaking, and social grace and to exchange ideas and information with colleagues.

Over 100 years ago, a few wholesalers and drugstore owners established the Boston Druggists Association. It now also includes educators, hospital pharmacists, members of the Board of Pharmacy, and representatives from industry. Socializing with pharmacists other than those in your specialty is a pleasant way to avoid professional myopia. The current president of the group is William Gouveia, our new ASHP Board member.

Participating in regional and national organizations gives you a chance to see how the profession is practiced outside your local community. Not too many years ago, I attended a meeting in a country where hospital pharmacists only worked on weekdays from 9 to 5. I was shocked to hear one speaker tell the audience that plans were afoot to bring 24-hour service, women, and generic drugs into pharmacy.

It is good to get a shock on occasion because otherwise you become mentally lazy and take the familiar for granted. For example, we accept as a norm what women have contributed to hospital pharmacy. Some, like the feisty Evlyn Gray Scott, the exquisitely organized Gloria Francke, and the lovable late Sister Gonzales, have been

Whitney Award recipients. In 1984, Mary Jo Reilly proved that the movement continues. We should also acknowledge contributions by others such as Ivey and Patrick.

In 1983, I was in China as a member of an IV Therapy Delegation. During the "show and tell" sessions, nurses would swarm around us because they had never before seen plastic bags and tubing or disposable needles. We take them for granted, but I still remember the excitement of sitting in as my predecessor, John Murphy, worked with a man who was developing disposable needles. Unfortunately, the developer lost his personal fortune before the needle was perfected. Obviously, the pursuit of excellence is not kind to everyone.

You could commiserate with early Whitney Award recipients who lived in a period of permanent austerity. Health care had a layered structure, and there were daily attempts to find funds to treat the indigent sick. The search was not always successful. It is some kind of social commentary that the American public had TVs years before it had Medicare.

An attempt to grow professionally is in effect a search for excellence. Perfection is sometimes mistaken for excellence. In striving to become perfect, people become discouraged. Seeking perfection is dangerous since you can never be satisfied with your performance and with time it leads to burnout. In the March 1986 issue of the *American Journal of Hospital Pharmacy*, Robert Williams says:

> *The pursuit of perfection is frustrating, neurotic, and a terrible waste of time. The pursuit of excellence is gratifying, healthy, and productive.*

Williams' article is recommended reading for everyone and should be mandatory reading for all who are interested in effective leadership.

In industry, IBM is frequently cited as the hallmark of excellence. Many, including people who work for IBM, believe that its most important asset is respect for the individual. All managers pay lipservice to this philosophy, but under duress it may well be forgotten. I am reminded of a prizefighter who gets hurt and forgets his fight plan and all of his hours of training. If he does not get things into focus quickly, he will lose the contest. Although DRGs and fiscal restraint have given new opportunities to pharmacists, the most common complaint I hear from health care workers is that managers have neglected their most important asset.

We all agree that continuing education is a pillar for professional growth, particularly with the information explosion being a part of our way of life. You are forced to pay attention to immediate problems but save some time for a specific topic that particularly appeals to you. Diligence in pursuing a "labor of love" allows you to grow intellectually, and you will be able to see exciting new horizons.

Those who urge you to be better quite often also suggest that you work on a topic of interest to them. It is tempting for me to use this occasion to suggest that you should study how to control infusion rates by programming drug half-lives and patients' biofeedback into a computer. Or you could study solubility problems that arise from concentrating drug solutions for microinfusions. Should we also use solvents other than water? What an amazing coincidence if we should both be interested in the same problems. No need to ask you because somewhere, someone is already toiling in the vineyards looking for answers to these and other perceived problems.

In *Ulysses*, Tennyson says: "I am a part of all that I have met." I have worked in Maine, Connecticut, and Massachusetts and have been on the faculties of three colleges of pharmacy. I could not begin to tell you about all the wonderful people I have worked with or the pleasure students have given to me over the years. Being with someone like Bouchard, Godley, Heller, Fish, Pierpaoli, or Zilz is always stimulating, productive, and enjoyable. These names come immediately to mind, but there are many others.

Let me tell you about just two people I have worked with. A young methods engineer came into our department fresh from college. His youthful enthusiasm and educational background caused the staff to look at their routine in an entirely new way. It wasn't long before he was contributing in the area of materials management. From there he established the country's first hospital Laboratory of Industrial Engineering. He now has his own company on the West Coast.

I am proud to tell you the next story, but it is also a little embarrassing. A young Latvian lady who joined us as a secretary always seemed to be taking a course at one of the many schools in the Boston area. Only when she asked for a couple of hours off one day did I learn that she was graduating from Harvard. So much for the myth that I have an interest in personnel.

The point is that each one kept chipping away at professional growth and, like compound interest, over a period of time the results are impressive.

If you are a part of all that you have met, logic dictates that you are a part of others. May I suggest that you be tolerant of others who at the moment hold an opinion different from yours. John Locke said: "New opinions are always suspected and usually opposed." Each recipient of the Whitney Award had his or her own strong personality, and there can be no doubt that some of their opinions were opposed. Yet each one had the courage to face rejection and the tenacity to persevere. They would also state their beliefs publicly. Francke had the courage to present provocative and controversial opinions and then stride down from the podium, leaving the audience buzzing. You don't have to be that dramatic, but if you don't speak out no one will know what you believe in.

I doubt that many of you have thought much about the dual role of journal editors. You are all familiar with their unpleasant task of rejecting certain submitted papers so that only those of the highest caliber are published for your reading pleasure. But they also have a role in recognizing new ideas and different approaches to old problems and in encouraging inexperienced or unsuccessful authors to submit their work for the rest of us to share. I appreciate the courtesy and encouragement given to me by Editors Francke, Provost, and Davis.

When you want to talk with someone about medication errors, you would think of Ken Barker; drug information, Paul Parker; organizational affairs, Joseph Oddis; clinical pharmacy, Donald McLeod; computers, William Gouveia; nuclear pharmacy, Ronald Callahan; and IV incompatibilities, Lawrence Trissel. Each one of them nurtured an innovative idea and, despite an incessant demand for their time and the constant clamor for conformity, each devoted much time and energy to his respective area of interest. Each was blessed with one or more of the points we have outlined this evening.

In addition to the ways that we have looked at, you may have others that work for you to attain that nice warm inner feeling of accomplishment. Public recognition then becomes frosting on the cake. The frosting is delicious!

Thank you for a most pleasant evening.

John W. Webb retired as the Director of Pharmacy at Massachusetts General Hospital, Boston, in 1983.

1987

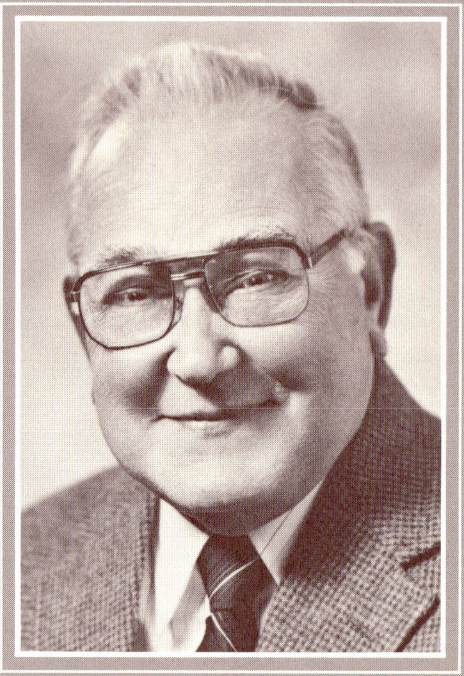

JOHN J. ZUGICH

"ASHP and its practitioners have developed a noble tradition for pharmacy."

INTIMATIONS ON A PROFESSION: RETROSPECT AND PROSPECT

The intent of the Harvey A. K. Whitney lecture series, now in its 37th year, is to serve as a partial chronicle of the history and culture of institutional pharmacy in the United States. The evolution and development have involved many men and women whom I shall refer to as "pathfinders"—people who lived the history.

My presentation will center on some observations about a few early developments and the meaning of these developments to the present environment. Some suggestions on unfinished business will be made.

Harvey A. K. Whitney was an original and creative pathfinder in practice and in his broad outlook for the profession. Working with him daily was infectious and inspiring for a lifetime.

"Uncle Harvey," or the "Chief" as we knew him, would have blessed a short break at an Annual Meeting such as this one, as a change from science and business, to look broadly at what has made a group "tick" with some success. He would have endorsed a little pause for reflection on some values and roots as he may have seen them. Our 45 years of existence as a Society should allow us to look back and make some judgments.

The hospital pharmacy movement within an older pharmacy profession has had its own distinct historical turning points. Joseph A. Oddis referred to four stages of the American movement in his Whitney Award lecture. Other stages have developed.

In my own lifetime, I have been privileged to be part of three of the stages, including what I would call the "joy of development" and the "pain of adversity." As an officer of ASHP, I found joy in helping our Society, after five years, finally establish a headquarters in Washington; volunteers were replaced by a paid staff, persons who came from hospital pharmacy ranks. There were many satisfactions like that for us all.

Pain came when we learned of the Society's financial deficit. We tried, with other executive officers, to achieve long-range solutions. This mixture of joy and pain, in retrospect, developed in me a lifelong "labor of love" attitude towards the profession, as cloying as that phrase may sound. Involvement brought that commitment.

From each evolutionary stage, certain characteristics developed that may have remained for the profession and the Society to recognize today. Without any modern fashionable jargon, these characteristics can be described as simple "fundamentals" stemming from the thinking of many early pathfinders.

Before we move into heavier material, let us pretend that we are not pharmacists but are outsiders looking at a group. We shall test a few areas to see where that group of professionals came from and where they are in 1987. Then we shall examine the significance of these areas.

One characteristic of a profession is that it has its own special body of knowledge. The evolution of hospital pharmacy literature is a major resource and strength.

We are now a long way from the early pathfinders, Harvey Whitney and Leo Mossman, who personally pecked at the typewriter to communicate "tips of the trade" and editorials. The sporadic, two-page, green stenciled publication had a proud masthead proclaiming, "Official Bulletin of the American Society of Hospital Pharmacists." From the beginning, these pathfinders intended that this medium would be the added "glue" to bind people and aspirations together for professional development. Because of that belief, many decisions were made along the way to keep the medium alive.

Having passed through many growing stages, the *American Journal of Hospital Pharmacy* is the official centerpiece today—the "flagship" publication. By all professional measures, it continues to advance in its literary quality, content, and range of technical information. The significance of the *Journal* is that it has greatly enriched the body of specialized pharmacy information while meeting the practitioner's needs in various historic periods.

Some people say that hospital pharmacy, to become a "profession" in itself, depends on pharmacy in general for its theory base. Who knows but that the developing specialized body of knowledge may eventually lead to that final rung, which would be the evolution of our own theory base, distinct for institutional pharmacy, and support yet unforeseen functions and techniques. It is visionary but intriguing!

The quality of editorials in the *American Journal of Hospital Pharmacy* has its own significance. The editorials appear to me, as a reader, to have great value for today's busy practitioners by summarizing contemporary issues, all expressed in fundamental and simple terms. Of equal importance is that the editorials serve as a major communication link for a huge membership to achieve a unity of purpose. This unity of purpose has been regarded as unique to, and the hallmark of, hospital pharmacy among all of American pharmacy practice areas. Some people contend that this consensus, cultivated very diligently, has historically been the energizing influence for the rapid developments in this pharmacy practice area.

The body of knowledge continues to grow through a supplemental support system of many official Society publications and programs for the practitioner. This support system serves a paramount need for frontline pharmacists, who increasingly require knowledge and information as their compounding role fades. Major advances in this support system are the innovative uses of the latest in computer technology and the beginning of consumer-designed information to extend the mission of the "safe and appropriate use of drugs" into the hands of the public.

Two programs in the support system deserve a nod in view of their track records. One is *International Pharmaceutical Abstracts*, which abstracts over 600 worldwide pharmaceutical, medical, and health care publications. No practitioner could do that alone. The other program is the *American Hospital Formulary Service Drug Information*. In my judgment, it is the outstanding contribution of the Society to American hospitals, other health professionals, and patients for the "safe and appropriate use of drugs." Most hospitals in the United States subscribe to this publication year after year, signifying its value in providing detailed information on practically every drug in the United States. The *American Hospital Formulary Service Drug Information* now has had more than 25 years of broad national acceptance. It extends the profession's mission through thousands of people in most American hospitals. That is involvement in our mission!

These foundations have expanded the body of knowledge for hospital pharmacy and have kept pace with related, rapid advances in health sciences and health care—no mean feat.

A profession that attempts to achieve a unity of purpose develops order through some formal organization.

ASHP developed its thrust in the "American way," using scattered volunteers for the initial five years. These hospital pharmacy volunteers, with working officers and committee members, were the "staff." ASHP has evolved today into a sophisticated and refined organization, with more than 100 staff people supporting 22,000 members. The form of the organization has changed over the years to fit different times. But each age has its fashions, concepts, values, and aspirations. The formal organization must adapt. With its record of above-average resiliency, ASHP stays viable regardless of changes in the players and pathfinders.

The early pathfinders applied some simple fundamentals to the organization of effort for the Society. One of these fundamental ideas was that ASHP would do for the practitioner what the practitioner could not do for himself. By providing information and knowledge for the profession, educating working practitioners, and stimulating the organization's evolving public influence and credibility, ASHP has achieved this goal.

Another fundamental was that the "network" of state groups in a formal organization is the primary area for action (the grassroots). Here, health-service-oriented goals are proved. In addition, ASHP appears to have made a conscious and deliberate effort over the years to value the importance of each member and the affiliated organization as the real epicenter for promoting and advancing standards and public service, rather than establishing a central power base, except as it serves to establish unity of purpose.

Today, we can see the growth (and retention) of a total of 49 state chapters, some having their own staff. They maintain constant relationships with the national core. ASHP Board and staff last year made outreach–personal contact visits to 33 of the 49 state chapters. In addition, regional sessions were held across the country for a two-way exchange of information and attitudes on current issues.

What about the signs of support being returned from the grassroots? The two-way liaison and local support appear to be working well. One piece of evidence is the reported 85% response from members on recent national surveys issued from ASHP headquarters. Another piece of evidence was demonstrated at this Annual Meeting. As many as 90 points or current issues and policies surfaced for review through different councils or groups (the formal organization), as officially recorded in the House of Delegates report.

An outside estimate of the formal organization would show that it is in touch with those older precepts, or fundamentals, and that it has strong participation from members, with genuine support from the grassroots. These characteristics must be guarded as a legacy for future pathfinders and leaders.

Institutional pharmacists and their Society have been cited by pharmacy media reports as "pharmacy's most dynamic group." It is interesting how the informal and social organization contributes one or two characteristics to this description.

Those of us who were on the faculty of the first "refresher course" or "institute," held at the University of Michigan in 1946, saw 136 hospital pharmacists almost euphoric about the new learning experience, not because of the faculty but because of the ability to "interchange information"—the announced purpose of the institute. The new format also stimulated hospital pharmacists because it was a departure from the traditional American convention program for professionals. It was a first in the pharmacy field. It was all learning, scheduled for 4½ to 5-day sessions from 8:30 to 5 and again from 7 to 9, with educational lectures, "show and tell" hands-on demonstrations, and spirited panel–audience interchanges. There were purposely scheduled periods when people could cluster and "jawbone." These "rap sessions" helped to develop changes in patterned behavior and attitudes—a prime goal of the educational sessions.

One characteristic of these meetings has been described as a literal "self-awakening," a self-motivation to reevaluate the standards of service the hospital practitioner provided (or the employer permitted to be provided). Additionally, in the informal contact with peers and in some "smoke-filled rooms," other ideas arose concerning service improvements that could be introduced and achieved back home.

A second observable characteristic of the informal sessions was described by Sister Mary Florentine and Clifton J. Latiolais in their Whitney Award lectures as the "enthusiasms," "verve," "vigor," and "dedication" that the groups generated. A practitioner's view was expressed as follows: The most valuable thing I got out of the meetings was when I got together with my friends and we talked till the wee hours of the morning on what we heard and how we could use it back home.

The informal, programmed time helped stimulate motivation and that initial self-awakening spark to improve services. The purposely limited size of the institutes (125–135 attendees) fostered the intimate interchange of information.

Time and growth factors have changed the way such educational sessions are conducted. Today, for example, the ASHP Midyear Clinical Meeting attracts the largest gathering of pharmacists in the United States and the world—as many as 10,000.

We trust the human spirit to achieve self-awakening, and we hope that self-motivation still accompanies the educational benefits derived from the meetings, despite the large attendance. Only the individual participant can answer that question.

Hospital pharmacy has taken the responsibility to "train its own" to provide skilled professionals. Like its companion profession—medicine—pharmacy's early philosophy maintained that "the hospital is the college," not the lecture room or laboratory bench alone. From the days of Edward Spease and Harvey A. K. Whitney, it took over 40 years of advocacy by institutional pharmacists before colleges of pharmacy fully accepted that premise.

Some of us early "interns" experienced the positives and negatives along the way, such as misgivings about being considered "cheap labor" for the hospital; the voluntary long hours on call; the timid and frightening curiosity of our first "post" (autopsy) or surgical procedure as we stood beside the pathologist or surgeon; the initial thrills of around-the-clock association with medical residents, including both work (ward rounds) and play (billiards and squash) as we lived side by side in the "interns' quarters"; and the attendance in the amphitheater with more than 100 house staff physicians at clinicopathological or specialty conferences. These events represented some learning experiences Whitney and others thought important for future hospital pharmacists.

Across the United States, these early prototype "nonacademic internships" had individual characteristics and variations, as designed by the pathfinder preceptors like Whitney. Yet all of the internships in hospital pharmacy then could be counted on two hands. Today, the growth and achievement are astounding to me. There are a reported 188 ASHP-accredited residency programs for pharmacy in hospitals. In one year, 1986, 400 graduates completed ASHP-accredited residencies. There have been 4000 graduates from those foundations of "training our own." Higher standards have gradually evolved, including formal visiting teams for accreditation according to refined guidelines.

The residency program has provided a major foundation and stimulus for the refinement and long-term continuity of improved practice standards for institutional pharmacy. Not all of the early visions of supplying manpower from this source have been achieved; but trainees, ever since the initial programs, have had national influence in the hospital pharmacy movement, in the affairs and events of American pharmacy in general, and in the pace-setting hospitals in the United States. The residency program has proved, over the long term, hospital pharmacy's special commitment to ensuring the continued education of skilled professionals.

One of my most vivid recollections of the evolution and development of the hospital pharmacy movement is the continuing influential leadership and commitment of women.

The Catholic Sisters provided some of the greatest impetus and spirit of enthusiasm for the profession and the development of programs. Many turned their pharmacies in Catholic hospitals upside-down to provide advanced services following their participation in institutes. Their presence was prominent in state affiliates and ASHP committees and as ASHP officers, and they contributed much volunteer time. Their contribution to American pharmacy, largely through ASHP, has not been told fully.

Women were in leading roles in the 11 city and state hospital pharmacy associations even before ASHP started. They were among the strongest advocates for standards and national development. Did you know that of the charter members of this Society, almost 50% were women hospital pharmacists?

Women continue to be elected to key officer positions at both state and national levels. The headquarters of the Society continues to have women with high levels of management ability in positions of influence.

Some of the most lasting contributions, far beyond the call of duty, were made by women pathfinders. Many foundation stones of today's Society programs, systems, and literature were first laid by the creativity and labor of these women. The place of women in the affairs of the profession and in leadership contributions is an accomplishment few other professions can match as an historical record.

Evolutionary development would have been slowed greatly without the economic organizational development of ASHP and the stewardship of this development to date. The method of funding the profession's Society has been a potent force, allowing the rapid evolution and expansion of programs and staff support and the development of a sophisticated formal organization.

What I call the "economic organization" stemmed from the following philosophy held by many pathfinders: Limit the burden of members' assessments or dues whenever possible to increase to the maximum the practitioner enrollment and thus professional participation.

From 1200 members, a $3900 yearly fund limit, and a deficit in 1947, annual funds now in eight figures have evolved through the efforts of many pathfinders. In 1986, the income for the Society's annual operating fund reached an amazing $12.3 million; but more amazing is that almost 90% of it came from income sources other than membership dues (e.g., publications, investments, and continuing-education programs).

What are the fruits of such an economic structure?

Two-thirds of all income is ploughed into education and professional information (professional services); almost one-third goes into what we termed unity of purpose (policy development). These accomplishments support the earlier ideals about the real place of the formal organization.

The favorable and successful economic picture, as well as the continuing good management of it, places many new horizons within reach. One new horizon is the sending of added leadership into the international arena. A favorable economic picture will allow for fuller participation now on a worldwide basis to help improve health care and to work on pharmacy standards.

The results of promoting creative income sources (other than membership assessments or dues) for the Society have been unusually successful, with prudent direction. This strong funding base has led to extraordinary accomplishments and to accelerated developments for institutional pharmacy and its practitioners.

A few characteristics have been examined that make up part of our history. In a short time, historically speaking, some noteworthy accomplishments and developments have occurred. This prompts me to suggest as "intimations" some unfinished business for the profession as we adjust our focus towards "pharmacy in organized health care settings" as the more recent orientation.

My first suggestion is that the formal organization, ASHP, should consider moving more heavily to another level. ASHP should develop stronger credibility, more influence, and added recognition at the level of public policy developments concerning total health care, not just pharmacy.

This level of involvement would be a new horizon, beyond issues of safe and appropriate use of drugs, although these factors would be included. It would entail helping to resolve the broader health care needs and issues of the public. It would mean joining and participating with newly identified leadership groups that clearly will affect health care and national health policies, institutions, and programs. For example, ASHP should collaborate closely with selected professional groups such as hospital administrators (e.g., American College of Health Care Executives and American Hospital Association), leading physician groups, health agencies (voluntary and government), and others. A close collaboration should exist with formal organizations that have similar stated goals of becoming more involved at the public policy level. It is my belief that hospital pharmacy "movers and shakers" are ready to handle this new horizon.

Taking this direction would mean involvement at both community and national levels through the ASHP's existing network organization. It would not mean just a liaison approach or propaganda, public relations, lobbying, protectionism, or establishment of speakers' bureaus to build credibility but would include strong participation leading to the introduction of new ideas for the public health and welfare. It would require new emphasis on an external, outward-looking approach, commitment, and the necessary energy beyond that required for current internal professional priorities.

An accepted and a followed ethic is a core characteristic for a profession. Such an ethic is my second suggestion.

Over the history of the hospital pharmacy movement, little or no direct attention has been given, to my knowledge, to a deliberate implementation of our own written set of principles for the specific guidance of institutional practitioners. I now suggest this approach.

The mechanisms, accountability, and responsibilities of a professional organization have not been established for the elimination of substandard practitioners and practices. I now suggest this approach also.

The environment of "organized" health care settings can have its own distinct conflicts of interest and deviations from ethical standards. Dealing with problems as they arise under a generic code for all of pharmacy will underline the need for our own standards specifically for institutional pharmacy.

I contend that a professed, guiding ethic is one of the most important foundations yet to be developed for refinement of our profession.

My third and last suggestion for unfinished business is the prompt preparation of a documented history of ASHP and the hospital pharmacy movement since 1952. I understand that this suggestion may be implemented in the future. The availability of first-source people and documents becomes more important as time goes by and recollections fade.

But the major part of this suggestion is that the history (stated facts, events, dates, names) include a strong parallel component of human and social interpretations, centering on how key events came about. It should include the values, ideas, beliefs, attitudes, customs, morals, behaviors, traditions, patterns, and systems that practitioners as a group, and the pathfinders, attached to their profession during certain periods. This history would begin to emphasize the foundations of a cultural perspective, along with the purely historical facts and events.

We have available the outstanding work that Gloria Niemeyer, Alex Berman, and Don Francke produced in *Ten Years of the American Society of Hospital Pharmacists.* It is, in my estimation, a fascinating recorded history—a legacy. With their in-depth interpretations, insights, and analyses of key events, the authors leave us with a deeper understanding of the heritage of hospital pharmacy for the years 1942–1952. We have had nothing comparable since 1952, a 35-year gap.

Bill Moyers, one of our contemporary documentary historians, said: "The future being a mystery excites, but the past instructs."

And now I must say adieu to a profession of the heart. Our professional group has shown an enviable record of refinements. We have touched on just a few. ASHP and its practitioners have developed a noble tradition for pharmacy, and a special dignity of their own, in practices and professional conduct. We all turn now to the young practitioners who are the pathfinders among us today. They are taking up the responsible stewardship and commitment—ever onward in spirit and energy.

Harvey A. K. Whitney and his contemporaries would have said: "Ladies and gentlemen—plus ultra! Press ahead and beyond to your own new horizons!"

Adieu. Thank you for the honor.

John J. Zugich retired as the Associate Hospital Director at the University of Michigan Hospital, Ann Arbor, in 1975.

1988

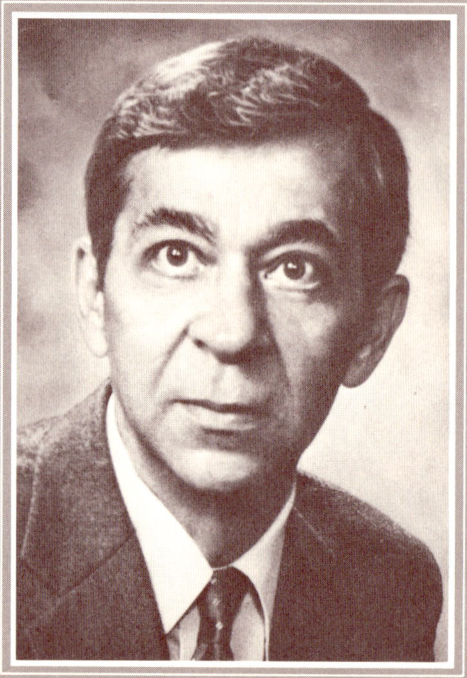

JOE E. SMITH

"We need leaders who can guide a pharmacy staff to assume new roles and higher professional responsibilities."

LEADERSHIP IN A CLINICAL PROFESSION

I am deeply honored, and I humbly thank the past recipients of the Harvey A. K. Whitney Lecture Award and the Southeastern Michigan Society of Hospital Pharmacists for choosing me, a practitioner, for this distinction.

I admit to experiencing what Dr. Pauline Clance described as the "imposter phenomenon."[1] Even when others proclaim your accomplishments, there is a feeling that any success you have realized must be due to some mysterious bit of luck or breaks and hard work but not a result of your own ability. You feel that others may have been misled into believing that you are more capable and knowledgeable than you really are and sooner or later the mask will be removed, exposing the real you.

I attribute any professional success I have had to knowing how long it takes to succeed and being persistent. Even a stopped clock is right twice a day, and after some years it can boast of a long series of successes.

I claim few personal accomplishments, but I do concede that anyone who survives being named Joe Smith deserves a little credit.

When Joe Oddis called to give me the great news, which elevated me right up through the roof, he quickly brought me back to earth with this comment: "Yes, Joe, it's a great trip, but there is some baggage that goes with it. You have to deliver the Whitney Award Lecture." That was certainly a sobering thought. It has indeed become a challenge and, I have since come to realize, an opportunity—an opportunity to raise your level of awareness or concern for some issue that I think is important to the profession.

It took only a small amount of time and thought to come up with a long list of problems that the profession needs to address, and the list swelled as I got ideas from the many friends I have spoken to recently. As the list of problems grew and I was becoming more depressed, I kept having to remind myself that we have faced problems like these in the past and have dealt with them rather effectively.

In fact, I feel very good about what the profession has accomplished. In the last 25 years, the profession has changed from one that was product and materials management oriented to one that is truly clinical and patient oriented. I feel fortunate that the greater part of my career has taken place during that period of time. So, I have looked for a subject through which I can express that good feeling about ourselves, one that has significantly contributed to that success and would symbolize it. And I have chosen to dedicate my lecture to accredited residency programs.

Harvey Whitney himself was one of our greatest preceptors, and from the well-designed internship program he began in the early 1930s at the University of Michigan Hospital came equally great preceptors such as Don Francke, Paul Parker, Clif Latiolais, George Phillips, and many others.

One of the most common characteristics among the Whitney Award recipients has been their contribution to the profession through the preceptorship of residency programs. Indeed, the first thought that comes to mind when the names of many of them are mentioned is of their legendary residency programs.

Residency programs and the accreditation process have been a strong force to bring about change in hospital pharmacy. I believe that residency training is the single most important activity initiated from within the profession itself that has advanced hospital pharmacy practice. Changes in practice have often been driven by influences from outside (e.g., nursing shortages, federal capitation grants for medical education, Joint Commission on Accreditation of Healthcare Organization standards, and a more litigious society). But the initiation of residency training and the accreditation process came from within the practice of hospital pharmacy itself.

This year is the silver anniversary of ASHP-accredited residency programs. Residency accreditation was initiated in 1962; in early and mid-1963, some site surveys were conducted; in December 1963, a few programs were accredited. Jefferson's was the first program surveyed and among the first accredited, I'm proud to say. Its accreditation, however, did not go without sharp criticism from the surveyors, John Oliver and Paul Parker. The program was cited, for example, for continuing to use cardboard slide boxes to dispense medications, and it did not go unnoticed that the department had only two dispensing pharmacists for a 736-bed hospital.

It was not uncommon in those days for preceptors to have to justify residency programs through the provision of a variety of services, and Jefferson was no exception. Twenty-four-hour service was accomplished by the rotation of residents on night shifts. As one means of justifying their existence, pharmacy residents provided, in addition to normal pharmaceutical services, inhalation therapy to all patients from 5 p.m., when the regular therapists went home, until 8 the next morning. Unusual services did not end there. Since the pharmacy was located in the basement alongside the morgue, the residents were assigned to release bodies from the morgue to undertakers during the night shift.

From beginnings that were tied strongly to personal preceptorship by a few of the profession's leaders, residency programs have grown in number and have become highly organized and often specialized to meet the changing needs of the profession. There are now 196 accredited programs, including 36 advanced clinical residencies and 35 advanced specialty residencies. More than 3000 pharmacists have completed accredited residency programs, and over 400 are currently completing them each year.

It is in these structured programs that we can best communicate values, philosophy, and a vision of the profession. The young professional, encouraged by a mentor, begins a process of introspection in which he tests his own abilities and limits and develops ethical standards and a philosophy of practice.[2] During this transition from a theoretical base to a professional practice, the resident also develops an attitude—a habit, if you will—of lifelong searching and learning. A culture develops around these residency programs that breeds commitment and exploration, and from the programs flow highly energized and motivated people with high individual and professional goals. Those who have been a part of this culture go on to build programs and similar cultures in other hospitals.

Supplying the profession with mature, highly skilled clinical and managerial practitioners is, without question, the primary value of residency programs, and assuring the quality of such programs is the primary purpose of the accreditation process. However, the importance of residency programs and the accreditation process to the advancement of professional practice has not been fully appreciated. That culture that develops around residency programs also breeds innovation and advancement in hospital pharmacy practice. The residents and others in the department who become a part of the culture help to keep these programs on the cutting edge of professional practice.

There is another force at play here that drives these programs to higher levels of excellence; that is the accreditation process itself. There are many elements to this dynamic process that make it effective, but the most important, I believe, is the existence of written standards defining the level of pharmacy practice that must be in place in that hospital before it can be accredited. The services are defined at a level that you and I would consider state of the art. Programs strive to meet these standards and become accredited. Subsequently, the ASHP Commission on Credentialing raises the level of standards as the state of the art changes, so that by the time the next survey is conducted the program has new goals to meet, and the cycle repeats itself. This never-ending challenge to meet higher and higher standards stimulates pharmacies with residency programs to advance pharmacy services.

We have 25 years of exceptional achievement through residency programs behind us. What is in store as we go for the golden anniversary? Before I share some thoughts on the role experiential training might play in the future, I would like to make some comments on the way we determine what that role will be.

Before we can rationally plan for the educational and training needs of future hospital pharmacists, we need to identify what it is that they will be doing. Since it takes 5–10 years to get any changes made in our educational system, we ought to be planning ahead at least that far. Dr. Henry Manasse, Dean of the College of Pharmacy at the University of Illinois, cautioned recently that:[3]

We must focus our attention on the necessity and mechanism for rational (manpower) planning. To date, there has not been a rational planning mechanism, and indeed, a consensus does not exist about the nature of the required manpower force.

If the profession is to be responsive to the manpower needs of the future, a rational planning process must be developed. Only four times in this century has the profession made any attempt to examine, analyze, and make recommendations for the profession in general and pharmaceutical education in particular—the last time being in 1975. In 1984, there was an APhA Task Force on Pharmacy Education, but it limited its recommendations primarily to some specific curriculum changes and the Pharm.D. degree. Although its scope was limited, that Task Force did make several important recommendations.[4] It recommended that the six-year Pharm.D. program evolve as the desired goal, with the intent that the Pharm.D. become the sole entry-level degree for the practice of pharmacy. However, the APhA Task Force concluded that there was relatively little documentation of the utility and effectiveness of Pharm.D.-degree pharmacists in practice, particularly in community practice, and recommended an analytical study on this issue. It then offered this advice:

If the profession makes the decision to move to the recommended six-year Pharm.D. degree as the sole entry degree for practice, that decision must be based on sound, supportable reasons.

It concerns many of us that we are rushing along toward a Pharm.D. for everyone and have not shown that a sixth year of education improves the quality of professional practice in community pharmacy—the area into which 59% of our pharmacy graduates currently go. Pharm.D.-level education (and residencies) have made all the difference in the world in the quality of services that have evolved in hospital pharmacy, but evidence of similar improvements in patient care as a direct result of advanced education is lacking in the community setting. It is surprising to me that this situation exists when we have the perfect laboratory in which to test the thesis that a sixth year of education would result over the years in improved patient care in the community setting.

In California, most graduates of colleges of pharmacy have received the Pharm.D. degree for more than 25 years. We should be able to find some detectable difference in the level of professional services in community pharmacy in, for example, San Francisco versus Philadelphia, where almost no one with a Pharm.D. degree has gone into community practice. That we have not conducted such a study suggests that we already know what the results would be.

How we educate and train pharmacists for community practice is important to you and me as we plan for the education and training of hospital pharmacists—not because of any inherent need to tie them together but because of the pharmacy school and hospital resources that are consumed in the education and training of that large portion of college classes directing themselves towards a future in community practice. Many schools of pharmacy are finding it difficult to put together the faculty and facilities to meet the demand from all of the profession for a larger number of graduating pharmacists and the ever-increasing demand from hospital pharmacy, academia itself, and the pharmaceutical industry for yet more highly educated and skilled professionals.

It seems irresponsible for us to be caught up in this snowball that is gaining force and propelling us toward a Pharm.D. for everyone without better evidence that the vast resources that will be consumed in so doing will be justified in terms of our better serving important societal needs. The importance of resolving this issue alone speaks strongly to the need for the profession to develop a mechanism for rational manpower planning.

Another problem we face that calls for rational manpower planning is the widespread shortage of pharmacists. Over the last 11 years (1977–1987), a time when all sectors of the profession have been expanding rapidly, the total number of pharmacy graduates has declined from 8200 per year to 6073—a decrease of 2127 (26%). The problem can only increase because we are not now graduating, nor have we for several years, even enough pharmacists to replace those retiring or otherwise leaving the profession.

On one hand, we have created exciting, challenging jobs requiring highly skilled specialized professionals; on the other hand, the manpower problem is compounded by the fact that there is a continuing and pervasive use of overly qualified manpower in boring, unsatisfying jobs. As the users of health care become more organized, more and more pressure will be put on the health care industry to become more efficient. This is another reason for community and hospital pharmacy to reevaluate the way manpower is trained and utilized.

This is a major issue and one that needs to be addressed immediately. One approach would be to assemble representatives from appropriate sectors of pharmacy in a Hilton Head-type consensus-building conference on pharmacy manpower. However, if all were drawn together, I believe that they should separate into at least two groups to deal with the issues according to the unique needs for manpower and training of community and hospital pharmacy.

If given the opportunity to work with educators and other stakeholders to develop appropriate programs in which to educate and train future hospital pharmacists, what programs would we prescribe? To answer that question, we first have to define what our roles will be. Fortunately, we have already taken that step. At the Hilton Head Conference, we agreed that it is a fundamental purpose of the profession to serve as a force for safe and appropriate use of drugs and that a fundamental goal is to promote optimal use of drugs. We went further to say that we should continue to have ultimate responsibilities for drug distribution and drug control activities, but that those functions should be carried out by technicians.

The consensus and commitment made at this Conference have since been reaffirmed in a number of similar conferences at regional, state, and local levels. I believe that we had an understanding as we came to those conclusions as to what those clinical roles will be. If those clinical activities are the primary and fundamental roles of hospital pharmacists, then the basic goal of our instructional and training programs should be to impart to pharmacists the knowledge and skills needed to fill those roles.

As schools of pharmacy are currently structured, I believe that the only way this can be accomplished is through a six- or seven-year program. It appears that in the near future that level of education will become a reality, at least for hospital pharmacy, as schools continue to convert to the six-year, entry-level Pharm.D. program. If we can accept for a moment that that will be the basic educational background of hospital pharmacists in the future, what, if any, additional experiential training will be needed? The APhA Task Force on Pharmacy Education concluded that "mastery of the subject areas in the proposed core curriculum will enable a person to *become* a pharmacist, not to *be* a pharmacist at the time of initial entry into practice."

General residencies in hospital pharmacy have in the past successfully fulfilled this experiential need for many hospital pharmacists, as I mentioned earlier. In some programs, an emphasis has been placed on either management experience or clinical experience, but, by and large, generalists have emerged who could in fact go on to provide leadership in one or more areas of practice. This served well to bridge the gap between theory and practice when most graduates were B.S. or M.S. graduates, but how should our entry-level residency programs change to meet the needs of those who will be beginning a career in the near future?

What has changed about the practice is that we have become a clinical profession. We are in the process of changing educational programs to meet the needs of a clinical profession, and it seems reasonable that we must change the entry-level experiential program to meet the needs as well. We then need to strengthen within the experiential program the clinical knowledge and skills beyond those acquired in the Pharm.D. program. A resident should be able to mature in clinical practice under the preceptorship of an experienced clinical pharmacist. However, since this is an entry-level experience, the residency must also provide meaningful training in the other components of hospital pharmacy service: administration, drug distribution and control, drug information services, etc. Pharm.D. graduates must come to understand how clinical services are integrated with other pharmacy services to best meet the needs of a given institution. In a clinical profession, advancement of clinical practice must be the single most important mission, but all pharmacists in an institution must understand and be able to give support to all important goals of the pharmacy department.

Let me summarize the changes that are implied in this recommendation for an entry-level residency program in hospital pharmacy. The first is that training in clinical (general) practice become the focus of the program. Second, a Pharm.D. degree should be a prerequisite for entry into the program. Third, the training program should provide meaningful experience in the other important services and in the overall management of the department. And fourth, this generalist entry-level residency should be a prerequisite for advanced specialized residency programs. It is this level of training that we should set our sights on for all pharmacists who are preparing for a future in hospital pharmacy practice. As educators and practitioners in a clinical profession, we have the moral and ethical responsibility to students and young pharmacists to develop qualified sites for such training programs and to guide future hospital pharmacists into them.

Beyond this entry-level training program, there is a growing need for highly specialized clinical training programs. We already have 35 such programs, but my sense is that we need many more. I believe that there is now a much greater demand for highly specialized clinicians than we can supply, and the demand will likely increase.

Having described the education and training scenario that I think is needed to prepare the general and highly specialized clinical practitioners for tomorrow's hospital pharmacy practice, I'll push your indulgence a little further and propose a training program for highly specialized managers in a clinical profession. And the scenario will not be that much different from the first, since I believe that managers and leaders in a clinical profession require a solid foundation in clinical practice. Although we are already a clinical profession, we need leaders who can guide a pharmacy staff to assume new roles and higher professional responsibilities. Those leaders need personal clinical experience if they are to appreciate fully the scope and depth of a pharmacist's clinical potential.

Such understanding is essential to be able to visualize the potential and take advantage of opportunities that develop as the environment changes. Only by having faced clinical challenges and enjoyed the success of meaningful contribution to the resolution of clinical problems can one visualize the purpose and generate value in those activities. The leaders of a clinical profession must be committed to—almost obsessed with—the idea of clinical practice. And, most important, they will need to project that idea into images that create excitement in other people about that activity.

Those pharmacists who are qualified and interested in developing their future along managerial lines should complete the programs described in the above scenario through the post-Pharm.D., entry-level residency program. And then, just as their counterparts who want to prepare for specialized clinical practice enter specialized clinical residencies, management-oriented pharmacists should enter a specialized residency in administration in which they acquire the knowledge and skills needed to accomplish the human resource management responsibilities of a clinical department.

ASHP, through specialty administrative practice groups, must foster the advancement of this specialty practice and encourage the development of training programs to support it. Just as we need clinical specialty practice groups to focus efforts on advancing clinical specialties, we need an administrative specialty practice group composed of our best-trained and specialized managers to focus on advancing our management capabilities.

The purpose of my comments has been twofold. First, I asked you to recognize and be proud of the fact that we have reached a milestone in one of the most constructive areas of our professional activity—residency training and the accreditation process. Second, I asked you to explore with me some ideas for the kind of education and experiential training that we are going to need as we grow and mature as a clinical profession. I made the point earlier that factors in the external environment have contributed significantly to our phenomenal growth but that at least one major contributing factor—residency training and accreditation—came from within. Having expanded our thinking to include didactic training, I would like to add that the second major contributor to that success that has come from within the profession is clinical training through Pharm.D. programs. The combined efforts of schools of pharmacy and hospital pharmacies have given many pharmacists clinical knowledge and skills.

The knowledge and the expertise to apply it in the patient care environment are what have driven the changes that brought us to the point of having a clinical profession. Schools of pharmacy are building on that success and are preparing to supply us with more graduates with clinical knowledge. I would ask that we devote adequate effort and resources to developing quality residency training sites and promoting them to pharmacy graduates so that when we arrive at the golden anniversary of accredited residency training programs, we shall have as much pride in them as we have today.

It gives me great pleasure to express my thanks to the many who share this Award. It occurred to me recently that if I were to share the very generous honorarium that goes with this Award with all those who contributed significantly to it, we would each receive about 10¢. Many have helped me along the way. Those who deserve the greatest share, however, are those professionally committed, creative colleagues at Jefferson with whom I have had the pleasure and good fortune to work. Many are more intelligent and highly skilled than I; all are willing to share their strength and talent for the cause, always with cheer, optimism, and great expectations of each other. To those very exceptional people, my most sincere thanks!

I'll close with this thought from George Bernard Shaw:

I'm not a teacher; only a fellow-traveller of whom you asked the way. I pointed ahead—ahead of myself as well as of you.

(For the complete list of references cited, please see page 1681 of the *American Journal of Hospital Pharmacy,* Aug. 1988.)

At the time he received this award, Joe E. Smith was the Director of Pharmacy at Thomas Jefferson University Hospital, Philadelphia, Pennsylvania, and Clinical Professor at Philadelphia College of Pharmacy and Science.

1989

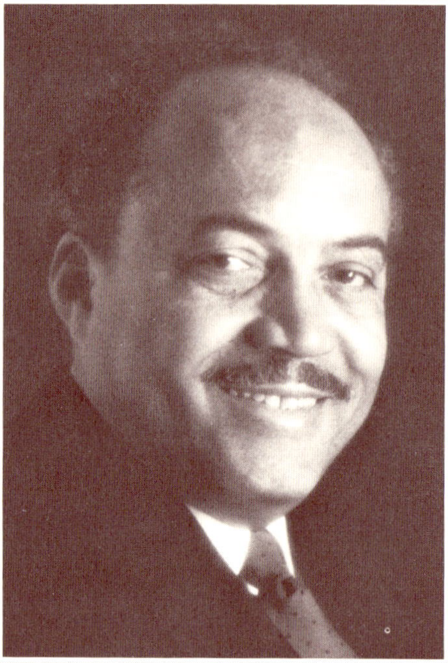

WENDELL T. HILL, JR.

"What we believe our profession to be determines what it is."

TAKING CHARGE OF THE PROFESSION

I am pleased and honored to have been selected to receive the 1989 Harvey A. K. Whitney Lecture Award and to have the opportunity to present the Whitney lecture for 1989. Receiving this Award is the highest point of my 39-year career in pharmacy. I wish to thank past recipients who voted for me, and I thank each of you personally for spending this evening with me in celebration of this important event. I thank Joe Oddis for his behind-the scenes magic and the ASHP staff for making this an enjoyable evening for my family and friends. And I thank many of you who have shared with me your personal expressions of congratulations, advice, and good will.

The purpose of my lecture is to motivate hospital pharmacists to take charge in the practice of pharmacy and to be committed to the highest conceivable standards of professional conduct. I challenge pharmacists to recognize that ideal professional practice begins with a personal commitment to excellence and integrity, a release of negative thoughts, and a thorough recognition that the high calling of pharmacy is an essential component of quality health care delivery.

Further, I challenge members of the profession to have complete conviction of, and determination for, maximum success and to understand that pharmacists alone are responsible for the status of the profession and are the only ones to change what needs to be changed. Professional change can occur when pharmacists become determined to make good things happen or when they allow others to make changes in the profession, good or bad. A central role of professional education, postgraduate education, inservice education, and continuing education is to institutionalize in the minds of pharmacists an attitude of service and excellence.

Willis Harman, Professor Emeritus of Engineering–Economic Systems at Stanford University, has written in his book *Global Mind*

Change that during the last part of the 20th century the world has been experiencing a basic mind change. He believes that the real action today is changing fundamental assumptions and that the key challenge is not to try to resist a change that may be inevitable but to go through the change with mutual cooperation and caring and with as little misery as possible.

Pharmacy, especially hospital pharmacy, has not escaped the forces of social, political, economic, and professional change. It is my thesis that these changes in public values make expert speculation about the future of pharmacy, especially hospital pharmacy, unreliable. Any assumption that history will prepare us for the future must be tempered by a recognition that events in the past were created in a different setting of public and private attitudes, values, and assumptions. Many of the assumptions and values that made life predictable in the past are changing.

People are no longer driven by traditional values such as a strict work ethic characterized by the dignity of labor, diligence, sobriety, and thrift. Waste, extravagance, and ostentation are no longer discouraged but rather are, at times, encouraged. Many people no longer assume that poverty is the result of individual failure. Many people no longer rely entirely on health care providers to remain healthy.

The Washington Post recently carried an article extolling the entrepreneurial success of a pharmacist who has generated a large annual income by supplying physicians with prepackaged prescription drugs for office dispensing. Not long ago, this enterprise would have been considered unethical and illegal by organized medicine and the public, and it still is despised in many pharmaceutical circles.

Since predicting the future of pharmacy is unreliable, it is necessary that pharmacists take another approach for securing an important role as health care providers. Success begins with the right kind of thinking. Success depends not so much on *what* people believe but that some belief exists—that we believe something, anything. If this is true, we had better believe good things for ourselves. Our belief determines our experience.

Examine the experience of hospital pharmacists. Most hospital pharmacists believe that they make important contributions to society; hence, ASHP has been said to be the most successful professional practitioner organization in pharmacy. Our success is controlled by how we think about the roles of pharmacists, by how pharmacists define success, and by our commitment to following successful principles. Our success is not controlled by what others think of us or even by changing social, political, economic, and professional circumstances. The professional pharmacist must always have in mind a clear purpose, especially while others may be confused, angry, frustrated, fearful, and defensive.

For a long time, the public and physicians told nurses that they should take orders from physicians; that worked as long as nurses went along with the program. Then one day some nurses said, "No more. We can be independent nurse practitioners." The result is current history. The public and most physicians today accept nurses as nurse practitioners, midwives, and so on. Psychiatrists were successful in establishing limits to the practice of psychology until psychologists had other ideas. The cases of acupuncturists, optometrists, social workers, and many others are similar.

Pharmacy almost stands alone today among health professions in permitting others to establish the scope and limits of professional practice. Notable exceptions within pharmacy include clinical pharmacists and hospital pharmacists.

What we as pharmacists believe our profession to be determines what it *is* (no more and no less). When we are dissatisfied with the state of affairs in pharmacy, pharmacists can examine the literature to find the cause in what pharmacists are saying to each other.

Not long ago, pharmacists were called druggists. Pharmacists decided that *pharmacist* is a superior designation. I seldom hear of druggists today. The magic of this concept is that no outside agency imposed this title on pharmacists—pharmacists did it themselves. Remember when Jere Goyan, as FDA Commissioner, tried to impose a drug counseling role on pharmacists? It did not work because most pharmacists could not see themselves in the patient-counseling role.

Only if we *think* such things as professional standards' review organizations, diagnosis-related groups, managed care, physician dispensing, and mail order pharmacies constitute threats to the practice of pharmacy will these agencies definitely cause us problems.

When we focus our attention instead on the health care delivery needs of the public that pharmacists are most suited to meet, and on meeting the challenges of providing pharmaceutical services that are attractive to the public, we shall have little time left to consider threats from perceived competitors, and they will appear less important in the total scheme of things.

I am not suggesting that we pharmacists ignore the world around us but rather that we recognize uncomfortable changes in popular attitudes about pharmaceutical services as indicators of unmet public demand that we can fulfill. We must mobilize our considerable intellectual resources to meet the public's need under new circumstances, no matter how much the health care environment changes.

The practice of pharmacy can conceptually be viewed as a continuum. Every pharmaceutical activity is part of, and inseparable from, that continuum. When pharmaceutical scientists consider the practice of pharmacy to be less important than research, they do harm to all of pharmacy. When clinical pharmacists separate themselves from other practicing pharmacists, all of pharmacy hurts. When pharmacist managers and owners separate themselves from other pharmacists economically, politically, and emotionally, all of pharmacy suffers. No useful purpose is served when pharmacists say that "counting and pouring" is a marginal task unworthy of the high calling of pharmacists or when they condemn the traditional product-related functions of the pharmacist.

Commonly accepted and easily understood ethical standards can create guidelines for successful practice in pharmacy. As a matter of professional viability at a time when public assumptions are changing, pharmacy is in great need of a revitalized interest in ethical standards of conduct. Hospital pharmacists have some work yet to do to establish a universal consensus for defining the ethical role for pharmacists in modern health care facilities.

Donald C. Brodie advised us that the principal role of the pharmacist is centered in "drug use control." From that simple principle flow all of the functions of the pharmacist. When all pharmacists come to accept drug use control as the primary ethic that drives pharmaceutical decisions, the public, the government, and other health care providers will respect that role for pharmacists, and pharmacists will be handsomely rewarded for their efforts. The secret is not that drug use control is a superior role for pharmacists, which it is; rather, the secret is that drug use control is a simple and understandable principle that leads to responsibility and accountability.

I propose that the ASHP limit its search for external conditions or influences as controlling factors for the future of pharmacy and look inward for a unifying principle to promote to pharmacists. It has worked for others, and it will work for pharmacy. Pharmacy must decide what its central role is in health care delivery before legislators, regulators, and managed care administrators establish a direction that we would like less.

Perhaps the greatest value in publishing the results of pharmacy practice studies measuring the value-added benefits of pharmaceutical services is in influencing pharmacists to have positive feelings about their contributions; the same might be true for measuring and reporting professional productivity of pharmacists.

The Society may wish to consider the establishment of local support groups that meet regularly to reinforce the ethics of pharmacy. ASHP's practice standards and the *American Journal of Hospital Pharmacy* could be reviewed by these discussion groups. The result would be wide acceptance and adoption of these valuable standards and guidelines. Witness the success of journal clubs, photography clubs, and others. Working together for a common ideal can produce amazing results. Imagine the effect if all pharmacists in a given community projected a common objective simultaneously, with conviction, determination, and commitment. There is no power strong enough to prevent success of the group. Skeptics and believers alike should try it.

People have told me that if I can change my thinking, I can change my life. I believe that if organized pharmacists can change their thinking, they can change their career opportunities.

At the time he received this award, Wendell T. Hill, Jr., was Dean of the College of Pharmacy and Pharmacal Sciences at Howard University, Washington, D.C.

1990

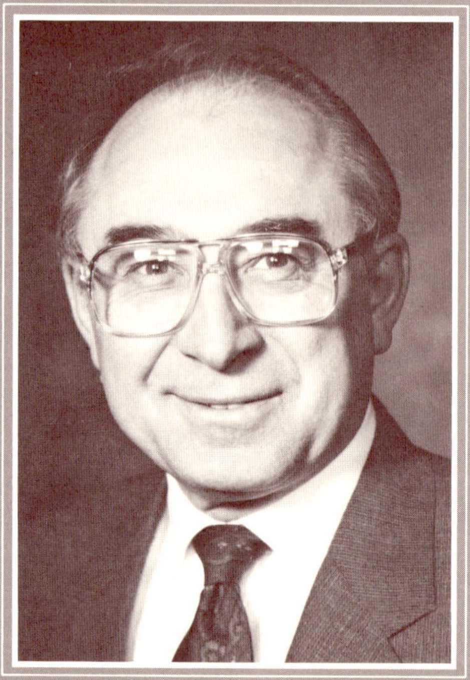

DAVID A. ZILZ

"Pursuit of individual independence is rapidly coming to a close as we move towards more interdependence."

INTERDEPENDENCE IN PHARMACY: RISKS, REWARDS, AND RESPONSIBILITIES

Receiving the Harvey A. K. Whitney Lecture Award is truly one of the highlights of my career. I am honored to receive this Award in 1990—four decades after the first Whitney Award, two and one-half decades after I entered pharmacy practice, and a decade after my ASHP presidency.

To recognize all of the individuals who have helped me in my professional and personal life would be impossible. Many are in this room, and I want to thank each of you for the opportunity to be a part of your hospital pharmacy network. It has been a pleasure as well as a great professional stimulus. As you know, the home base for my entire career has been at the University of Wisconsin; I have been fortunate to be at an institution with so many progressive, stimulating, positive-thinking, and caring people.

In trying to identify people, forces, or trends that affect our lives, we have to stop and consider longer time frames—such as decades. In particular, we need to examine areas that are in transition, whether in the world we live in, in our careers, in our practices, or in our lives.

This evening I shall discuss what I believe to be the beginning of an era in which the pursuit of individual independence is rapidly coming to a close as we move towards more interdependence. We may not recognize that as a trend yet; but I hope that when we look back a decade from now, we shall recognize success that resulted from our effective cultivation of interdependence in pharmacy.

First, let me define interdependence. *Webster's New World Dictionary* defines it as "dependence on each other or one another; mutual dependence."

Why do I think interdependence is so important? The late Ray E.

Brown, a renowned hospital administrator, said: "It is necessary to distinguish between prevailing winds and intermittent breezes." I think Brown's wise words are pertinent. We can see the "prevailing winds" of interdependence everywhere.

First, we see it in the political arena worldwide, most notably in Europe. The collapse of the Berlin Wall in November 1989 is a signal event in our lifetime, a dramatic happening beyond the wildest expectations of those individuals whose job it is to monitor and predict such events. Even casual observers of such events are speculating on the potential positive impact this new wave of interdependence will have on the future of the world.

This trend is also already well established in the worldwide marketplace. Most companies are talking about their "globalization" plans and the need for financial and sales dependency among countries throughout the world for growth and progress. It will probably never again be possible for a single country to be totally independent of all other countries. And when the Europe 1992 plan is unleashed, everyone that produces, buys, or uses products will be affected even more significantly. Even today we only have to pause for a minute to realize that not many large pharmaceutical companies have their home corporate offices in the United States.

The merging of two or more pharmaceutical companies is another form of interdependence, and that trend is well established. These joint ventures, mergers, or partnerships are not merely a matter of economy of scale but also a process for integrating different companies' individual strengths. The *Wall Street Journal* often identifies the synergy, or interdependence, created between two companies and how one company's marketing and sales force, joined with a second company's strength in research and worldwide distribution capabilities, results in a stronger, more successful new organization or venture.

We also see interdependence in pharmacy management arrangements. Again, various "partnerships"—large, integrated private health care companies, nonprofit service groups, and myriad other organizations and associations—are being created to "bond" individuals whose needs can best be met by becoming interdependent for the purpose of providing purchasing services, research networks, information support, and other activities that can no longer be carried out as successfully when those individuals act independently.

The last place we see increasing interdependence is in our daily work activities in our hospitals and individual practice settings. I think that physicians and pharmacists are, every year, becoming more comfortable with being interdependent on each other, and both are becoming more effective practitioners because of it. I, for one, am delighted to see the "prevailing winds" blowing in that direction.

We might ask what is driving this movement towards interdependence. Let me suggest three fundamental reasons.

First, modern communication technology has created worldwide linkages that facilitate—if not mandate—interdependence. These capabilities have removed previous barriers that would not have allowed the interactions, the transfer of information, or the global working relationships we see today. Technology will accelerate this trend, and we shall all become comfortable routinely receiving professional information from PharmNet, ClinNet, COMNET, and a variety of electronic consumer communications networks such as Prodigy, CompuServe, and (for us AARP members) SeniorNet, all of which will support virtually every aspect of our lives.

The second force is the explosion of "new knowledge," which is increasing at an accelerated rate—in fact, doubling every two or three years. It is now impossible for a single individual to stay current even in a narrow field. Therefore, to be even minimally effective, we must all become mutually dependent on each other for managing certain segments of that information and merging it with the knowledge of others.

The third force driving interdependence is based on one of Newton's well-known laws of nature: For every action there is an equal and opposite reaction. It follows that if one sector (the pharmaceutical industry) creates large and effective interdependent structures, then other sectors that interface with it must do likewise to retain a balance of power or influence. I believe that the pharmacy purchasing and services groups are driven by that phenomenon more than by any other factor, although it may not have been recognized at the time they were started.

Because hospital pharmacy has a long-standing tradition of exchanging ideas, information, and data, the concept is not new. The movement to more interdependence will be easier for us than for many others. I believe that the heritage of interdependence in hospital pharmacy—a great deal of it fostered by ASHP—has been the single most significant force in the profession's expanding influence over the use of drugs. As a result of this interdependence, hospital and clinical pharmacists in the aggregate, and therefore as individuals, have achieved far more influence than had ASHP not encouraged interdependence. Some of that open sharing of information may have decreased recently because of the competition between hospitals and groups, and we should from time to time remind ourselves of the long-term value of that sharing in the interdependent society.

With that influence, which continues to increase, come not only rewards but responsibilities and, perhaps, some profound risks as well. Let us consider some of these rewards and risks for clinical pharmacist researchers, clinical pharmacy practitioners, pharmacy administrative staff, and pharmacy organizations.

I am delighted to see clinically trained pharmacists becoming so influential in clinical research. They are actively participating in organizing, leading, and conducting this research. The current ASHP Spotlight Topic is research. The American College of Clinical Pharmacy has a major thrust this year, a series of educational programs that give pharmacists higher level skills in performing clinical research. Such efforts will enhance the ability of all interested members of the pharmacy profession to assume leadership in the total spectrum of drug-related activities.

The pharmacist's contribution to clinical research is increasingly respected and needed by the pharmaceutical industry. Because there is currently a reduction in the number of physicians being trained with such expertise, the industry will become even more dependent on pharmacists for clinical drug research in the future.

But what about the risks and the responsibilities that result from pharmacists' increased influence? One of the greatest potential risks is the risk of compromising ethical standards and integrity—for fear of losing the next grant or by making a presentation at a conference in return for financial gain or personal benefit. Some practitioners in medical specialties have bowed to that temptation and have lost credibility with their colleagues, other health care practitioners, and the ever-vigilant public. We must learn from their dilemma.

Many of you working for the pharmaceutical industry have assisted the pharmacy profession in a number of ways, in the practice setting and more recently in the research arena. You were pioneers in the companies, leading the way by convincing your executives of what a pharmacist trained in performing clinical research can contribute. Less than a decade ago, that funding for research was almost exclusively directed to medically trained individuals.

But we are now at a stage in our evolution when a word of caution is appropriate, and I solicit your support. Continue to influence those in your companies who may be misguided in meeting marketing needs at all costs to satisfy the short-term expectations of the stockholders. Continue your vigilance to reduce or remove any pressure on those performing clinical research so that they do not compromise good science by changing conclusions through "controlled release of information" in publications or their presentations at educational meetings to satisfy that marketing need. The long-term negative implications of such actions will be counter to the constructive interdependence that has been achieved thus far. It is in the best interest of everyone to sustain the integrity of the industrial–academic research enterprise.

Clinical pharmacists at the bedside have also achieved significant influence over the selection and use of drugs. This influence will increase as medical practitioners rely on their expertise and recommendations in the future. The long-term impact will be felt especially in academic centers or teaching hospitals because those institutions will affect the thought patterns of physicians and pharmacists in training.

I believe that there will be increasing pressure by some companies to convince clinical pharmacists to provide biased information to the prescriber, which would compromise their well-respected image. In the future, the companies will want and need to establish a closer relationship with clinical pharmacists because of their influence. This interdependence between the industry and the practitioners could easily result in principles and ethics being compromised for short-term gains.

Unprecedented influence has been achieved by group purchasing organizations as member hospitals have combined their purchasing volumes. It is now common for 10 or 20 individuals in just a few days to make awards valued at hundreds of millions of dollars worth of products. The stakes for the companies and the groups will be even higher in the future. Whereas drug budgets have been 5–7% of hospitals' total expenses in the past, it is now projected that by the mid 1990s 12–15% of the hospital budget will be for drugs.

The pharmaceutical industry will then become even more dependent on pharmacists to select their products because of the dollars involved. This scenario, in which significant sums of money are involved and the decisions are made by a few individuals, sets the stage for potential risks to the image of the entire profession of pharmacy. If only one or a few individuals were to choose personal gain through unethical actions in purchasing these drugs, the negative effect on our entire profession would be enormous, if not irreparable.

Only a decade ago, during the year of my ASHP presidency in 1980, a most dramatic event took place. The first genetically engineered product entered clinical trials. The product, of course, was human insulin. Since then, other major and innovative biotechnology products have reached the marketplace, and 100–150 are currently in the research pipeline.

Every segment of pharmacy—pharmaceutical education, the industrial–academic research enterprise, individual practitioners, pharmacy departments, purchasing groups, and professional associations and organizations—will be significantly affected by these products. The members of ASHP and affiliated state hospital pharmacy organizations will be a central focus of the biotechnology industry because their members will be the prime purchasers and users of these items.

Several factors related to biotechnology products set the stage for potential conflicts of interest and reduced ethical standards in the pharmacy profession. Because there are only a few of these biotechnology products to monitor, how well we handle them could serve as a gauge for the profession's ethical standards.

- Almost every item produced by biotechnology is relatively expensive. The cost per dose or annual cost for treatment is very high. There is a lot of money at stake for everyone: the producing and selling company and its stockholders, the prescriber and users, and the payers.
- Because most of these items are produced from proteins, they must be administered by injection and are likely to be used initially in hospitals or other organized health care facilities. Also, most of the diseases treated by these agents are managed primarily in acute care facilities.
- There is a considerable mystique about these entities and bewilderment as to what they do and the effect they will have on patient care.
- These products will probably continue for the foreseeable future to have only a single or a very limited indication, as in FDA-approved labeling; however, most will have other practical applications and are likely to be used for many other purposes. Further, different companies with the same products will strive to have different indications approved by the FDA, which will lead to confusion in our daily practice activities.
- Because these items are "new" moieties, there will be a need for considerable continuing education in the profession, a great deal of which will be done through national and state societies and organizations and their meetings.
- Many of these items will most likely be very visible to the public because they are unique. It appears that only a small number will be approved during the next couple of years; therefore, those entering the market can be easily monitored.
- There are relatively few individuals—including pharmacists—with substantial experience in the use of these items. The few who do have this expertise will be highly sought after for presentations and publications. The rest will, at best, have only superficial knowledge and will be seeking guidance and direction from the few "experts."

The current "prevailing winds" of the impact of biotechnology drugs will become a whirlwind within just a couple of years. The financial stakes are high, the potential uses are unlimited, the concepts and technology are confusing. Although some may consider it controversial, I believe that the time has come to establish a professional standard of conduct that all members of our profession should strive to attain. I remind you that the definition of ethics is "a study of the standards of conduct and moral judgment."

To address this issue, I encourage ASHP to create a commission on ethics, possibly in concert with the American College of Clinical Pharmacy, the pharmaceutical industry, and other organizations, especially medical societies. Medicine has already begun to address some of these issues, as has been noted in recent articles in medical journals. Because hospital-based pharmacists and physicians often jointly influence decisions on drugs through collegial interdependence in research, product selection, and management of drug therapy, it follows that both would mutually benefit from a collaborative effort.

Thomas S. Thielke, in his 1989 ASHP presidential address, stated the need for ASHP to work more aggressively with organized medicine in addressing issues of mutual interest. If ASHP were to take the lead and work with medicine to address the interdependent needs of the two professions and the pharmaceutical industry, it would clearly demonstrate ASHP's leadership on a multidisciplinary drug-related issue in organized health care settings.

Interdisciplinary guidelines and indicators would best serve the public, our professions, and the industry if they addressed the standards of conduct for the individual practitioner, for the hospital, and for professional associations.

If we are willing to take the initiative on establishing guidelines, several issues should be addressed. First, would our hospitals' Pharmacy and Therapeutics (P&T) Committees be willing to implement policies and procedures that require each voting member, as well as each individual who requests an expensive pharmaceutical or biotechnology product, to provide full disclosure of his or her relationship with the vendor or producer of the product? Under such policies, P&T Committees might ask the following questions:

- Has anyone involved with the request or the decision received financial support for research on the development of the product being considered for approval or for other products developed by that company?
- Which P&T Committee members are or have been on an advisory panel for the company whose product is being evaluated?
- Who is on the speakers' roster or has made presentations on that product or on behalf of the company that is selling the product?
- Who has attended a "conference" on that product for which the company has paid all expenses?

Next, the quality, sophistication, and integrity of the literature are important indicators of not only the competence of the clinical pharmacy investigators but the ethical standards they strive for in their work. Answers to the following questions must be able to stand the scrutiny of the most critical observers:

- Does the quality of the publications and the conclusions reached stand the test of time? In other words, will a retrospective analysis two to three years after the article is published reaffirm as accurate and pertinent the original article's conclusions regarding the uses of an item? It is important to remember that the labeling indications will be few but that the actual uses will be many.

- Are the conclusions reached in the nonrefereed and "throw-away" journals consistent with those appearing in refereed journals? If not, can it be concluded that some of the authors and our colleagues are compromising the standards of the entire profession by publishing for the purpose of personal gain? If they are guilty, what are we willing to do about it?
- Should authors declare when they are being paid for articles and are benefiting financially from writing them? If they are paid, should they declare who is reimbursing them and for how much?
- Are conclusions modified and published in different tabloids reaching different audiences, thereby creating confusing messages about the optimum therapeutic uses for these items? Promotional articles should be surveyed closely and caustically.

Finally, can the educational programming of our organizations withstand the scrutiny of society when the following questions are asked:

- Do individuals receive personal financial gain for developing, endorsing, or participating in educational programs?
- How many times a year does an individual appear on programs to "discuss" or promote a specific product?
- How often do "thought leaders" participate in educational programs, thereby implicitly or explicitly endorsing products or uses of specific products?
- How much of an organization's support for educational programming comes from industry, and does it influence the content of the programs and the potential use of products?
- Does an organization have written criteria and/or guidelines under which it will not accept an educational grant, and, if so, does it follow them explicitly?

I do not have all the answers to these questions, but I am convinced that we can wait no longer to establish a formal process to address them. Such a process could be the largest and least expensive insurance policy our profession ever invested in to ensure that interdependent facets in pharmacy (and medicine), as well as the pharmaceutical industry, meet society's expectations.

Some pharmacy organization must take the lead in addressing these issues soon, and I believe that organization should be ASHP.

We have talked thus far about the effect of past and future interdependence at a number of levels, but what about between pharmacists at the very personal level? It is here that I see the most significant long-term rewards if we can truly cultivate interdependence. Interdependence is being available to help an ambitious and energetic youth just starting a career who needs support in deciding which job to accept. It is being available to a professional friend who has lost his or her job, not because of lack of competence but because of circumstances in the hospital, or to one who is frustrated or "burned out" in a current position and does not know which way to turn.

Interdependence between colleagues in hospital pharmacy departments and colleges of pharmacy benefits both by providing the unique expertise of each group to support the missions of both. In far too many cases, we continue to deprive ourselves, our institutions, and our patients of benefits by failing to strive for interdependence—that is, mutual dependence—and instead continuing to seek independence, with the result of nonproductive conflict.

I have believed for a long time that there must be a unique interdependence between residents and the preceptors and leaders of hospital pharmacy residency programs. Good residency training requires a strong relationship between the preceptor and the resident or fellow. This is a model we should strive for throughout the profession; it is not seen to the same degree in any other sector of pharmacy.

I feel more strongly than ever that we shall never be able to optimize the contribution of our future practitioners unless individuals with experience in the profession constantly test the "prevailing winds" to see what new practice or career opportunities are on the horizon and then guide those future practitioners into those careers with the best long-term potential.

Perhaps the lack of interest by students in hospital pharmacy and specialty practice sites in clinical functions is because of confusion over too many available options, none of which is effectively portrayed. "We ain't seen nothin' yet" compared to the number of specialties and different practice sites that will be available in less than one decade, in the year 2000. A more organized process is needed for guiding young pharmacists to the most rewarding career opportunities.

Our colleagues in medicine have a long tradition of mentorship, encompassing several years of proceeding through a "coaching" hierarchy basically composed of specialists. The University of Wisconsin School of Medicine has gone a step further by selecting each year a renowned senior faculty person who spends the entire academic year with a class of medical students, attending all their classes and all their functions, and who is always available as a mentor. What an outstanding way to close out one's career: investing in the career satisfaction of future professionals by advising them on the many changes and opportunities they will have available.

We do not have such a system in pharmacy, but we could and should have because we are now at a stage in our clinical specialty evolution where we have almost as many specialty practice options as our colleagues in medicine.

Unfortunately, we still have senior pharmacy students who do not even know that there are residency programs or specialty practice opportunities available to them. Any school or college of pharmacy where that occurs in the 1990s is negligent in its responsibilities to the student and the profession for failing to advise the future practitioners and thereby depriving them of potential lifelong specialized career opportunities.

In conclusion, I believe successful leadership in every organization will be achieved by those with the ability constantly to identify new opportunities for interdependence. This requires identification of changing incentives for linkages in order to cope with the changing technology and ever-increasing volume of new knowledge. At the same time, these leaders must be able to conform to the highest ethical standards, which will require making critical judgments about those with whom to become interdependent.

Business has already recognized the need to establish a new, higher order of managerial skills and evaluative processes for their leaders to enable them to "network" differently and more effectively to meet the changing times.

Let us not wait too long to recognize that the changes we see in the need and desire for interdependence are brought on by the "prevailing winds" and are not "intermittent breezes" of the times, so that we shall be ready to proceed full sail ahead to maximize our profession and our lives.

At the time he received this award, David A. Zilz was the Administrator of Pharmacy, Respiratory Care Services, and Research Development at the University of Wisconsin Hospital and Clinics and a Clinical Professor at the School of Pharmacy, University of Wisconsin, Madison.

1991

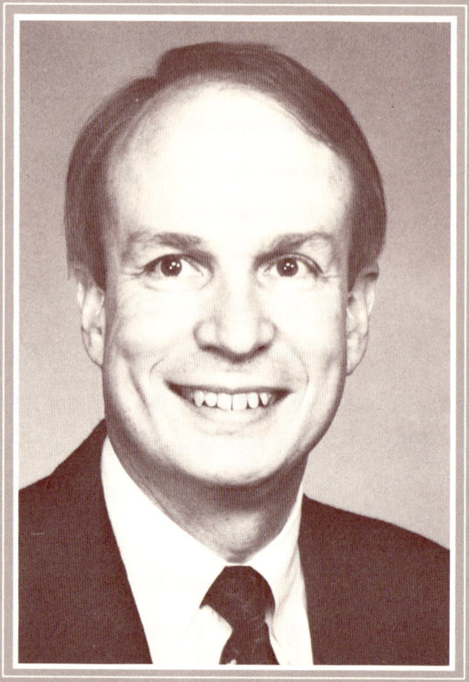

HAROLD N. GODWIN

"Converging paths have led to the profession's transition to pharmaceutical care."

TO A NEW BEGINNING FROM CONVERGING PATHS

I stand here in awe. Recognition by one's peers is the greatest recognition of all.

I wish to express my love and thanks to my family—Judy, Jennifer, and Paula—who have provided the supportive environment for me to achieve my professional goals and for my attempts to influence the profession. My thanks to Sara White, my colleague and confidant, and to my colleagues at the University of Kansas Medical Center and School of Pharmacy who provide a stimulating practice base on which to grow professionally.

A special recognition goes to all of the residents associated with my career who provide challenges, stimulation, and rewards in the process of developing leaders for the profession reaching for excellence. I also want to thank all of you here tonight and all who have sent notes and letters and made phone calls of congratulations. This experience is truly heart warming and humbling.

While I have had no direct link to the University of Michigan and Harvey A. K. Whitney, my preceptor and mentor, Clifton J. Latiolais, provided me with the influence and principles that are the legacy of the man we are honoring tonight. In preparing for this presentation, I read many of the previous addresses by Whitney Award winners. Indeed, the legacy lives! Previous Whitney addresses are thought provoking and provide a vision for the profession. Stephen Leacock once wrote, "It may be those who do the most, dream the most."

Napoleon said, "A leader is a dealer in hope." It is truly an honor to be associated with this collection of leaders and pathfinders.

The pharmacy profession is on the edge of a great new beginning. The near future will bring opportunities that, if recognized and seized, will change our health care system significantly. A new beginning! Wouldn't we all like to have a new beginning—knowing what we know now, retaining our insights, avoiding previous mistakes, and having the ability to do it right. So often we pass through time without the chance to start over—to reset the stage—or the ability to follow the correct path. Finding that path is the key, as Lewis Carroll knew:

One day Alice came to a fork in the road and saw a Cheshire cat in a tree. "Which road do I take?" she asked. His response was a question: "Where do you want to go?" "I don't know," Alice answered. "Then," said the cat, "it doesn't matter."

The pharmacy profession is facing a unique window of opportunity to meet a new societal obligation. Pursuit of this opportunity could represent a landmark akin to the differentiation of apothecaries from medical practitioners. As I reflect on our professional history and look at the signals in our profession today, I see evidence of a new horizon for pharmacy.

Historians tell us emphatically that we are leaving the industrial revolution and passing into an age dominated by science, technology, and knowledge. Never in history has knowledge been so central to the conduct of an entire society. The advent of the knowledge age and our rapidly changing environment will profoundly affect the profession of pharmacy.[1] The impact of the knowledge or information age on pharmacy has been recognized for years. In 1967, Donald C. Brodie, Whitney Award winner and pathfinder for the profession, used the term "drug use control" to describe a system of knowledge, skills, controls, and ethics that ensures optimal safety in the distribution and use of medications.[2] Drug use control became a central concept in the development of clinical pharmacy.

In 1972, the Millis Commission was created to examine the practice of pharmacy as an integral part of the health care system. Two years later, the Millis Commission reported that the main function of pharmacy centers on the discovery, interpretation, and dissemination of drug knowledge.

In 1985, ASHP held an invitational conference on directions for clinical practice in pharmacy, the famous "Hilton Head Conference." At Hilton Head, pharmacy leaders concluded that a commitment must be made to establish pharmacy as a true clinical profession.[3]

Since that time, there has been an evolution from Brodie's idea of drug use control to the philosophy of practice espoused by Hepler and Strand: pharmaceutical care.[4–6] Hepler first described pharmaceutical care at the Hilton Head Conference and later refined the concept in his paper entitled "Unresolved Issues in Pharmacy."[7,8] Pharmaceutical care is described as "the responsible provision of drug therapy for the purpose of achieving definite outcomes that improve a patient's quality of life. These outcomes are (1) cure of a disease, (2) elimination or reduction of a patient's symptoms, (3) arresting or slowing of a disease process, or (4) preventing a disease or symptoms."[4]

Pharmaceutical care is not practiced in isolation from other health professionals. Rather, it must be provided in collaboration with patients, physicians, nurses, and others. Pharmaceutical care should not be available only on the basis of patient need or when requested by the patient. Most importantly, the concept is not and must not be restricted to pharmacy practice in organized health care settings. Supporting the need for the provision of pharmaceutical care, Manasse[9,10] demonstrated the critical need for a system to improve medication use in society and to avoid medication misadventures.

Great interest in the concept of pharmaceutical care was demonstrated at the Pharmacy in the 21st Century Conference, held in October 1989. A conclusion of this Conference was that pharmacy practice needed a mission statement, for public declaration, that fostered such a concept.

This movement towards pharmaceutical care has prompted the American Pharmaceutical Association (APhA) to approve a new mission statement for the pharmacy profession, which states: "The mission of pharmacy is to serve society as the profession responsible for the appropriate use of medications, devices, and services to achieve optimal therapeutic outcomes." Further, a mission statement being drafted by the Joint Commission of Pharmacy Practitioners (JCPP) states that the "mission of pharmacy practice is to help people make the best use of medications."[11]

The specific elements of these mission statements are important. According to the APhA mission statement, "the mission of pharmacy is to serve society as *the* profession responsible for the appropriate use of medications...." The stated aim, "to achieve optimal therapeutic outcomes," dictates an important new responsibility and commitment by the profession. The mission statement suggests that pharmacy has a covenant with the patient to ensure the positive outcome of drug therapy. This applies to all of the pharmaceutical services (clinical and nonclinical) that are required and received by the patient to obtain the desired clinical outcomes of the use of drugs.

The provision of pharmaceutical care inherently means that the pharmacist is responsible for and is to be held accountable for a patient's achieving the desired clinical outcomes of the use of drugs. I like to describe the pharmacist's role as being a drug therapy manager. The physician still makes the diagnosis and prescribes drug therapy in broad terms. The pharmacist is responsible for managing that drug therapy to achieve optimal patient outcomes.

The recent concurrence of events is unequaled. The profession's leaders and organizations have reached consensus on the definition of pharmacy practice and the mission of the profession. Practitioner organizations have come from converging paths to agree on our profession's societal purpose and our new beginning. It is time to stop debating the future and to implement pharmaceutical care.

A number of activities are occurring that will accelerate the implementation of pharmaceutical care.

In addition to adopting a new mission statement for pharmacy, APhA has embarked on revalidation of its Standards of Pharmacy Practice. Revision of the standards will be based on assessments of practice by 5000 pharmacists. This summer, the first examination for the certification of specialized practitioners in pharmacotherapy will be administered by the Board of Pharmaceutical Specialties. This examination will assess the level of clinical knowledge of pharmacists and help to establish baseline expectations.

The American Association of Colleges of Pharmacy (AACP) has formed the Commission to Implement Change in Pharmaceutical Education. As this Commission continues its work, it is publishing a series of position papers. The first paper, "Mission of Pharmaceutical Education,"[a] states that pharmaceutical education is responsible for preparing students to enter into the practice of pharmacy and to function as professionals and informed citizens in a changing health care system. AACP is responsible for generating and disseminating new knowledge about drugs and about pharmaceutical care systems.

Pharmaceutical education promotes advances in pharmaceutical care by fostering postgraduate residencies and fellowships in clinical sciences and differentiated areas of pharmacy practice. Pharmaceutical education is also responsible to the profession and to society for generating new knowledge about drugs, drug products, drug therapy, and drug use through the conduct of basic and applied research. This position paper states that pharmacy practice is one means through which the profession delivers its knowledge and products to patients in society. Thus, the Commission stated its belief that the mission of pharmacy practice is to render pharmaceutical care.

The Commission's second paper, "Entry Level, Curricular Outcomes, Curricular Content, and Educational Process," states that "to enter practice is to render pharmaceutical care."[b] Students prepared at the entry level must be capable of coordinating and rendering pharmaceutical care. The Commission recommends that AACP member schools and faculty immediately commit themselves to curricular change that (1) engenders competencies and outcomes essential to pharmaceutical care and (2) strengthens the effectiveness of the process of pharmaceutical education. The stage is set for the colleges of pharmacy to meet the challenges of preparing the entry-level student to practice pharmaceutical care.

Another significant development in education is occurring. In 1989, the American Council on Pharmaceutical Education (ACPE) announced its intent to begin a 10-year review process to establish, as part of its periodic review of accreditation standards, revised standards that will reflect and respond to the mission set forth for pharmacy practitioners. This process is another sign that the profession is embracing the provision of pharmaceutical care.

ACPE also has said that it foresees the time when the accreditation standards will focus on a Doctor of Pharmacy program as the only professional degree program evaluated and accredited. Current standards consider both the B.S. and the Pharm.D. as entry-level degrees for pharmacist licensure. Standards that are consistent with the entry-level practitioner's ability to provide pharmaceutical care may become reality as soon as the year 2000.[c,d]

The first few years of the 10-year revision of standards will be devoted primarily to determining what competencies and curricular content are necessary for a generalist practitioner. The revision process provides for open hearings and for the submission of written comments on drafted or proposed revised standards. Unfortunately for the profession, at least one pharmacy trade association representing corporations that employ pharmacists, the National Association of Chain Drug Stores, is initially focusing efforts in opposition to this process based on the degree designation and the length of programs leading to the entry-level degree—elements of the standards that are to be determined after the establishment of competencies required for entry into the profession to practice pharmaceutical care.

The revised accreditation standards will represent competencies required for the entry-level generalist practitioner. While many Doctor of Pharmacy graduates up to now have practiced in specialized areas, the standards for the future will set entry-level competencies for practice. The standards will acknowledge the new mission of the profession and will focus on the provision of pharmaceutical care for all practice sites, including community practice.

Significantly, ACPE is also calling for opinions and recommendations about appropriate educational development for baccalaureate-degreed pharmacists already in practice (i.e., nontraditional educational approaches). It is equally important to develop and train existing practitioners to provide pharmaceutical care at all practice sites.

ASHP has a rich tradition of promoting pharmacy as a clinical profession through its *Statement on Long-Range Pharmacy Manpower Needs and Residency Training*, its residency accreditation standards, and the Hilton Head Conference and its state and local followup conferences. Continuing this philosophy, the ASHP House of Delegates has unanimously endorsed the concept of pharmaceutical care, reaffirmed support for the Doctor of Pharmacy as the single entry-level degree for practice, and endorsed the proposal for a clinical skills development program. Thus, ASHP continues to position itself well to help practitioners in organized health care settings to practice pharmaceutical care.

Thus, converging paths have led to the profession's transition to pharmaceutical care. What of the future? Einstein once said, "I never think of the future. It comes soon enough." We have a great future ahead of us because of what is behind us. H. G. Wells wrote, "The past is but the beginning of a beginning." We must move rapidly from the frontiers of the past to the new frontiers of the future.

With all of the signs and signals pointing to the correct path, we can no longer afford to debate the future; we must implement pharmaceutical care. Our challenge is not concept, not philosophy, not agreement with the mission statement for the profession; rather, it is implementation. The implementation of pharmaceutical care is the most important challenge the profession has faced in this century. Pharmacy is committed to this end. Implementation must occur at all levels of pharmacy practice—hospitals, HMOs, nursing homes, community practice sites of independent pharmacies, professional pharmacies, and chain pharmacies.

There is an urgency for implementation of pharmaceutical care. Joseph Califano, former Secretary of Health, Education, and Welfare, recently stated that pharmacists' monopoly over dispensing should be eliminated. His comments reinforced the uninformed perception that pharmacy services are rooted in self-interest rather than in consumer protection.

What must be done to accomplish our goals on a timely basis? Each professional organization must make pharmaceutical care a priority, not merely rhetoric.

The JCPP must move beyond adopting the philosophy of pharmaceutical care; it must commit to implementing pharmaceutical care. The value of the mission statement drafted by JCPP is that it is aimed at society rather than the profession: "The mission of pharmacy practice is to help people make the best use of medications." JCPP could best serve the profession by aggressively marketing this mission—or patient expectation concept—to the public. We need a unified national campaign depicting the value-added pharmaceutical services that we call pharmaceutical care.

APhA must continue to focus on its newly adopted mission statement. It must not only revalidate the Standards of Pharmacy Practice but continue to measure the levels of practice to determine the current contributions of pharmacy practitioners, their potential, and their limitations in providing pharmaceutical care. We need a continuing analysis of the services provided by our nation's pharmacists, parallel to ASHP's national survey of hospital pharmaceutical services.

Probably most important, APhA needs to promote postgraduate residency training programs aimed at developing and providing pharmaceutical care to patients in all settings. We must expand model practices that depict value-added pharmaceutical services, the drug knowledge component of pharmaceutical care. The concept of the office-based family pharmacist, pioneered by Eugene White, must be adopted. APhA must grasp the opportunity to establish the pharmaceutical care concept in relation to the Omnibus Budget Reconciliation Act of 1990 mandate for patient counseling and drug use review by 1993.

ACPE must continue to seek input from the profession and practitioners as it receives, analyzes, and produces the competency requirements for entry-level practice of providing pharmaceutical care. The focus for the first few years of the 10-year revision process must be on the competency requirements and not the title of the degree or the length of the program. ACPE should seek input and formulate sound and efficient educational pathways for current practitioners who need to develop their practice competencies to meet the goal of providing pharmaceutical care to all patients.

AACP must receive, debate, and act on the recommendations of the Commission to Implement Change in Pharmaceutical Education to ensure that the academic process is consistent in meeting the needs of the graduate entering the practice of pharmaceutical care.

ASHP has been a leader in promoting the concept of clinical practice for the profession. Through its strategic planning process, it has identified in advance many of the changes in the health care arena. The Hilton Head Conference nurtured the early development of the concept of pharmaceutical care. Now, ASHP must take a leadership role in the implementation of pharmaceutical care. Attention must shift from the ASHP strategic planning process to an expedited process for strategic implementation.

ASHP should convene a followup national conference on the issues of implementing pharmaceutical care in organized health care settings. Such a forum would be appropriate during ASHP's 50th anniversary celebration in 1992. As we recognize ASHP's half century of progress, we should chart a course for the implementation of pharmaceutical care by the turn of the century. This would give our members an opportunity for a renewed commitment to reaching higher practice goals.

After such a national conference, I recommend that ASHP create a commission to implement pharmaceutical care in organized health care settings. This commission should have the highest priority for professional development and programming. Timetables would be set and an action plan would be carried out. This commission should identify methods for implementing pharmaceutical care at all practice sites, develop educational mechanisms to ensure that all current practitioners are capable of providing pharmaceutical care, assist colleges of pharmacy with electronically mediated educational methods for developing clinical practice skills and clinical practice experiences, develop strategies to remove the barriers to pharmaceutical care, and foster research programs that demonstrate the cost-effectiveness of pharmaceutical care.

Why create a commission rather than just follow the regular policy implementation process of the ASHP councils and Board of Directors? A commission would be better able to focus continually on the mission of implementation, respond to the urgency for implementation of pharmaceutical care, and commit to reaching closure on this vital task. Creation of a commission would also signal to the profession and the public that ASHP is dedicated to this cause. This concept of creating a commission could be reviewed and debated at the proposed 1992 national conference for implementing pharmaceutical care.

What issues confront us in the implementation of pharmaceutical care? First, there is a need for commitment by the individual practitioner and the management of each department to support this cause. The concept will have to be marketed not only to our patients but to other health care professionals as well.

To meet the challenges of being responsible for optimal therapy outcomes, our practitioners are going to need more training and confidence in patient-assessment techniques. Programs for training in primary care skills and patient monitoring, such as the ASHP Foundation's anticoagulant clinic traineeship program, should be expanded.

Patient medication compliance is also critical for achieving desired therapeutic outcomes. Efforts should be made to mandate pharmaceutical manufacturers to provide unit-of-use packaging and packaging that encourages patient compliance.

We need to press on for standardized education and recognition of technicians, and we must expand automation in our pharmacy systems so that much of the current pharmacist labor force can be redeployed into providing pharmaceutical care.

Electronic patient medication databases must be developed to provide information for both acute and ambulatory care. Mechanisms must be developed so that patients' medical data can be shared by all providers of pharmaceutical care.

These are but a few of the issues that will need to be addressed by the commission.

Back to ASHP initiatives. ASHP must ensure that pharmacy practice in organized health care settings is meeting the accepted standard of practice for patient care, including both clinical and nonclinical practices. I refer to data suggesting that intravenous admixture programs and drug distribution services still do not meet the standards of practice in many of our nation's hospitals. Pharmaceutical services meeting the standards of practice in all areas are mandatory as we move into providing pharmaceutical care for all patients.

ASHP states that it represents pharmacists in organized health care settings, encouraging them to provide high-quality pharmaceutical services that foster the efficacy, safety, and cost-effectiveness of drug use. However, most of ASHP's efforts and services have been aimed at practitioners in acute care hospitals. ASHP must give the same priority to the establishment of pharmaceutical care in all organized health care settings such as managed care organizations, nursing homes, ambulatory care pharmacies, and home health care pharmacies. ASHP must accelerate the previously recommended "name identity change" from the American Society of Hospital Pharmacists to ASHP.[12] A revised mission statement should proclaim that ASHP represents pharmacists providing pharmaceutical care in organized health care settings.

ASHP must examine its current organizational structure to validate that it is providing appropriate services and representation for all practitioners in organized health care facilities. Membership programs should promote the provision of pharmaceutical care at multiple levels and all sites of activity. The current organizational structure, which attempts to meet the needs of generalists, members who identify themselves by practice interest, and members of specialty practice groups, should be reevaluated to ensure that the depth and breadth of membership needs of all differentiated practitioners are recognized and met.

ASHP has been the preeminent professional organization providing educational services to its members and the profession. Given the importance of the implementation of pharmaceutical care, ASHP should prioritize and accelerate the clinical skills development project. In fact, using its expertise, ASHP should develop curricular resources via electronic media to meet the needs of the practitioner to practice pharmaceutical care. Likewise, ASHP should use its resources and extensive experience in residency training to develop a cadre of practitioner educators to provide experiential opportunities through which practitioners can improve their clinical skills.

During the implementation of pharmaceutical care, the different pharmacy degrees and different levels of pharmacy practice will be a problem. Current practitioners are legitimately concerned about their professional status and value. We must recognize that pharmacy is in a transitional mode, and we must not dwell on such differentiating issues. I urge ASHP to encourage employers recruiting practitioners to not use the term "clinical pharmacist only" or "Pharm.D. only," but rather to indicate that the qualifications for employment include the ability and expertise to practice pharmaceutical care. The profession must quickly adapt to the educational requirements for entry-level practice. But in this transitional time, we must recognize the important contributions of those pharmacists who have achieved distinction as clinical practitioners the "old-fashioned way," by self-development.

We know the direction we must follow. Mark Twain said, "Even though you are on the right track, you get run over unless you can move down that track." Implementation of pharmaceutical care is imperative. It is the profession's destiny. William Jennings Bryan once wrote, "Destiny is not a matter of chance, it is a matter of choice, it is not a thing to be waited for, it is a thing to be achieved." The profession as a whole is positioned to achieve our destiny. To a new beginning!

(For the complete list of references cited, please see page 1703 of the *American Journal of Hospital Pharmacy*, Aug. 1991.)

At the time he received this award, Harold N. Godwin was the Director of Pharmacy at the University of Kansas Medical Center, Kansas City, and Associate Dean and Professor and Chairman of the Pharmacy Practice Department at the University of Kansas School of Pharmacy, Lawrence.

INDEX

(Prepared, in part, by Betsy L. Allan and Valorie J. Wilkins, Hospital Pharmacy Residents, North Carolina Memorial Hospital, Chapel Hill)

Abbott parenterals, 187
Academy of Medicine of Toledo and Lucas County, 63
Accountability, 237
Accreditation of residencies, 121, 345, 355, 383
Administrators, hospital, 11
Adverse reactions, 131, 137, 179, 245, 287, 301
Advisory Panel on Hospital Practices, 187
Ambulatory patient care, 225, 245, 253, 261, 301
American Association of Colleges of Pharmacy (AACP), 383
American College of Clinical Pharmacy, 371
American College of Hospital Administrators, 47, 101
American College of Surgeons, 3, 17, 31, 47, 63
American Council on Pharmaceutical Education (ACPE), 209, 383
American Hospital Association, 3, 47, 93, 111
American Hospital Formulary Service, 93, 111, 187, 199, 225, 345
American Journal of Hospital Pharmacy, 81, 93, 111, 121, 137, 171, 187, 199, 225, 345
American Medical Association, 3, 47, 93, 147
American Pharmaceutical Association, 3, 17, 23, 37, 47, 75, 81, 93, 111, 171, 199, 209, 217, 383
American School of Hospital Pharmacy (American College of Hospital Pharmacists), 3, 225
American Society of Hospital Pharmacists (ASHP), 17, 23, 31, 37, 47, 63, 75, 93, 101, 111, 121, 137, 157, 171, 187, 199, 209, 225, 237, 245, 253, 261, 271, 315, 327, 345, 383
    Personnel Placement Service, 187
    Statement of Guiding Principles on the Operation of the Hospital Formulary System, 315
    Statement on Clinical Functions in Institutional Pharmacy Practice, 301
    Statement on Goals for Hospital Pharmacy, 171
    Statement on Long-Range Pharmacy Manpower Needs and Residency Training, 383
    Statement on the Pharmacy and Therapeutics Committee, 315
    Statement on Unit Dose Drug Distribution, 271
Andrews, Marvin "Jack," 81
Annual institutes, hospital pharmacy, 121
Apothecaries, 245
Apple, William S., 327
Archambault, George, 63, 81
Aseptic technique, 187
Audit of pharmaceutical services in hospitals, 111, 157, 315
Autoclave, 131
Automation, 111, 121, 171, 187, 271, 301

Babcock, Kenneth B., 93
Barker, Ken, 187, 245, 339
Baxter solutions, 187
Becker, Irwin, 17
Bergen County Pharmaceutical Association of New Jersey, 47

Berman, Alex, 37, 111, 121, 345
Bezold, Clement, 301
Biotechnology, 371
Board of Pharmaceutical Specialties, 383
Boards of pharmacy, 47, 81, 111, 121, 209, 225, 287
Boston Druggists Association, 339
Bowles, Grover, 131, 217, 339
Brodie, Don, 339, 365, 383
Brookings Institution, 271
Brooks, Carl, 187
Brown, Ray E., 371
Bruch, Carl, 187
Bryan, William Jennings, 383
Budget, 121, 253
Bulletin of American Society of Hospital Pharmacists, 3, 17, 31, 37, 63, 75, 81, 111, 131, 199, 345
Bulletin of the American College of Surgeons, 17

Califano, Joseph, 383
Callahan, Ronald, 339
Cardiopulmonary resuscitation, 261
Carroll, Lewis, 383
Catholic Hospital Association, 93, 111
Center for Disease Control, 187
Centralized drug system, 237, 287
Churchill, Sir Winston, 37
Clance, Pauline, 355
Clark, Don, 81
Clarke, Donald A., 63, 75
Clinical clerkship, 287
Clinical drug research, 287, 327, 383
Clinical educator, 209, 237, 383
Clinical practice, 147, 163, 171, 209, 217, 225, 237, 245, 253, 287, 355, 371, 383
Clinical research, 371, 383
Commission on Credentialing, ASHP, 355
Commission on Goals of American Society of Hospital Pharmacists, 209
Commission on Pharmaceutical Services to Ambulant Patients by Hospitals and Related Facilities, 261
Commission to Implement Change in Pharmaceutical Education (AACP), 383
Communication, 37, 225
Community pharmacists, 111, 187, 225, 287, 355
Compatibility of injectables, 131
Compliance, 217, 253
Compounding, 47, 111
Computers, 261, 271, 287, 315
Consultation, 225, 245
Continuing education, 37, 209, 225, 237, 287, 339
Corporations for profit, 271
Corresponding Society of Hospital Pharmacists, 81
Cost justification, 237, 253, 287, 315
Cousins, Norman, 75
Crout, Richard, Jr., 187
Cutter solutions, 187
Cybernation, 301

Daniels, Troy C., 17
Data processing, 121, 137, 163
Decentralized pharmacy services, 111, 237, 271, 287, 315
Deprofessionalization, 225
Detailmen, 147, 225
Dewey, John, 75
Disaster preparedness committees, 93
Discharge drug counseling, 287
Dispensing, 3, 47, 121, 171, 225, 261
Douglas, May, 187
Downs, George, 187
Drug-induced diseases, 287
Drug information, 23, 147, 315
Drug information centers or specialists, 3, 131, 137, 171, 179, 225, 237, 253, 261, 271, 287, 315
Drug interactions, 237
Drug product defect reporting program, 187
Drug product information forecasting, 187
Drug research reports, 187
Drug room, 3
Drugs, cost of, 147
Drugstore, 3, 17
Drug treatment plan, 245
Drug use control, 365, 383
Drug utilization review, 147, 253, 301

Eckel, Fred, 271
Education, pharmacy, 11, 23, 101, 111, 121, 137, 163, 225, 237, 253, 287, 327, 339, 345, 371, 383
Einstein, Albert, 383
Electronic communications networks, 371
Erskine, John, 37
Ethics, 365, 371
Ethics, Code of, 47, 111, 225, 245, 345
Expense management, 287

Experiential training, 355, 383
Externship, 171

Fellowships, 47
Finer, Herman, 75
Fischelis, Robert, 225
Flack, Herbert, 131, 237, 327, 339
Floor stock, 37, 237
Florentine, Sister Mary, 345
Food and Drug Administration, 187, 287
Food and Drug Laws, 121
Formulary, 3, 17, 23, 63, 93, 101, 121, 179, 187, 199, 237, 287
Formulations, 131
Forum of Hospital Pharmacists, 81
Foster, Thomas A., 315
Francke, Don, 3, 31, 37, 63, 81, 93, 111, 131, 171, 199, 225, 301, 315, 339, 345, 355
Francke, Gloria Niemeyer, 17, 31, 63, 81, 93, 339, 345
Franklin, Benjamin, 47
Frazier, Walter, 81, 93, 131, 199
Fuqua, Robert S., 81, 253
Futurism, nonpharmacy, 137, 271, 301

Generics, 63, 93, 179, 261
Godley, Leo, 63, 187
Goldsmith, Jeff, 301
Goldsmith, Maury, 81
Gonzales, Sister M., 339
Gouveia, William, 339
Government Accounting Office (GAO), 271
Goyan, Jere, 365
Graduate study, 3, 17, 47, 111
Gray, William, 17
Griffenhagen, George, 217
Griffith, Ivor, 17
Gross, Mason, 47
Group purchasing programs, 287

Hamilton, Harold, 187
Hansen, Hans T. S., 17, 37, 93
Harman, Willis, 365
Harris Amendments (1962) to Food and Drug Act, 147
Hartford Foundation, 187
Harvey A. K. Whitney Lecture Award, 17, 23, 31, 37, 47, 75, 81, 93, 101, 111, 131, 171, 187, 199, 237, 253, 345
Health maintenance, 301
Health maintenance organizations, 179, 225, 287
Henry, Robert, 187
Hepler, C. D., 383
Hewitt, Hildreth Whitney, 199
Hickenall, Louis, 81
Hilton Head Conference, 355, 383
Home health care programs, 47, 261
Hospital pharmacy administration, 101
Hospitals, history of, 23, 63, 137, 253, 345
Hospitals as a business, 23
Howiler, Ben, 81
Hudson, Paul Raymond, 17

Image of pharmacy, 23, 121
Incompatibilities, 287
Industry, pharmaceutical, 111, 171, 225, 261, 371
Institutes of hospital pharmacy, 93, 345
Insurance, health, 287
Interdependence, 371
Interdisciplinary team, 147, 237
International Pharmaceutical Abstracts, 187, 225, 345
Internships, pharmacy, 3, 23, 31, 47, 63, 75, 101, 111, 121, 137, 171, 199, 209, 345
Intravenous medication, 131, 187, 287, 315
Inventory control, 121
Investigational drugs, 81, 93
In vitro control procedures, 187

Jang, Ray, 187
Jenkins, Glenn, 93
Joint Commission of Pharmacy Practitioners (JCPP), 383
Joint Commission on Accreditation of Healthcare Organizations, 355
Joint Commission on Accreditation of Hospitals, 47, 93, 137, 237, 245
Joseph, Earl, 301

Kazin, Louis, 47
Kelly, E. F., 81
Kennedy, John F., 101, 121
Knapp, D. A., 225
Kossler, Bert, 187

Lager, Roger, 17, 81
Landeen, Hazel, 75
Lapidus, Jules, 327
Large volume parenterals, 187
Latiolais, Clifton, 101, 171, 327, 339, 345, 355, 383
Lauve, Albert, 327
Leacock, Stephen, 383
Leadership, 37, 345, 355

Lesse, Stanley, 301
License, 47, 93, 171
Literature, professional, 121, 163, 345

MacEachern, Malcolm, 17
MacIver, Robert, 47
Mail order prescriptions, 93
Management, pharmacy, 121, 253, 287, 355, 371
Manasse, Henry, 355, 383
Manpower planning, 355
Manufacture, 3, 17, 47, 121, 131, 287
Marquand, Roger, 17
Martinez, Brenda, 187
Masefield, John, 37
Master degree in hospital pharmacy, 3
Masur, Jack, 47
Mattei, Tom, 217
Maxmen, Jerrold S., 301
McMahon, John Alexander, 315
Medicaid, 225, 287
Medication errors, 137, 187, 245, 271, 287, 315
Medication history, 163, 179, 217, 245, 261, 301
Mergers, pharmaceutical companies, 371
Michigan Society of Hospital Pharmacists, 11, 23, 37, 81, 93, 101
Midyear Clinical Meeting, 225, 245
Mill, John Stuart, 23
Miller, John, 17
Miller, Lloyd, 101, 187
Millis Commission, 383
Minimum Standards for Internships in Hospitals, 3, 93, 111
Minimum Standards for Pharmacies in Hospitals, 31, 37, 81, 93, 101, 111, 121
Mission statement, 383
Monitoring drug therapy, 301
Mooney, James D., 75
Mordell, J. Solon, 23, 75, 81
Morrison, Jack, 81
Mossman, Leo, 75, 199, 345
Moyers, Bill, 345
Muldoon, Hugh, 47
Murphy, John T., 339

Naisbitt, John, 301
Napoleon, 383
National Advisory Council on Allied Health Manpower, 209
National Association of Chain Drug Stores, 383
National Drug Clerks Journal, 17
National health insurance, 3
National Institutes of Health, 187
Neumann, Ellsworth T., 339
Newton, Issac, 371
Nonprescription medication, 47, 179, 271
Nonproprietary names, 121

Oddis, Joseph A., 187, 199, 345, 355, 365
Ohio Society of Hospital Pharmacists, 75
Oliver, John, 355
Organizations, 383
Osler, Sir William, 101
Ostomy care, 261
Outpatients, 3, 47, 121, 271
Overeducation, 163, 179

Parenterals, 237
Parker, Paul, 339, 355
Patient education, 237, 245, 253, 261, 271, 287, 301
Patient interviews, 147, 179, 237, 245
Patient orientation, 187, 217, 237
Patient package inserts, 261, 271
Patient–pharmacist relationship, 179
Patient profiles, 261, 315
Payment programs, 147
Pediatric dosage calculations, 287
Pellegrino, Edmund, 209
Personnel, 121, 163, 287
Pharmaceutical care concept, 383
Pharmaceutical evaluation, 121
Pharmaceutical Manufacturers Association, 187
Pharmaceutical research, 17, 47, 121, 327
Pharmacist, community, 137, 147, 187, 261, 287
  future of, 301, 365
  future of hospital, 365, 383
  hospital, 3, 31, 47, 63, 111, 131, 157, 187, 209, 245, 261, 287, 327, 339, 345
Pharmacist prescribing, 261, 301
Pharmacokinetics, 245, 261
Pharmacokinetic service, 287
Pharmacy, history of, 81, 121, 137, 271, 345
  organized, 23, 37, 101, 171, 287, 327, 345
Pharmacy and Therapeutics Committee, 3, 17, 23, 63, 93, 101, 147, 187, 199, 237, 253, 287, 371
Pharmacy in the 21st Century

Conference, 383
Pharmacy practice, 121, 171, 245, 261, 383
Pharmacy Practice newsletter, 245
Pharm.D. degree, 101, 171, 253, 355, 383
Phillips, George L., 339, 355
Physical pharmacy, 111
Physicians, future of, 301
Point-Rating Plan, 31, 63
Poison treatment pharmacist, 225, 261
Policy Analysis Laboratory (PAL), 271
Pope, Louise, 187
Porter, Robert M., 3, 17
Practitioners, 121, 147, 163
Preceptors, 355
Prepacking, 47
Prepaid health care plans, 93
Pricing schedule, 37
Principles of Medical Ethics of American Medical Association, 47
p.r.n. drugs, 287
Procedural manuals, 63
Professional growth, 339, 345
Professional organizations, 339, 345, 383
Professionalism, 17, 121, 131, 225, 261, 287, 339, 345
Program planning, 121
Provost, George, 187, 217, 225
Pseudopharmacy, 271
Public Health Service, 187
Public policy issues, 315, 345
Purdum, W. Arthur, 37, 253, 301

Quality assurance programs, 187
Quality control, 121, 253
  newsletter, 187
  purchasing, 101

Radioisotope medications, 93
Reamer, I. Thomas, 63, 75, 93, 111, 253
Recruitment, 101
Registration, pharmacist, 137
Reilly, Mary Jo, 187, 339
Reinhardt, Max, 47
Repackaging, 187, 287
Research, clinical, 11, 47, 147, 327
Research, role of, 327
Residency programs, 101, 121, 137, 199, 225, 253, 287, 345, 355, 383
Residency training, 355, 383
Responsibility, professional, 23, 37, 81, 327, 383
Roberts, Eldon, 81
Roberts, Jonathan, 47
Satellite pharmacy, 287
Schon, Svend Aage, 101
Schools of pharmacy, 3, 17, 23, 31, 75, 111, 171, 209, 225, 261, 287, 327
Schweiker, Richard, 271
Schweitzer, Albert, 75
Scott, Evlyn Gray, 37, 63, 75, 93, 131, 339
Self-education, 31
Self-help in health care, 301
Self-medication, 147, 271
Self-rating of pharmacists, 81
Shaw, George Bernard, 355
Smith, William E., 301
Society of Apothecaries of England, 245
Spease, Edward, 31, 37, 63, 75, 81, 93, 315
Special Conference on Drug Information Services, 315
Special interest groups, 245, 327
Specialties, pharmacy, 225, 253, 261, 327
Specialty practice groups, 355
Sprowls, Dean, 81
Stability, 187
Standards for hospital pharmacy orientation programs, 101
Standards of Pharmacy Practice (APhA), 383
Sterile products, 47, 121, 199, 217
Stevenson, Robert Louis, 93
Stimson, Russell, 75
Stockert, Geraldine, 75
Stolfi, Julius, 217
Strand, L. M., 383
Strip packaging, 111
Study Commission on Pharmacy, 225, 245, 287, 315
Substitution, 47
Swallow, Edward, 17

Task Force on Continuing Competence in Pharmacy, 209
Task Force on Pharmacy Education, APhA, 355
Technicians, 31, 171, 225, 261, 287
Therapeutic levels, 245
Thielke, Thomas S., 371
Third-party payers, 287
Thomas Jefferson University Hospital, 355
Thudium, John, 199
Toffler, Alvin, 261, 271
Tousignaut, Dwight, 187, 301
Toxicity, 287

Training of hospital pharmacists, 121, 345
Trissel, Lawrence, 339
Twain, Mark, 383

Unit dose, 111, 131, 187, 217, 237, 245, 271, 287, 315
United States Pharmacopeia, 3, 187
Utah Society of Hospital Pharmacists, 37

Van Dyke, Henry, 111
von Plessen, Baroness I., 63

Walters, Carl, 217
Wang, R. I. H., 245
Wells, H. G., 383
Werble, Wallace, 187
White, Sara, 383
Whitney, Harvey A. K., 3, 11, 17, 23, 31, 37, 63, 75, 81, 93, 101, 111, 121, 131, 137, 157, 199, 261, 301, 315, 339, 345, 355
Whitney–Spease Scholarship, 81

Zopf, Louis, 75
Zugich, John, 199